The Royal Marsden Hospital

manual of

Clinical Nursing Procedures

second edition

D1354353

The Royal Marsden Hospital

manual of
Clinical
Nursing
Procedures

second edition

edited by

A. Phylip Pritchard BA, RGN, RMN
Assistant to the Director of
In-Patient Services/
Chief Nursing Officer

and

Jill A. David MSc, RGN, HV, CertEd, MIBiol
Director of Nursing Research

Foreword by

Robert Tiffany OBE, RGN, RCNT, FRCN
Director of In-patient Services/
Chief Nursing Officer

Harper & Row, Publishers
London

Cambridge
Mexico City
New York
Philadelphia

San Francisco
São Paulo
Singapore
Sydney

First edition published 1984
Reprinted 1989

Harper and Row Ltd
Middlesex House
34–42 Cleveland Street
London
W1P 5FB

British Library Cataloguing in Publication Data

The Royal Marsden Hospital manual of clinical nursing
procedures 2nd ed.
1. Medicine. Nursing – Manuals
I. Pritchard, A Phylip (Albert Phylip)   II. David, Jill A.
III. Manual of clinical nursing policies and procedures.
610.73

ISBN 0-06-318404-4

Typeset in Baskerville 9/11pt by Inforum Ltd, Portsmouth.
Printed in Great Britain at the Alden Press, Oxford

Contents

Contributors

Judith M. Bibbings RGN, DipN, FETC, Sister (Gastro-intestinal/Genito-urinary Unit)

Jill A. David MSc, RGN, HV, CertEd, MIBiol, Director of Nursing Research

Barbara Dicks RGN, RM, Regional Nurse (Continuing Care), North-East Thames Health Authority

Sarah Hart RGN, Clinical Nurse Specialist (Control of Infection/Radiation Protection)

Rachel Hair RGN, DipN, FETC, Senior Nurse (Neuro-oncology Unit)

Elizabeth A. Houlton BNurs, RGN, NDH, HV, Senior Nurse (Community Liaison/Self-Care Unit)

Nest Howells BSc, RGN, DipN, Information Officer, Cancerlink

Jennifer M. Hunt MPhil, RGN, FRCN, Nursing Officer, Department of Health and Social Security

Maureen Hunter, BSc, SRD, Chief Group Dietitian

Elizabeth M. Janes, BSc, RGN, SRD, Dietitian

Catherine Miller, RGN, FETC, Senior Nurse (Continuing Care Unit)

Cathryn Newton BA, RGN, DipN, formerly Senior Nurse (Gastrointestinal/Genito-urinary Unit)

A. Phylip Pritchard BA, RGN, RMN, Assistant to the Director of In-patient Services/Chief Nursing Officer

Helen Roberts RGN, Senior Nurse (Head and Neck Unit)

Tim Root BSc, MPS, Group Pharmacist

Miriam Rushton MSc, RGN, DipN, FETC, Senior Nurse (Gynaecology Unit)

Mave Salter RGN, NDN, CertEd, (Clinical Nurse Specialist (Stoma/Incontinence Care)

Valerie D. Speechley RGN, RCNT, DipN, Clinical Nurse Specialist (Intravenous Therapy)

June Toovey RGN, Sister (Intravenous Therapy Team)

Robert Tunmore BSc, RGN, RMN, Clinical Nurse Specialist (Psychological Support)

Anne Topping BSc, RGN, Senior Nurse (Gastro-intestinal/Genito-urinary Unit)

Valerie A. Walker BSc, RGN, Research Sister, Pain Clinic, Department of Anaesthetics, Leeds infirmary

Isobel White RGN, RSCM, DipLS, Research Sister (Continuing Care Unit)

Karen A. Wright RGN, RCNT, DipN, FETC, formerly Research Assistant, Nursing Research Unit

Foreword

It is with enormous pleasure that I once again write a foreword to The Royal Marsden Hospital Manual of Clinical Nursing Procedures.

Little did we realise in September 1984, with the publication of the first edition, that following the success of that venture four years later we would be asked to prepare a second edition of this work. It is personally gratifying that this should be so for it confirms recognition by the nursing profession as a whole of the value of my colleagues' work. The manual has been found to be both useful and interesting and has become a valuable resource for individuals and organizations alike.

It is our belief that this new edition is even better than the first and that it will continue to assist nurses to base their clinical practice on sound and, whenever possible, research-based principles. We are eternally indebted to those of you who have taken the time and made the effort to write to us pointing out our mistakes and offering your suggestions for improvement and we have endeavoured to incorporate these in the revised text. Again, the second edition, like the first, is not a 'final' document. If you have more information to support or challenge any of our statements, please let us know so that we can incorporate them in the third edition which is already in preparation!

Robert Tiffany
Director of In-Patient Services/
Chief Nursing Officer

Acknowledgements

Our debt to our contributors will always remain. They have given of their time and expertise willingly and have borne our editorial activities with exemplary fortitude. Medical and paramedical colleagues have also given valuable advice and support while without the assistance of the staff of the libraries of the Royal College of Nursing and the Institute of Cancer Research this project would have floundered.

We are grateful to Lynne Montgomery upon whom has fallen the bulk of the responsibility for typing the manuscript, for her skilled work and unending patience and we also thank the members of staff at Harper & Row for their help and encouragement.

A. Phylip Pritchard
Jill A. David
1988

Introduction

The format of the second edition of The Royal Marsden Hospital Manual of Clinical Nursing Procedures remains as for the first, i.e. every procedure has two sections:
1 Reference material
2 Guidelines
while some procedures also have a third section devoted to nursing care plans.

Reference Material
The reference material is a short review of the literature and other relevant material. Wherever possible research findings have been utilized. A reference list is included at the end so that you know where our information came from, and to assist you in looking up the topic if you need more detailed information.

Guidelines
The guidelines gives you a list of the equipment needed, followed by a detailed, step-by-step account of the procedure, plus the rationale for the method proposed.

Nursing Care Plan
The nursing care plan gives a list of the problems which may occur, their possible causes and proposals for solving them. Items from this sheet can be used on the patient's own nursing care plan.

Some of the procedures have been rearranged in order to bring related topics together. This applies specifically to the procedures on Blood pressure, Pulse, Respirations and Temperature which will now be found under the general heading of Observations. Similarly many of the procedures associated with radio-active implants will now be found under the general heading of Radioactive implants. The procedure on Barrier nursing has been expanded to include material on infectious diseases. The majority of the procedures have been either rewritten or considerably updated. The remainder are little changed from those found in the first edition. This is due mainly to the fact that we were unable to discover relevant new material on these topics. However, in the interests of knowledge, we would love to be proved wrong and so, as in the Introduction to the first edition and to echo the sentiments found in the Foreword to this edition, we urge you to send us your criticisms and suggestions. The 'final' document is far from seeing the light of day.

A. Phylip Pritchard
Assistant to the Director of In-patient Services/
Chief Nursing Officer
Jill A. David
Director of Nursing Research

1

Abdominal Paracentesis

Definition

Abdominal paracentesis is used for the insertion of solutions into, and the withdrawal of fluid from, the peritoneal cavity.

Indications

Abdominal paracentesis is indicated under the following circumstances:

1 to obtain a specimen of fluid for analysis;
2 to relieve pressure when abdominal fluid interferes with respiration or bladder function or is compressing the abdominal viscera and blood vessels;
3 to insert substances such as radioactive gold colloid or cytotoxic drugs (e.g. bleomycin) into the peritoneal cavity;
4 to achieve regression of serosae deposits responsible for fluid formation.

REFERENCE MATERIAL

Abdominal paracentesis is normally performed by a doctor assisted by a nurse. It is an invasive procedure performed at the patient's bedside.

The procedure is most frequently performed for diagnostic purposes. The removal of large amounts of peritoneal fluid is not routine because of the danger of inducing hypovolaemia, hypokalaemia and hyponatraemia. Immediately after removal of large amounts of peritoneal fluid, fluid moves from the vascular space and reaccumulates in the peritoneal cavity so that the problems that occurred before the procedure was performed reappear. In addition, ascitic fluid contains proteins, and body proteins in an already debilitated patient will be further depleted after abdominal paracentesis.

Anatomy and physiology

The peritoneum is a semipermeable serous membrane consisting of two separate layers:

1 parietal layer: this layer lines the wall of the abdominal cavity;
2 visceral layer: this layer covers the organs contained within the abdominal cavity.

Those organs completely surrounded by peritoneum will be suspended from the posterior abdominal wall by a double fold of the membrane. It is in this way that a mesentery or fold of the peritoneum by which the intestine is attached to the posterior abdominal wall is formed. It is between these two layers that the blood vessels reach the organs, for the abdominal aorta and its branches lie outside the peritoneal cavity.

The stomach, intestines (except for the duodenum and rectum), liver and spleen are almost completely surrounded by peritoneum. The duodenum, rectum and pancreas are covered only on their anterior surfaces.

The pelvic peritoneum is continuous with that of the rest of the abdominal cavity. It covers the front aspects of the rectum. In the male it passes forwards over the posterior and anterior surfaces of the bladder to become continuous with that on the anterior abdominal wall. In the female it passes from the rectum over the posterior and anterior surfaces of the uterus before reaching the bladder.

Functions of the peritoneum

1 The peritoneum is a serous membrane which enables the abdominal contents to glide over each other without friction.
2 It forms partial or complete cover for the abdominal organs.
3 It forms ligaments and mesenteries which help keep the organs in position.
4 The mesenteries contain fat and act as a store for the body.
5 The mesenteries can move to engulf areas of inflammation and this prevents the spread of infection.

6   It has the power to absorb fluids and exchange electrolytes.

References and further reading

Phipps, W.J. *et al.* (1986) *Medical–Surgical Nursing: Concepts and Clinical Practice* 3rd edn, C.V. Mosby, St Louis.

Sears, W.G. and Winwood, R.S. (1985) *Anatomy and Physiology for Nurses*, 6th edn, Edward Arnold, London.

Wolff, L. (1983) *Fundamental Nursing: The Humanities and the Sciences in Nursing*, 7th edn, J.B. Lippincott, Philadelphia.

GUIDELINES: ABDOMINAL PARACENTESIS

Equipment
1   Sterile abdominal paracentesis set containing forceps, blade holder, swabs, towels, suturing equipment, trocar and cannula, rubber tubing to attach to the cannula and guide fluid into the container
2   Sterile dressing pack
3   Sterile receiver
4   Sterile gloves
5   Sterile specimen pots
6   Local anaesthetic
7   Needles and syringes
8   Antiseptic solution
9   Plaster dressing or plastic spray dressing
10   Large sterile drainage bag or container
11   Gate clamps.

Procedure

Action	Rationale
1 Explain the procedure to the patient.	To obtain the patient's consent and co-operation.
2 Ask the patient to void his/her bladder.	If the bladder is full there is a chance of it being punctured when the trocar is introduced.
3 Ensure privacy.	
4 The patient should be sitting in an upright or Fowler's position.	Normally the pressure in the peritoneal cavity is no greater than atmospheric pressure but, when fluid is present, pressure becomes greater than atmospheric pressure. This position will then aid gravity in the removal of fluid and the fluid will drain of its own accord until the pressure is equalized.
5 The procedure is performed by a doctor: (a) The abdomen is prepared aseptically and draped with sterile towels. (b) Local anaesthetic is administered. (c) Once the anaesthetic has taken effect the doctor makes an incision approximately halfway between the umbilicus and the symphysis pubis on the midline of the abdomen. (d) The trocar and cannula are inserted via the incision and the rubber tubing is attached to the cannula. (e) The trocar is removed.	To prevent local and/or systemic infection. The peritoneal cavity is normally sterile. To minimize pain during the procedure and thus ensure maximum co-operation from the patient. To avoid puncturing the colon.

6   If the cannula is to remain in position, sutures will be inserted and a supportive dry dressing applied and taped firmly in position.

To prevent trauma to the patient.
To prevent local and/or systemic infection

7   A closed drainage system is now attached to the cannula.

A sterile container with a non-return valve is necessary to maintain sterility.

8   Monitor the patient's vital signs and observe his/her peripheral circulation.

To monitor any reaction to the procedure. There may be major circulatory shifts of fluid which may precipitate a 'shock syndrome'. The sudden release of intra-abdominal pressure may cause vasodilation and a fall in blood pressure.

9   Apply a gate clamp to the tubing of the drainage system.

To exercise some control by maintaining a steady rate of flow. Approximately 1 litre can be removed safely before reducing the rate of flow.

10 Monitor the patient's fluid balance. Encourage a high protein and high calorie diet.

After removal of large amounts of peritoneal fluid, fluid moves from the vascular space and reaccumulates in the peritoneal cavity. Ascitic fluid contains protein in addition to sodium and potassium. Problems of dehydration and electrolyte imbalance may be present.

11 When the cannula is withdrawn, apply a sterile topical swab to the wound.

To maintain asepsis and protect the wound.

NURSING CARE PLAN

Problem	Cause	Suggested action
Patient exhibits 'shock syndrome'.	Major circulatory shift of fluid or sudden release of intra-abdominal pressure, vasodilation and subsequent lowering of blood pressure.	Clamp the drainage tube with a gate clamp to prevent further fluid loss. Record the patient's vital signs. Refer to the medical staff for immediate intervention.
Cessation of drainage of ascitic fluid	Abdomen is empty of ascitic fluid.	Check with the total output of ascitic fluid given on the patient's fluid balance chart. Measure the patient's girth; compare this measurement with the pre-abdominal paracentesis measurement. Suggest to medical staff that the cannula should be removed. Discontinue the drainage system.
	Patient's position is inhibiting drainage.	Change the patient's position, i.e. move the patient upright or onto his/her side to encourage flow by gravity.
	The ascitic fluid has clotted in the drainage system.	'Milk' the tubing. If this is unsuccessful, change the drainage system aseptically.

Problem	Cause	Suggested action
Signs of local or systemic infection.	Bacterial invasion at site of abdominal paracentesis cannula.	Obtain a swab from the site of the cannula for cultural review. Apply a dry dressing. Refer to the medical staff.
Cannula becomes dislodged.	Ineffective sutures, trauma or infection at the puncture site.	Obtain a swab for culture. Apply a dry dressing. Inform the medical staff.

2

Aseptic Technique

Definition

Aseptic technique is a method used to prevent contamination of wounds and other susceptible sites by ensuring that only sterile objects and fluids come into contact with these sites and that the risk of contamination is minimized.

Indications

Aseptic technique is intended to prevent infection of a wound or susceptible site due to:

1 the size, position or nature of that wound or site, e.g. recent surgical incisions;
2 increased susceptibility of the host to infection, e.g. neutropenia or cachexia;
3 environmental factors, e.g. high humidity or other infected patient.

REFERENCE MATERIAL

The literature shows that a significant number of patients acquire some type of wound infection during their stay in hospital. Not only does this cause unnecessary suffering, but it may also result in extended periods of hospitalization. Because aseptic procedures are used as a method of preventing wound infection, it is essential that they are both sound in theory and are carried out correctly.

Qualified nurses within any one hospital often demonstrate different aseptic techniques according to their training schools, practical experience, etc. It must be emphasized, however, that the success of the aseptic technique depends not on the type of procedure used but rather on how well the principles of asepsis are adhered to.

Principles of asepsis

The aim of using an aseptic technique is to prevent the spread of infection by direct or indirect transmission. When dressing a wound, the most usual means of

infection spread are as follows:

1 the hands of the staff involved;
2 inanimate objects, e.g. instruments and clothes;
3 dust particles or droplet nuclei suspended in the atmosphere.

HAND WASHING

Hand washing greatly reduces the risk of infection transfer but studies have shown that this is rarely carried out in a satisfactory fashion. Fox (1974) showed that most nurses missed some part of their hands while washing and that right-handed people washed the left hand more thoroughly and vice versa. Areas where organisms may shelter include the wrists, under fingernails and under rings.

Transient bacteria can be almost completely removed from the hands by soap and water washing (Lowbury *et al.*, 1974a). Conversely, soap and water do not reduce the number of resident bacteria by any significant amount. Resident skin flora, such as *Staphylococcus aureus*, are most effectively removed by rubbing the hands with an alcoholic solution of chlorhexidine, such as Hibisol. Lowbury et al. (1974b) showed that rinsing the hands with alcoholic chlorhexidine 0.5% removed more resident skin flora than washing the hands with a chlorhexidine 4% detergent wash, such as Hibiscrub.

It is suggested that a preparation such as Hibiscrub is used for cleaning physically dirty or contaminated hands while a preparation such as Hibisol should be used for disinfecting clean hands immediately prior to carrying out an aseptic technique. If a nurse has physically clean hands, he/she will not need to wash them during the aseptic procedure but should use a preparation such as Hibisol whenever disinfection is required, e.g. after opening the outer wrappers of dressings. This will also remove the need for the nurse to leave the bedside during the procedure to wash his/her hands at a basin, unless they become physically contaminated with blood, pus, excreta, etc. (assuming that adequate washing facilities are not available within the area where the procedure is being carried out).

It should be noted that preparations such as Hibiscrub may cause skin reactions in some people; in these cases soap and water may be used. Caution is required, however, if this method is adopted as the sludge or moist soap under the bar often becomes contaminated. A preparation such as Hibisol contains emollients that prevent drying of the skin.

CLEANING INANIMATE OBJECTS
The sterile field and instruments
All instruments, fluids and materials that come into contact with the wound must be sterile if the risk of contamination is to be reduced. The central sterile supplies department should normally provide all sterile instruments. In the event of supplies being short or in an emergency, it is acceptable to disinfect a clean instrument, such as a pair of scissors, by immersing it completely in alcoholic chlorhexidine 1 in 200 (70%) for 5–10 minutes.

Any equipment that becomes contaminated during the procedure must be discarded. On no account should it be returned to the sterile field.

The dressing trolley
The trolley should be washed every day with detergent and water. It should not need cleaning between dressings unless a surface becomes physically contaminated since organisms cannot survive on cold, smooth, dry surfaces. The sterile field, usually made of thick waxed paper, will not allow the passage of organisms through it. Trolleys used for aseptic procedures must not be used for any other purpose.

MASKS, GOWNS AND APRONS
The purpose of a mask is to protect the patient against organisms dispersed from the upper respiratory tracts of the staff. Masks used in operating theatres are usually of the 'deflector' type and are impervious to large droplets from the user's mouth. The use of paper masks on the ward, however, is not recommended, as their value is limited. 'Experimental studies and trials have shown that masks contribute little or nothing to the protection of patients in wards against infection and their routine use for aseptic ward procedures, including postoperative dressings, is therefore unnecessary' (Lowbury et al., 1975).

It would seem that a greater reduction of droplet dispersion of organisms could be achieved by staff not talking unnecessarily during dressing procedures. Ideally, no staff with respiratory tract infections or sore throats should perform dressings. Nurses without infections who are likely to cough or sneeze while carrying out an aseptic procedure, e.g. sufferers from hay fever, should wear surgical masks to reduce the risk of droplet dispersion.

Nurses' clothing does become contaminated with organisms from the ward and from the nurses themselves. The front of the uniform is the area most likely to be contaminated, so it is advisable for nurses to wear protective clothing during aseptic procedures. This also prevents the transfer of bacteria from the uniforms to the patients.

Cotton material, because of its weave, allows bacteria to pass through it. It is therefore recommended that a disposable plastic apron, impermeable to bacteria, is worn during aseptic procedures. Aprons should be discarded after any dirty or infected dressing.

AIRBORNE CONTAMINATION
The spread of infection is most likely to occur in a large open ward and ideally dressings should all be performed in a properly ventilated room. Many dressings, however, are carried out at the patient's bedside; in such cases ward cleaning should cease at least 30 minutes before, and curtains should be drawn at least 10 minutes before a dressing is begun. To reduce opportunities for airborne contamination to a minimum, a wound should be exposed for the shortest time possible, dirty dressings being placed carefully in a bag, preferably plastic, which is sealed before disposal (Lowbury et al., 1975). Clean wounds should be dressed before contaminated wounds. Colostomies and infected wounds should be dressed last of all to minimize environmental contamination and cross-infection.

A potential source of infection can be the water in which flowers or pot plants stand; these must be removed from the bedside before screens are closed. Air movement should be kept to a minimum during the dressing. This means that adjacent windows should be closed and the movement of personnel within the area discouraged. The use of an alcohol-based hand wash solution at the bedside is advantageous as it reduces the air movement created by a nurse in leaving the cubicle to go to a sink; it also shortens the time that a wound is left exposed.

SELECTION OF HAND HYGIENE PREPARATIONS IN GENERAL USE
ANTISEPTIC SKIN CLEANSERS
Hibiscrub
This is a cleansing solution containing chlorhexidine gluconate 4%. This solution should be used instead of soap as a preoperative scrub or disinfectant wash for hands and skin.

Betadine

This is a surgical scrub containing povidone-iodine 7.5% in a non-ionic detergent base. Betadine should be used as a preoperative or pre-procedural scrub for hands and skin.

WIDE-SPECTRUM MICROBICIDES
Hibisol

This is a solution containing chlorhexidine gluconate 0.5% in isopropyl alcohol 70% with emollients. Hibisol may be used in undiluted form for hand and skin disinfection.

Manusept

This is an antibacterial hand rub containing triclosan 0.5% and isopropyl alcohol 70%. Manusept should be used for disinfection and for preoperative and pre-procedural hand preparation

CHLORHEXIDINE IN SPIRIT SPRAY
Hibispray

This is a preparation of Hibitane in a spray containing chlorhexidine gluconate 0.5% and isopropyl alcohol 70%. This spray may be used as a disinfectant on clean, dry surfaces.

References and further reading

Fox, M.K. (1974) How good are hand washing practices? *American Journal of Nursing*, Vol. 74, pp. 1676–8.

Hayward, M.P. (1980) An experimental study to determine the efficiency and effectiveness of a simplified dressing procedure, BSc Thesis, Leeds Polytechnic.

ICI (1981) *ICI Antiseptics in Practice*, ICI Pharmaceuticals Division.

Lascelles, I. (1982) Wound dressing techniques, *Nursing*, Vol. 2, no. 8, pp. 217–19.

Lowbury, E.J. *et al*. (1974a) Disinfection of hands: removal of transient organisms, *British Medical Journal*, Vol. 2, pp. 230–3.

Lowbury, E.J. *et al*. (1974b) Preoperative disinfection of surgeons' hands: use of alcoholic solutions and effects of gloves on skin flora, *British Medical Journal*, Vol. 4, pp. 369–72.

Lowbury, E.J. *et al*. (1981) *Control of Hospital Infection – A Practical Handbook*, 2nd edn, Chapman and Hall, London.

GUIDELINES: ASEPTIC TECHNIQUE

Equipment

1 Sterile dressing pack containing gallipots or an indented plastic tray, wool balls, topical swabs, disposable forceps, dressing towel, sterile field, disposable bag
2 Fluids for cleaning and/or irrigation
3 Hypo-allergenic tape
4 Appropriate hand hygiene preparation
5 Disposable plastic apron.

Any other material required will be determined by the nature of the dressing: special features of a dressing should be referred to in the patient's nursing care plan.

Procedure

Action	Rationale
1 Explain the procedure to the patient.	To obtain the patient's consent and co-operation.
2 Screen the bed and position the patient comfortably so that the dressing is easily accessible without unduly exposing the patient.	To allow dust and airborne organisms to settle before the wound and the sterile field are exposed.
3 Wash your hands with an appropriate solution such as soap and water or Hibiscrub.	
4 Put on a disposable plastic apron.	

5   Place all the equipment required for the dressing on the bottom shelf of a clean dressing trolley.

6   Take the trolley to the patient's bedside, disturbing the screens as little as possible.

To minimize airborne contamination.

7   Open the outer cover of the sterile dressing pack and slide the contents on to the top shelf of the trolley.

8   Open the sterile field using the corners of the paper only. Using the forceps in the pack, arrange the sterile field with the handles of instruments in one corner.

So that areas of potential contamination are kept to a minimum.

9   Attach a plastic disposal bag to the side of the trolley, below the level of the top shelf.

So that any contaminated material is below the level of the sterile field.

10   Open the other sterile packs, tipping their contents gently onto the centre of the sterile field. Pour lotions into gallipots or an indented plastic tray.

11   Loosen the old dressing gently, touching only the hypo-allergenic tape, etc. securing it.

So that the dressing can be lifted off easily with forceps.

12   Clean your hands with an alcohol-based hand wash solution, such as Hibisol.

Hands may have become contaminated by handling outer packets, etc.

13   Using forceps or sterile disposable gloves if the dressing is large or bulky, remove the old dressing and discard it with the forceps or gloves, into plastic bag.

14   Clean the wound as necessary, working from the inside to the outside of the area and dealing with the cleanest parts of the wounds first.

To minimize the risk of spread of infection from a 'dirty' to a 'clean' area.

15   Apply the new dressing with forceps and fix it in place with hypo-allergenic tape, etc. There is no need to use forceps for securing the dressing as the wound is now covered.

16   Make the patient comfortable and ensure that the dressing is secure.

The dressing may slip or feel uncomfortable as the patient changes position.

17   Fold up the sterile field, place it in the plastic disposal bag and seal the bag before moving the trolley.

To prevent environmental contamination.

18   Draw back the curtains.

19   Dispose of waste in appropriate bags.

20   Check that the trolley remains dry and physically clean.

3

Barrier Nursing and Care of the Infectious Patient

BARRIER NURSING

Definition

Barrier nursing involves the use of practices aimed at controlling the spread of, and destroying, pathogenic organisms. These practices may require the setting up of mechanical barriers to contain pathogenic organisms within a specified area.

Indication

Barrier nursing is required under the following circumstances:
1 to prevent the spread of infection from patients with communicable diseases (i.e. contagious diseases such as glandular fever, or infectious diseases such as chicken pox);
2 to prevent the spread of infection from patients infected with organisms which are resistant to the usual range of antibiotics; such as methicillin-resistant *Staphylococcus aureus* (MRSA);
3 to protect those patients whose susceptibility to infection is increased (protective isolation or reverse barrier nursing).

REFERENCE MATERIAL

Most precautions against transferring infection demand more effort, take more time and cost more than the comparable procedures in normal circumstances.

For the infected patient the consequences can be considerable and may include the following:
1 delayed or prevented recovery;
2 increased pain, discomfort and anxiety;
3 extended hospitalization, which has implications for the patient, the family and the hospital;

4 psychological stress as a result of long periods spent in isolation.

Sources of infection
SELF-INFECTION (ENDOGENOUS INFECTION)
Self-infection results when tissue becomes infected from another site in the patient's body. The normal microbial flora of the human body consists largely of the organisms in the alimentary tract, upper respiratory tract and female genital tract and on the skin. This flora may include versatile pathogens (e.g. *Stephylococcus aureus*) that may cause disease in almost any tissue as well as others (e.g. micrococcus species and diphtheroids) which are usually of very low pathogenicity; many organisms exist with capabilities between these extremes.

CROSS-INFECTION (EXOGENOUS INFECTION)
Cross-infection may be caused by infection from patients, hospital staff or visitors who are suffering from the relevant disease (cases) or who are symptomless carriers. Food and the environment may also be factors in cross-infection.

Routes and reservoirs of infection
A reservoir of infection is anywhere where organisms can survive and multiply. For infection to occur there has to be a route of transmission between the reservoir and the susceptible host. Routes of spread include:

DIRECT CONTACT
Careful hand washing by every grade of health care attendant is essential as hands have been identified as a major route in the transmission of infection (Casewell and Phillips, 1977). Studies have also shown that this

procedure is not carried out effectively (Albert and Condie, 1981; Gidley, 1987). (Further information on hand washing can be found in the procedure on aseptic technique, pp. 5–6).

AIRBORNE

Organisms can be transmitted in dust or skin scales carried by air. This is likely to occur during procedures such as bed making when particles may land directly on open wounds or puncture sites. Airborne infection may also occur through droplet infection. Water from nebulizers or humidifiers may be contaminated by Pseudomonas species. Fine droplet spray from ventilation cooling towers or showers contaminated with *Legionella pneumophila* has also been shown to be a hazard (Ayliffe *et al.*, 1982).

FOOD BORNE

Food poisoning occurs when contaminated foods are ingested, Salmonella species being one of the most common causes.

BLOOD BORNE

Blood, or blood-stained material, is potentially hazardous transmitting infection through inoculation accidents, existing breaks in the skin, gross contamination of mucous membranes, sexual activity or, prenatally, from mother to baby.

INSECT BORNE

Although disease transmitted by biting insects is not a major problem in the United Kingdom, insects, such as cockroaches, can carry pathogenic organisms on their bodies and in their digestive tracts. This may infect the hospital environment which includes food and sterile supplies.

Note: Water in flower vases usually contains a range of Gram-negative organisms, including Escherichia, Klebsiella, Pseudomonas and Serratia species, but the importance of this as a source of infection is uncertain.

Types of isolation
SOURCES ISOLATION (BARRIER ISOLATION)

This form of isolation, i.e. physical isolation of the patient, is applied to patients who are infected and are hazardous to others. The need for isolation is determined by the ease with which the disease can be transmitted in hospital and, if it is transmittable, by its severity.

PROTECTIVE ISOLATION (REVERSE BARRIER NURSING)

Patients whose susceptibility to infection is increased

may require isolation for their own protection as an alternative to, or as well as, antibiotic treatment. The decision to use isolation is influenced by the individual circumstances and by the available facilities. Control of Infection Group, Northwick Park Hospital and Clinical Research Centre (1974) has outlined in detail the indications for protective isolation.

Design and construction of isolation accommodation

The literature agrees that good isolation practice is more efficacious in a well-designed building. Easy, direct and short-distance access to patients' supplies and facilities reduces the nursing load, thereby allowing more time to be devoted to the observation of the correct isolation procedures.

Barrier nursing may be achieved in a variety of ways:
1   purpose-built units;
2   plastic isolators;
3   single rooms.

PURPOSE-BUILT UNITS

A purpose-built unit will include a filtered air supply, a series of single rooms with integral toilets and showers, a hatch system for the aseptic transfer of equipment into the room without affecting the air pressure in the room and facilities for providing clean or sterile food. Entry to such rooms should also be restricted with protective robing areas for all those who need to enter these areas. Evidence that this form of isolation is more effective than other techniques is inconclusive (Jameson *et al.*, 1971; Yates and Holland, 1973). Buckner *et al.* (1978), however, demonstrated that patients in laminar airflow rooms had significantly less incidence of septicaemia than patients in the control group. Among the practical disadvantages of these units is the cost of building and maintaining them, the latter requiring a high staff/patient ratio.

PLASTIC ISOLATORS

An isolator consists of a framework erected around a bed from which a PVC tent is suspended. The tent has an air supply attached which keeps the whole inflated. A positive air pressure is usually maintained within the isolator. In some cases, for example when nursing patients with Lassa fever, the pressure within the isolator is slightly below atmospheric pressure which prevents the escape of any infected particles. Although patients may feel a strong sense of containment within the isolator, this system does have the advantage of achieving high standards of bacteriological control and can be assembled and dismantled rapidly.

SINGLE ROOMS (ON GENERAL WARDS)

The decision to isolate a patient will be influenced by the availability of facilities as well as by the physical condition of the area where the isolation is to take place. In determining the most suitable area, a number of criteria need to be met. Among these are the relative cleanliness of the ward, the standard of domestic services support, the microbiological status of the other patients and the anticipated length of the isolation.

General principles of barrier nursing

The main emphasis for successful barrier nursing procedures is on hand washing and protection of clothes. Several general principles need to be adhered to if effective barrier nursing is to occur. Every effort must be made to ensure that instructions are kept simple and realistic. Regular assessment and evaluation of the situation must take place to ascertain whether barrier nursing continues to remain the most appropriate form of care.

HAND WASHING

Washing the skin removes harmful organisms quickly. Studies of hand washing by nurses and others, however, have shown that this procedure is not carried out efficiently. The use of disinfectants improves the cleaning process, although no method of chemical disinfection will produce a sterile hand. Soaps and detergent emulsions containing hexachlorophane build a protective barrier in the skin against Gram-positive organisms. A solution which is now widely used is one containing 4% chlorhexidine (Hibiscrub). A convenient and effective disinfectant for the hands is 70% alcohol with the addition of enough glycerine to prevent excessive drying of the skin. Washing in running water is essential. Basins should be deep enough to contain any splashing water and should be plugless. Taps should not be operated by hand but by elbow, knee or foot as appropriate.

CLOTHING AND GOWNS

Lidwell et al. (1974) have shown that disposable plastic gowns that cover the parts of the body that come into the closest contact with the patient reduce contact transfer substantially. Ayton (1984) discusses this area in more detail.

CAPS, MASKS AND FOOTWEAR

There is evidence that hair picks up bacteria readily from the environment. Because the head is moved directly above the patient it should be covered when a high degree of patient protection is necessary. If caps are to be used effectively they must cover all the hair.

Masks can be worn to protect the wearer or the patient. The wearer will only be protected if the mask fits the face closely.

Evidence that floors and footwear contribute to the risk of infection is, at present, inconclusive.

BATHING

There is no evidence to date to show that showering is more effacious than bathing.

FOOD

Sterile water should be available if required. Complete food sterilization is not required except for the most stringent germ-free conditions.

WASTE

Plastic bags have simplified and improved methods of disposal of waste, but care is needed to ensure that the bags are closed correctly. Separate routes for entry into and exit from the isolation area are the ideal. If this is not possible, correct bagging must be adhered to scrupulously. Any waste should be clearly labelled before leaving the isolation area. Bedpans and urinals should be bagged within the isolated area after use and then sent to be washed and sterilized.

NOTIFICATION OF INFECTION

If bacteriological analysis identifies an organism which necessitates barrier nursing, swift communication and action are needed to instigate this. Any problems may be discussed with the microbiologist or infection control nurse.

ISOLATION OF THE PATIENT

Effective barrier nursing practice is most easily achieved by isolating the patient in a single room with:
1   an anteroom area for protective clothing;
2   hand washing facilities;
3   toilet facilities.
However, with good technique an area in the ward away from especially vulnerable patients can be used.

INFORMING THE PATIENT AND VISITORS

Careful explanation to the patient is essential so that he/she can co-operate fully with the restrictions. The nurse should be sensitive to the psychological implications of being labelled 'infectious' and being confined in isolation. The patient's visitors must also be informed why the barrier nursing restrictions are necessary. Visitors may be allowed into the room, but only at the discretion of the bacteriologist. They must be taught to observe the correct procedures for entering and leaving the room. As children are more susceptible to infection than adults, any visit by a child should be discussed with the appropriate personnel.

DOMESTIC STAFF

The domestic manager must be informed as soon as barrier nursing is commenced. He or she will then provide the ward domestic with written instructions.

The ward domestic staff must clearly understand why barrier nursing is required and should be instructed on the correct procedure. The nursing staff must check that the ward domestics understand and are following their instructions correctly. If the patient is in a single room, a mop, cleaning fluid and disposable cloths should be kept in the room solely for this patient's use. If the patient is in a general ward, special care must be taken with the cleaning so that potentially infectious material is not transferred from the area around the infected patient to other patient areas. The infected patient's area must be cleaned last and separately.

STAFF ALLOCATION

A minimum number of staff should be involved with an infected case. The nurse concerned with the infected patient should not also attend to other susceptible patients. If barrier nursing is for an infectious disease, it is preferable that only personnel who have already had the disease should attend this patient.

The protection of staff against the risk of infection is one of the main functions of the occupational health department. This department offers an immunization and counselling service.

References and further reading

Albert, K.A. and Condie, M.S. (1981) Handwashing patterns in medical intensive-care units, *New England Journal of Medicine*, Vol. 24, pp. 1464–66.

Ayliffe, G.A.J. (1983) Epidemiology, in W.C. Noble (ed.) *Control of Hospital Acquired Infections*, Update Publications, Guildford, pp. 12–18.

Ayliffe, G.A.J. and Lowbury, E.J.L. (1982) Airborne infection in hospital, *Journal of Hospital Infection*, Vol. 3, pp. 217–40.

Ayliffe, G.A.J. et al. (1984) *Hospital-acquired Infection: Principles and Prevention*, John Wright, Bristol.

Ayliffe, G.A.J. et al. (1984) *Chemical Disinfection in Hospitals*, Public Health Laboratory Service.

Ayton, M. (1984) Protective clothing – what do we use and when, *Journal of Infection Control Nursing*, Vol. 25, pp. 5–7.

Bagshawe, K.D. et al. (1978a) Isolating patients in hospital to control infection. Part I. Sources and routes of infection, *British Medical Journal*, Vol. 2, pp. 609–12.

Bagshawe, K.D. et al. (1978b) Isolating patients in hospital to control infection. Part II. Who should be isolated, and where? *British Medical Journal*, Vol. 2, pp. 684–6.

Bagshawe, K.D. et al. (1978c) Isolating patients in hospital to control infection. Part III. Design and construction of isolation accommodation, *British Medical Journal*, Vol. 2, pp. 744–48.

Bagshawe, K.D. et al. (1978d) Isolating patients in hospital to control infection. Part IV. Nursing procedures, *British Medical Journal*, Vol. 2, pp. 808–11.

Bagshawe, K.D. et al. (1978e) Isolating patients in hospital to control infection. Part V. An isolation system, *British Medical Journal*, vol. 2, pp. 879–81.

Buckner, C.D. (1978) protective environment for marrow transplant recipients: a prospective study, *Annals of Internal Medicine*, Vol. 89, no.6, pp. 893–901.

Casewell, M. and Phillips, I. (1977) Hands as route of transmission for Klebsiella species, *British Medical Journal*, Vol. 2, pp. 1315–17.

Control of Infection Group, Northwick Park Hospital and Clinical Research Centre (1974) Isolation system for general hospitals, *British Medical Journal*, Vol. 1, pp. 41–4.

Gidley, C. (1987) Now wash your hands, *Nursing Times* 83 (29): 40–2. Infection Control Nurses' Association (1976) Stirling Conference of the Infection Control Nurses' Assocation, Kimberley Clark.

Jameson, B. et al. (1971) Five year analysis of protective isolation, *Lancet*, Vol. i, pp. 1034–40.

Lidwell, O.M. et al. (1974) Transfer of micro-organisms between nurses and patients in a clean air environment, *Journal of Applied Bacteriology*, Vol. 37, no. 4, pp. 649–56.

Taylor, L.J. (1978) On evaluation of hand washing techniques, *Nursing Times*, Vol. 74, no. 2, pp. 54–5.

Yates, J.W. and Holland, J. (1973) A controlled study of isolation and endogenous microbial suppression in acute myelocytic leukaemia patients, *Cancer*, Vol. 32, pp. 1490–8.

GUIDELINES: BARRIER NURSING

Equipment

1   Isolation suite if possible
2   All items required to meet the patient's nursing needs during the period of isolation, such as crockery, linen, instruments to assess vital signs, etc.

Procedure

PREPARATION OF THE ISOLATION ROOM

Action	Rationale
1 Place a barrier nursing sign outside the door.	To inform anyone intending to enter the room of the situation.
2 List requirements for personnel before entering and after leaving the isolation area.	
3 Remove all non-essential furniture. The remaining furniture should be easy to clean and should not conceal or retain dirt or moisture either within or around it.	To minimize the risk of furniture harbouring microbial spores or growth colonies.
4 Stock the hand basin with a suitable antiseptic solution, e.g. Hibiscrub, and paper towels for staff use.	Facilities for hand washing within the infected area are essential for effective barrier nursing.
5 Place a yellow rubbish bag in the room on a foot-operated stand. The bag must be sealed before it is removed from the room, either by knotting (polythene bags) or by stapling the top (paper bags).	For containing contaminated rubbish within the room. Yellow is the international colour for clinical waste.
6 Place a container for 'sharps' in the room.	To contain contaminated 'sharps' within the infected area.
7 When the 'sharps' container is full it must be placed in a yellow polythene bag, securely sealed and sent for incineration.	To minimize the risk of leakage from the 'sharps' safe.
8 Keep the patient's personal property to a minimum. Advise him/her to wear hospital clothing. All belongings taken into the room should be washable, cleanable or disposable.	The patient's belongings may become contaminated and cannot be taken home unless they are washable or cleanable. Anything else may have to be destroyed.
9 Provide the patient with his/her own thermometer and sphygmomanometer, water jug, glass and tray, and all items necessary for attending to personal hygiene.	Equipment used regularly by the patient should be kept within the infected area to prevent the spread of infection.
10 Keep dressing solutions, creams and lotions, etc. to a minimum and store them within the room.	All partially used materials must be discarded when barrier nursing ends (sterilization is not possible), therefore unnecessary waste should be avoided.
11 Set up a trolley outside the door to hold plastic gowns, gloves, an appropriate antiseptic solution and spare recording charts, e.g. for fluid balance.	If equipment is readily available staff are more likely to use it.

ENTERING THE ROOM

Action	Rationale
1 Collect all equipment needed.	To avoid entering and leaving the infected area unnecessarily.
2 Roll up long sleeves to the elbow.	To protect clothing from contamination.
3 Put on a disposable plastic apron when there is no risk of airborne transmission of organisms or when close contact with the patient is not anticipated.	A plastic apron is inexpensive and adequate to protect clothing from contamination in most situations.
4 Put on a disposable gown for close work, e.g. lifting or bed making.	To protect clothing from contamination to shoulders, arms and back. Cotton gowns are an ineffective barrier against bacteria, particularly when wet.
5 Put on a disposable, well-fitting mask if there is a risk of airborne spread, i.e. (a) Smear-positive pulmonary tuberculosis patient with a productive cough. (b) Patient with heavy colonization of MRSA of nose, skin, hair, etc. (c) Meningococcus meningitis.	To reduce the risk of inhaling organisms.
6 Put on disposable overshoes *only* if there is a risk of serious shedding of infected skin scales onto the floor, i.e. the patient with exfoliative dermatitis who has been shown to be a heavy shedder.	Putting on and taking off overshoes is likely to contaminate the hands thus increasing the risk of contact, transmission of infection.
7 Put on a disposable paper cap *only* when procedures such as bed making are being undertaken for patients who, for example, are heavily colonized with MRSA.	There is some evidence to show that hair picks up bacteria readily from the environment. Because the head is often moved directly above a patient it should be covered in certain circumstances to prevent cross-infection.
8 Safety glasses, visors and goggles should be put on only when blood splashes are expected, e.g. during haemodialysis or when the patient is hepatitis B positive.	To give protection to the conjunctiva from blood splashes.
9 Only put on disposable gloves if you are intending to deal with blood, excreta or contaminated material.	To reduce the risk of contaminating your hands. Over-use of disposable gloves may ultimately detract from the importance of hand washing.
10 Enter the room, shutting the door behind you.	To reduce the risk of airborne organisms leaving the room.

ATTENDING TO THE PATIENT

Action	Rationale
1 *Meals* Meals should be served on disposable crockery and eaten with disposable cutlery if deemed necessary by the bacteriologist. Disposable and uneaten food should be discarded in the appropriate bag.	Contaminated crockery is a potential disease vector. Cleaning of same may be difficult and time consuming.

2 *Non-disposable Crockery* A personal water jug, glasses and tray should be kept at the bedside. These, and any other non-disposable crockery, should be washed separately from the rest of the ward's utensils, preferably in a dishwasher with a hot disinfecting cycle.

Separation of contaminated crockery reduces the risk of the spread of infection in washing-up water.

3 *Excreta* Ideally a toilet should be kept solely for the patient's use. If this is not available, a separate bedpan or urinal and commode should be left in the patient's room. Gloves must be worn by staff when dealing with excreta. Bedpans and urinals should be bagged in the isolation room, emptied and then washed in a bedpan washer, then dried and returned immediately to the patient's room.

To minimize the risk of infection being spread from excreta, e.g. via a toilet seat or a bedpan.

4 *Accidental spills* Any suspected contaminated fluids must be mopped up immediately and the area cleaned with disinfectant.

Damp areas encourage microbial growth and increase the risk of spread of infection.

5 *Bathing* An infected patient must be bathed last on the ward. Clean the bath after the previous patient and after the infected patient. If the patient has infected lesions, disinfectant may be added to the bath water, e.g. Steribath or Hibiscrub. Salt is not a disinfectant and has little antibacterial effect.

Leaving the bath dry after disinfection reduces the risk of microbes surviving and infecting others. Bacteria will not grow on clean dry surfaces.

6 *Dressings* Aseptic technique must be used for changing all dressings. Waste materials and dirty dressings should be discarded in the appropriate bag. Used lotions, creams, etc. must be kept in the room and not used for other patients.

Aseptic procedure minimizes the risk of cross-infection. Lotions and creams can become easily contaminated.

7 *Linen* Place linen in a polythene bag which must be tightly secured before it leaves the room. Just outside the room place this bag into the routine dirtly linen bag which must be secured tightly and not used for other patients. These bags should await the laundry collection in a safe area.

Holding dirty linen in a polythene bag confines organisms and allows staff handling the linen to recognize the potential hazard.

8 *Waste* Yellow bags should be kept in the room for disposal of all the patient's rubbish. The bag's top should be sealed by knotting or stapling before it is removed from the room. If the waste is from patients with hepatitis B infection the yellow bag should be labelled accordingly.

Yellow is the international colour for clinical waste. Virus can survive in blood for some time.

LEAVING THE ROOM

Action

Rationale

1 Wash your hands with gloves on. Remove the gloves and discard them in the appropriate bag. Wash your hands again with an appropriate antiseptic solution.

Pathogenic contamination of gloves will be minimized before they are discarded.

2 Remove your gown and discard it in the appropriate bag. Wash your hands again with an appropriate antiseptic solution.

Hands may be contaminated by a dirty gown.

Action	Rationale
3 Used gowns should-not be re-used.	Mistakes are made if gowns have to be re-used, particularly as staff find it hard to distinguish the inside/outside of a gown. If the gown is worn inside out uniforms can be contaminated.
4 Leave the room, shutting the door behind you.	
5 Rinse your hands with an alcohol-based hand wash solution, such as Hibisol.	To remove pathogenic organisms acquired from such items as the door handle.

CLEANING THE ROOM

Action	Rationale
1 Domestic staff must understand why barrier nursing is required and should be instructed on the correct procedure.	To reduce the risk of mistakes and to ensure that barrier nursing is maintained.
2 The area where barrier nursing is being carried out must be cleaned last.	To reduce the risk of the transmission of organisms.
3 Separate cleaning equipment must be kept for this area.	Cleaning equipment can easily become infected. Cross-infection may result from shared cleaning equipment.
4 Members of the domestic services staff must wear gloves and plastic aprons.	To reduce the risk of cross-infection.
5 *Floor* (hard surface) This must be washed daily with a disinfectant as appropriate. All excess water must be removed.	Daily cleaning will keep bacterial count reduced. Organisms, especially Gram-negative bacteria, multiply quickly in the presence of moisture.
6 After use, the bucket must be cleaned, dried and stored within the barrier nursing area.	Bacteria will not survive on clean dry surfaces.
7 Ideally, mop heads should be laundered in a hot wash daily. When this is not possible, the mop must be washed, rinsed, all excess water removed and stored with the mop head uppermost to allow for quick drying within the barrier nursing area.	Mop heads become contaminated easily.
8 *Floor* (carpet) An infected patient may have been admitted into a room with a carpet. A vacuum cleaner should be used which is fitted with an efficient filter. After use the dust bag must be changed and the brush head washed and dried.	Vacuum cleaning reduces the dust thus reducing organisms.
9 On discharge, the carpet must be steam cleaned.	Bacteria can survive in dust trapped in the carpet fibres. The heat of the steam will kill these bacteria.
10 Furniture and fittings should be damp dusted using a disposable cloth and a detergent solution or a disinfectant if appropriate.	To remove any organisms.

11 The toilet, shower and bathroom area must be cleaned at least once a day using a non-abrasive hypochlorite powder or cream. A disinfectant will only be required if soiling of the area has occurred.

Non-abrasive powders or creams preserve the integrity of the surfaces. These areas rapidly recontaminate after cleaning and routine chemical disinfection is of little value and should be saved for terminal cleaning.

TRANSPORTING INFECTED PATIENTS OUTSIDE THE BARRIER NURSING AREA

Action

1 Inform the department concerned about the diagnosis.

2 Arrange for the patient to have the last appointment of the day.

3 Provide the department concerned with the necessary gloves and aprons.

4 Any porters involved must be instructed and given the necessary gloves, together with cleaning equipment for the trolley or chair.

5 The nurse should escort the patient.

Rationale

To allow other departments time to make their own arrangements.

The department concerned will then be empty of other patients; time can be allowed for special cleaning or disinfecting; hospital corridors, lifts, etc. are usually less busy at this time of day.

Protection and reassurance of porters are necessary to allay fear and to minimize the risk of the infection being spread to them.

To ensure the necessary precautions are maintained.

DISCHARGING THE PATIENT

Action

1 Inform the bacteriologist when the patient is due for discharge.

2 The room should be stripped and aired. All textiles must be changed and curtains sent to the laundry.

3 Impervious surfaces, e.g. lockers, stools, blinds and thermometer holders, should be washed with soap and water.

4 The floor must be washed and dried thoroughly.

5 If the room is known to be contaminated with blood or blood-stained excreta from hepatitis B-positive or HIV antibody-positive individuals, a hypochlorite solution, such as Domestos or Milton, should be used.

6 If the room has been used by a patient with an enteric infection, a clean soluble phenolic should be used.

Rationale

The bacteriologist will advise on any special precautions.

Curtains readily become colonized with bacteria.

Wiping of surfaces is the most effective way of removing contaminants. Relatively inaccessible places, e.g. ceilings, may be omitted; these are not generally relevant to any infection risk.

To remove any organisms present.

To remove the source of potential contamination.

To remove the source of potential contamination.

ANTIBIOTIC-RESISTANT ORGANISMS

Definition
The term 'antibiotic resistance' denotes a strain of bacteria that is not killed or inhibited by antimicrobial agents to which the species is generally sensitive.

REFERENCE MATERIAL
The importance of antibiotic-resistant organisms cannot to be overemphasized. Patients who are immunocompromised, debilitated or with open wounds are at particular risk and deaths have occurred (Hone *et al.*, 1981; Bradley, 1985). Bacterial resistance to antibiotics may take many years to develop as in the case of the gonococcus. Strains resistant to penicillin G only appeared after 25 years of use (Sparling *et al.*, 1976). Methicillin-resistant *Staphylococcus aureus* (MRSA), however, was first reported in 1961 (Jevons) only two years after the drug's clinical introduction. MRSA is now increasing with some hospitals reporting its frequenty as high as 20–40% of all *Staphylococcus aureus* identified (Ayliffe, 1985).

The widespread and often indiscriminate use of antibiotics for prophylactic and veterinary purposes, as well as the inappropriate selection of antibiotics, are believed to be important factors in the development of resistant forms of bacteria (Swan Joint Committee, 1969; Garrod, 1972). The transmission of genetic material between bacteria by conjugation has been well documented (Jaffe *et al.*, 1980; Mendoza, 1985) and this conjugation accounts in part for the rapid spread of resistance with mutation, transformation and transduction also involved (Sande and Mandell, 1980).

The consequences of a patient being infected with a resistant form of bacteria are demanding in terms of increased length of stay, costs of care and treatment (Grazebrook, 1986).

Theoretically, any organism can develop antibiotic resistance. In practice, however, two groups present the major problem: Gram-negative bacteria and *Staphylococcus aureus*.

GRAM-NEGATIVE BACTERIA
Gram-negative bacteria normally inhabit the gut but cause infections in the urinary tract, respiratory tract and wounds. Outbreaks of resistant forms have been reported (Casewell, 1982; Dance, 1987) which may be the consequence of excessive use of broad-spectrum antibiotics. Pseudomonas species may cause particular problems. This organism can multiply in warm, moist conditions and has been identified in eye drops, soap solutions, lotions and in the tubing used for ventilators and incubators. This is particularly difficult because of the shortage of drugs which are effective against resistant forms of Pseudomonas species.

STAPHYLOCOCCUS AUREUS
Staphylococcus aureus is also a normal human inhabitant, and large numbers of the organism being found on the skin and mucosa. Carriers and patients infected with resistant forms of MRSA need to be identified and the extent of colonization of the nose, perineum, wounds, skin lesions, indwelling catheters and tracheostomies (Ayliffe, 1986). Contacts of infected patients or staff should be screened to prevent spread and staff found positive should go off duty until treatment results in negative swabs. Infected patients should be barrier nursed (see p. 9) and only transferred within or between hospitals under close supervision. All staff concerned should be informed that the patient has MRSA. Prompt barrier nursing may limit the spread of MRSA (Selkon *et al.*, 1980) but the resistant strain is very difficult to eradicate. Barrier nursing should, therefore, continue for the entire time the patient remains in hospital even when specimens are negative. The presence of MRSA should be documented in the patient's records to alert staff should readmission be necessary (*Journal of Hospital Infection*, 1983).

References and further reading
Ayliffe, G.A.J. (1985) Guidelines for the control of epidemic methicillin-resistant *Staphylococcus aureus*, *Journal of Infection*, Vol. 7, pp. 193–201.

Ayliffe, G.A.J. (1986) Guidelines for the control of epidemic methicillin-resistant Staphylococcus aureus, *Journal of Infection*, Vol. 7, pp. 193–201.

Bradley, J.M. (1985) Methicillin resistant *Staphylococcus aureus* in a London hospital, *Lancet*, Vol. i, pp. 1493–5.

Casewell, M.W. (1982) The role of multiply resistant coliforms in hospital acquired infection, *Recent Advances in Infection*, Vol. 2, pp. 31–50.

Casewell, M.W. (1986) Epidemiology and control of the modern methicillin resistant staphylococcus, *Journal of Hospital Infection*, Vol. 7 (Suppl.A), pp. 1–11.

Crow, A.W. *et al.* (1979) A nosocomial outbreak of infection due to multiply resistant *Proteus mirabilis*, *Journal of Infectious Disease*, Vol. 139, pp. 621–7.

Dance, D.A.B. (1987) A hospital outbreak caused by a chlorhexidine and antibiotic resistant *Proteus mirabilis*, *Journal of Hospital Infection*, Vol. 10, pp. 10–16.

Garrod, L.P. (1972) Causes of failure in antibiotic treatment, *British Medical Journal*, Vol. 4, pp. 473–6.

Grazebrook, J. (1986) Counting the cost of infection, *Nursing Times*, Vol. 83, No.6, pp. 24–6.

Hone, R. *et al.* (1981) Bacteraemia in Dublin due to gentamicin resistant *Staphylococcus aureus, Journal of Hospital Infection* Vol. 2, pp. 119–25.

Jaffe, H.W. *et al.* (1980) Identity and interspecific transfer of gentamicin resistant plasmids in *Staphylococcus aureus* and *Staphylococcus epidermidis, Journal of Infectious Diseases* Vol., 141, p.738.

Jevons, M.P. (1961) Celberin resistant staphylococci, *British Medical Journal,* Vol. 1, pp. 124–5.

Journal of Hospital Infection (1983) Methicillin resistant *Staphylococcus aureus, Journal of Hospital Infection,* Vol. 4, pp. 327–9.

Keane, C.T. (1983) Evidence for the dispersion and evolution of R. Plasmids from *Serratia marcescens* in a hospital, *Journal of Hospital Infection,* Vol. 6, pp. 147–53.

Mendoza, M.C. (1985) Evidence for the dispersion and evolution of R. Plasmids from *Serratia marcescens* in hospital, *Journal of Hospital Infection,* Vol. 6, pp. 147–53.

Sande, M.A., and Mandell, G.L. (1980) Chemotherapy of microbial diseases, in L.S. Goodman *et al.* (eds.) *The Pharmacological Basis of Therapeutics,* Macmillan, London.

Selkon, J.B. *et al.* (1980) The role of an isolation unit in the control of hospital infection with multi-resistant *Staphylococcus aureus, Journal of Hospital Infection,* Vol. 1, pp. 41–6.

Sparling, F.P. *et al.* (1976) Antibiotic resistance in the gonococcus in D. Schlessinger (ed.) Microbiology, American Society of Microbiology.

Swan Joint Committee (1969) *Use of Antibiotics in Animal Husbandry and Veterinary Medicine,* HMSO, London.

HEPATITIS A

Definition

Hepatitis A is an acute infectious disease caused by hepatitis A virus (HAV).

REFERENCE MATERIAL

Hepatitis A is spread predominantly by the faecal–oral route, and has been associated with:

1 contaminated water, milk and food;
2 breakdown of sanitary conditions;
3 ingestion of raw or undercooked shellfish harvested from contaminated water;
4 travel to areas of the world with poor hygienic conditions;
5 institutionalized children and adults;
6 male homosexuals, when infection is related to high degree of promiscuity, and the practice of oral/anal and genital/anal intercourse.

Hepatitis A virus can be detected in faeces during the incubation period which averages 30 days (range 15–45 days), and the early symptomatic phase of the disease. From then the number of virus particles in the stools usually decreases and consequently may not be detectable at the time of onset of jaundice.

Antibodies to HAV can be detected serologically. This is the best means to diagnose reliably and follow the course of hepatitis A illness.

Antibodies to HAV (anti-HAV) are present in the serum by the time on onset of illness, and consist of both the 1gG and 1gM class. After 3–12 months 1gM anti-HAV disappears whereas 1gG anti-HAV persists in high titre and is associated with lifelong immunity.

Generally HAV produces an acute, self-limiting disease, which characteristically has an acute sudden 'influenza-like' onset with:

1 myalgia;
2 headache;
3 fever;
4 malaise;
5 jaundice.

The mortality rate is low, being less than 0.5%. Unlike hepatitis B, hepatitis A does not lead to chronic hepatitis or to a chronic carrier state.

All family and close personal contacts must receive 2–5 ml of immune serum globulin (1sG) as soon as possible after exposure, ideally within 7–14 days. After treatment protection lasts for 4–6 months (DHSS, 1984).

References and further reading

Department of Health and Social Security (1984) *Immunization Against Infectious Disease,* DHSS, London.

Francis, D.P. and Maynard, J.E. (1979) The transmission and outcome of hepatitis A B and non A, non B review, *Epidemiologic Review,* Vol. 1, p. 17.

Garey, L. and Holmes, K.K. (1980) Sexual transmission of hepatitis A in homosexual men, incidence and mechanism, *New England Journal of Medicine,* Vol. 302, p. 435.

Hadler, S.C. *et al.* (1982) Risk factors for hepatitis A in day care centres, *Journal of Infectious Diseases,* Vol. 145, p. 255.

Rakela, A. *et al.* (1978) Hepatitis A virus infection in fulminant hepatitis and chronic active hepatitis, *Gastroenterology,* Vol. 74, p. 879.

GUIDELINES: HEPATITIS A

OUTPATIENT

Action	Rationale
1 It is not usually necessary to admit the individual to hospital.	Self-limiting disease.
2 Patient education is essential and must include advice on good personal hygiene and careful hand washing.	Limits the spread of the virus. Careful hand washing removes contamination from hands.
3 Separate soap, flannel and towel must be provided.	To minimize the risk of infection being spread via equipment used for hygiene purposes.
4 Meticulous cleaning of bath, wash basin and toilet.	To remove contamination.
5 Bath and wash basin must be allowed to dry after use.	Viruses will not survive on clean dry surfaces.
6 Soiled bedlinen and underclothing should be given a hot wash.	To remove contamination.
7 Refrain from intimate kissing and sexual intercourse while symptoms are present.	To prevent cross-infection.
8 Avoid contact with susceptible persons, i.e. very young, old or those with debilitating illness.	To reduce the likelihood of infection.
9 Crockery and cutlery must be washed and rinsed in hot water.	Heat destroys the virus.

INPATIENT

Action	Rationale
1 Whenever possible, the patient should have medical or surgical treatment postponed under he/she is symptom free.	Medical and surgical treatment will debilitate the patient further and recovery will be slower.
2 Ideally the patient should be discharged.	Cross-infection is less likely to occur at home among fit, healthy persons.
3 A single room with separate toilet should be made available for the patient.	Although patients are no longer excreting the virus once they have become symptomatic, there are always exceptions.
4 Blood, secretions and excreta (particularly faeces) must be handled using plastic apron and gloves.	To prevent cross-infection.

Note: For further information on barrier nursing, see pp. 9–17.

NON-A NON-B HEPATITIS

Definition

Since the introduction of radioimmunoassays for the diagnosis of hepatitis B and A virus infection, the existence of a third hepatitis virus, called non-A and non-B (NANB), has become apparent (Prince *et al.*, 1974).

REFERENCE MATERIAL

There are no accepted serological tests for NANB. Diagnosis is achieved by excluding infections associated with NANB. These include symptoms associated with hepatitis A, hepatitis B, cytomegalovirus, Epstein–Barr virus, toxic and drug-induced liver injury (including alcoholic liver disease), circulatory abnormalities, shock, sepsis, biliary tract disease and metabolic liver disease (Dienstag, 1983).

Non-A and non-B hepatitis has been shown to occur in patients who have received:

1 blood transfusions;
2 clotting factors for coagulation disorders;
3 haemodialysis;
4 outbreaks of epidemics in tropical areas;
5 sporadic cases with no identifiable cause.

Transmission appears to be similar to that of hepatitis B, i.e. principally through blood and blood products. There is an increased incidence in drug addicts due to the sharing of contaminated needles and syringes (Bamber and Thomas, 1983). There is evidence, however, of sporadic cases with no obvious contributory factors (Farrow *et al.*, 1981).

The incubation period is estimated at 6–8 weeks followed by clinical features similar to hepatitis B, although as a rule acute illness tends to be less severe.

Despite its relatively mild, often asymptomatic and anicteric presentation during acute infection, NANB may progress to chronic liver disease. The prognosis is ultimately good except in patients who are immunosuppressed. These succumb to liver failure.

Treatment involves responding to the signs and symptoms as they occur. Liver transplantation is the treatment of the future for patients with liver failure.

It is essential that safe techniques are used at all times when in contact with blood and body fluids.

Human immunoglobulin can be used to give prophylactic protection.

References and further reading

Bamber, M. and Thomas, H.C. (1983) Acute type A, B and Non-A Non-B Hepatitis in a hospital population in London clinical and epidemiological features, *Gut*, Vol. 24, pp. 561–4.
Dienstag, J.L. (1983) Non-A Non-B Hepatitis recognition epidemiology and clinical features, *Gastroenterology*, Vol. 85, pp. 439–62.
Dienstag, J.L. *et al.* (1977) Non-A Non-B post transfusion hepatitis, *Lancet*, Vol. i, pp. 560–2.
Farrow, L.J. *et al.* (1981) Non-A Non-B hepatitis in West London, *Lancet*, Vol. i, pp. 982–4.
Inarson, S. *et al.* (1973) Multiple attacks of hepatitis in drug addicts, *Journal of Infectious Disease*, Vol. 12, pp. 165–9.
Prince, A.M. *et al.* (1974) Incubation post transfusion hepatitis without sero-logical evidence of exposure to Hepatitis B virus, *Lancet*, Vol. i, p. 241.
Wong, O.C. *et al.* (1980) Epidemic and endemic hepatitis in India: evidence for a Non-A Non-B Hepatitis virus aetiology, *Lancet*, Vol. ii, pp. 876–8.

GUIDELINES: NON-A NON-B HEPATITIS

The procedure should be as for hepatitis B (see pp. 23–27).

HEPATITIS B

Definition

Hepatitis B is a serious infectious disease which is associated with necrosis and inflammation of the liver. It is relatively uncommon in the United Kingdom.

REFERENCE MATERIAL
Epidemiology

Hepatitis B virus infection is caused by the transfer of the virus from an infected individual or article to a susceptible individual via the blood. The virus has also been detected in saliva and semen. This transfer normally occurs through one of the following means:

1 accidental inoculation;
2 an existing break in host skin;
3 spillage into the eyes or mouth;
4 perinatal.

Infectivity

An individual with acute hepatitis B is probably most infectious during the late incubation and prodromal periods. The incubation period of hepatitis B is about 2–5 months. There are three patterns of clinical response:

1 some 30–40% of adults develop clinically apparent hepatitis;

2   some 50–60% of adults remain asymptomatic but show serological evidence of infection;
3   some 5–10% of adults develop chronic infection (HBs Ag carrier state). Between 40 and 50% of those with chronic HBV infection will die of that infection from cirrhosis or hepatocellular cancer (Short and Jones, 1987).

Infections with hepatitis B virus are generally mild, presenting as a flu-like illness, approximately half of known cases being accompanied by jaundice. There is a fatality rate, however, of less than 1% and deaths are mainly due to fulminating liver failure. In the United Kingdom only 0.1% of the population are carriers. Less than 5% of infections in the United Kingdom progress to the carrier state. This state occurs most frequently after inapparent infections without a history of jaundice and which are often only detected on routine screening for other procedures, such as blood donation.

Diagnosis

Diagnosis is confirmed by blood test, i.e. a virological test requiring 10 ml of clotted blood. Three antigen–antibody systems are recognized as serological markers for the diagnosis of present or past infection with hepatitis B virus:
1   hepatitis B surface antigen (HBs Ag) denotes current hepatitis B infection. Antibody to hepatitis B surface antigen (anti-HBs) denotes past infection and immunity to further infections;
2   antibody to hepatitis B core antigen (anti-HBc) denotes present or past hepatitis B virus infection and very high levels are found in hepatitis B surface antigen carriers;
3   hepatitis Be antigen is detected both in the early period of acute hepatitis B infection and in some carriers. During recovery from an acute infection HBe Ag is usually replaced by anti-HBe (e antigen carriers are more infectious than surface antigen carriers).

Screening policy for hepatitis B surface antigen

Screening of the entire hospital patient population would be an effective way to identify hepatitis B infection, but this would be costly and time consuming in terms of the benefits derived. It is important, however, to screen patients before their admission to a transplant or renal unit (Tedder, 1980).

In general, the best compromise is to test those patients belonging to groups in which there is a high prevalence of hepatitis B. These include the following persons:
1   all new admissions who currently live or were born in countries where there is a high prevalance of hepa-

titis B, such as the developing countries;
2   drug addicts;
3   male homosexuals;
4   mentally subnormal patients in institutions;
5   multiple transfusion patients;
6   all patients acutely or recently jaundiced;
7   tattooed individuals.

Immunization and vaccination

Prophylactic measures are the only means of combating the disease to date since no safe and effective antiviral agent for the treatment of hepatitis B infection has been discovered.

Specific hepatitis B immunoglobulin derived from the plasma of donors with a high titre of anti-HBs has been available in the United Kingdom since 1971 (British Medical Journal, 1982). It shows no benefit for the treatment of fulminant acute hepatitis B infection (Annals of Internal Medicine, 1977) but provides benefit for post-exposure prophylaxis after inoculation accidents, cuts/abrasions or splashes of blood from a hepatitis B-positive patient into the eye or the mouth.

The Medical Research Council report (1980) describes a low (3%) incidence of subsequent hepatitis B infection when specific hepatitis B immunoglobulin had been given prophylactically. Department of Health and Social Security guidelines (1984) advise that immunoglobulin should be given as soon as possible after the incident – preferably not later than 48 hours after.

There are two types of hepatitis B vaccine available – a genetically engineered vaccine and a plasma-derived vaccine. The Immunization Practices Advisory Committee (US Department of Health and Human Services, 1987) states that these are comparable.

Between 1980 and 1984, 364 cases (131 nurses) of acute clinical hepatitis B in health service staff in the United Kingdom were reported. Eighty (20%) of these individuals acquired the infection while working abroad (Polakoff, 1986). This would seem to support the World Health Organization's recommendations that health care personnel in contact with blood or sharp instruments and needles should be immunized (Short and Jones, 1987).

PREVENTION OF HEPATITIS B IN HEALTH CARE WORKERS

Safe technique is essential when in contact with blood and body fluids regardless of whether the patient is hepatitis positive or negative. Dienstag and Ryan (1982) have shown that general ward nurses are at no greater risk of acquiring hepatitis B than the general population.

EMPLOYMENT OF HBs AG PERSONS

Tedder (1980) discusses the problem of carriers of HBs

Ag who want to return to full-time employment, particularly those whose carrier state lasts for many years or possibly for the rest of their lives. Guidelines are available to those individuals working in the health service (Department of Health and Social Security, 1981).

PATIENT EDUCATION

The Department of Health and Social Security (1984) recommends that individuals found to be HBs Ag carriers should be counselled about the ways in which hepatitis B may spread and the precautions which can be taken to reduce the risk to others. It stresses that unnecessary restrictions and precautions may cause distress and should be avoided.

References and further reading

Annals of Internal Medicine (1977) Acute hepatic failure study group. Failure of specific immunotherapy in fulminant type B hepatitis, *Annals of Internal Medicine*, Vol. 86, pp. 272–77.

British Medical Journal (1982) Use of immunoglobulin with high content of antibody to hepatitis B surface antigen (anti-HBs), *British Medical Journal*, Vol. 285, pp. 951–4.

Department of Health and Social Security (1981) *Hepatitis B and NHS staff*, (CMO (81) 11), HMSO, London.

Department of Health and Social Security (1984) *Guidance for Health Service Personnel Dealing with Patients Infected with Hepatitis B Virus*, (CMO (84) 11, CNO (84) 7), HMSO, London.

Department of Health and Social Security (1987) *Decontamination of Equipment, Liver or Other Surfaces Contaminated with Hepatitis B or Human Immunodeficiency Virus* (HN (87) 1), HMSO, London.

Dienstag, J.L. and Ryan, D.M. (1982) Occupational exposure to hepatitis B virus in hospital personnel: infection or immunization, *American Journal of Epidemiology*, Vol. 115, pp. 22–9.

Medical Research Council and Public Health Laboratory Service (1980) The incidence of hepatitis B infection after accidental exposure and anti-HBs immunoglobulin prophylaxis, *Lancet*, Vol. i, pp. 6–8.

Polakoff, S. (1986) Acute viral hepatitis B: laboratory reports 1980–4, *British Medical Journal*, Vol. 293, pp. 37–8.

Short, R. and Jones, G. (eds.) (1987) *Hepatitis B and Nursing in the U.K.* Report from the Wembley Conference (of the Royal College of Nursing Safety Representatives), Mark Allen Publishing, London.

Tedder, R.S. (1980) Hepatitis B in hospital, *Journal of Hospital Medicine*, Vol. 23, no. 3, pp. 266, 274–6, 278–9.

GUIDELINES: HEPATITIS B

Procedure

Action	Rationale
1 The patient may be nursed on an open ward unless there is a high risk of blood contamination of the ward environment.	If adequate precautions can be adhered to on an open ward, there is no need to isolate the patient.
2 The patient must be assessed daily to establish accurately any sites of bleeding. Changes in the patient's condition should be recorded in his/her care plan.	Sites of bleeding must be identified in order that the appropriate precautions can be taken.
3 An individual container for disposing 'sharps' must be kept for the patient. The container must be labelled 'High Risk' and when half full it must be sealed and put into the appropriate bag. The bag is then securely sealed, marked 'High Risk' and sent for incineration.	Contaminated 'sharps' are a potential inoculation hazard to others, so particular caution must be taken in handling them. Overloaded 'sharps' containers may cause needles to pierce the walls of the container or even protrude through the top.
4 A personal disposable bag should be kept on a regular holder with a lid for the patient's disposable waste. When full this should be securely closed, marked 'High Risk' and sent for incineration.	To confine potentially contaminated material, e.g. blood-stained tissues.

Action	Rationale
5 The patient's personal hygiene equipment must be clearly marked and kept at the bedside.	To prevent accidental use of equipment by others.
6 Used linen that is not blood-stained is placed in the ward linen bags in the usual way.	Linen free from blood stains is not contaminated and may be dealt with in the normal manner.
7 The patient should use the ward bath or shower last and the area must be thoroughly cleaned afterwards.	To allow time for cleaning before the area is used by others.
8 During venepuncture or other procedures likely to cause bleeding, furniture, bedding and clothing in the adjacent area should be protected with polythene sheeting.	To prevent contamination of the environment with spilled blood.
9 All staff involved with the patient should cover any cuts or grazes on their hands with waterproof dressings.	Broken skin provides a portal of entry for the hepatitis virus in the event of contact with the patient's blood.
10 Routine daily cleaning procedures may be carried out as normal. Domestic staff are advised to wear gloves. It should be ascertained that domestic staff understand the potential hazard associated with blood contamination.	Explanation is necessary as the domestic staff may not understand the hazards involved or may over-react to the situation.

ACCIDENTAL INOCULATION OR SPILLAGE OF BLOOD

Action	Rationale
1 Any accident involving skin penetration or heavy contamination of abraded skin or mucosal surfaces of staff should be recorded on an accident form and taken to bacteriology immediately. If the risk of infection from this incident is high, hepatitis B immunoglobulin must be given within 48 hours.	To protect personnel. To comply with legal and/or hospital requirements.
2 Blood spillage onto unbroken skin should be washed off with soap and running water. A scrubbing brush should not be used as this could break the skin. Complete an accident form, as above.	To remove the source of potential contamination.
3 Accidental inoculation sites should be cleaned under running water, encouraged to bleed freely and then sealed. Complete an accident form, as above.	Bleeding helps 'wash' the inoculated virus out of the system.
4 Blood spilled on hard surfaces must be wiped up immediately with paper towels and the area washed well with a solution such as glutaraldehyde.	To prevent viral spread. Dried blood remains infectious for several days.
5 Linen stained with blood should be treated as infected linen.	Blood-stained linen is highly infectious.

PRECAUTIONS IF BLEEDING IS PRESENT

Action

Rationale

1   Disposable pillowcases and sheets must be used if there is a likelihood of blood spillage. A plastic pillowcase must be used to protect the pillow.

Blood-stained linen is highly infectious. Disposable linen is therefore cheaper and more practical.

2   If bleeding is present in the mouth:
  (a)   Use disposable crockery and cutlery and discard, with any uneaten food, into the disposal bag at the bedside.
  (b)   Keep a personal food tray and water jug at the bedside.
  (c)   Disposable mouth-care equipment, sputum pot and tissues should be kept at the bedside.

The sputum may be contaminated with blood from the mouth, therefore precautions must include avoiding contact with the patient's sputum.

3   If haematuria or melaena is present:
  (a)   Wear plastic gowns and gloves when handling excreta.
  (b)   Keep a toilet and handbasin for the patient's sole use, if practicable.
  (c)   If a toilet is not available for the patient's sole use, bedpans or urinals must be used. These should be washed in the usual manner in the bedpan washer and dried carefully. They should then be placed in the appropriate bag, marked 'High Risk', stapled securely and sent to the central sterile supplies department for autoclaving.

Blood present in the urine or faeces makes the patient's excreta a potential source of hepatitis B contamination.

4   If the patient has a wound or a break in the skin:
  (a)   Cover the area adequately so that there is no seepage.
  (b)   Used dressings should be securely sealed in a plastic bag before being disposed of in the appropriate bag.
  (c)   All tapes, lotions and creams are kept solely for the patient's use.
  (d)   The dressing trolley must be cleaned carefully before re-use.
  (e)   Metal instruments should be cleaned scrupulously with soap and water and soaked in a solution such as glutaraldehyde for 3 hours. Instruments are then placed in the appropriate bag, marked 'High Risk', which is securely stapled shut and sent to central sterile supplies department.

To prevent the spread of the virus from dried or fresh blood. It should be remembered that dried blood can remain infectious for several days.

OTHER HOSPITAL DEPARTMENTS

Action

Rationale

1   All departments and staff involved with the patient must be made aware of the diagnosis.

To allow them to make their own precautionary arrangements.

Action	Rationale
2 All request cards to be labelled appropriately.	To alert the receiving department of the diagnosis.
3 All specimens to be labelled appropriately and correctly bagged. (For further information on specimen collection see p. 335.)	To alert the receiving department of the diagnosis and prevent contamination of the environment.
4 If a patient who is bleeding has to be transported elsewhere, the porter involved should be provided with the following: (a) disposable gloves and aprons; (b) disposable trolley sheets or chair covers; (c) cleaning equipment for the trolley or chair prior to use by the next patient.	To prevent the contamination of the porter or other patients.

DEATH OF A PATIENT WITH HEPATITIS B

Action	Rationale
1 There should be minimal handling of the body.	To reduce the risk of infecting the nursing staff.
2 Nurses should wear disposable plastic aprons and gloves when handling the body.	
3 The body should be totally enclosed in a plastic bag specifically designed for highly contagious patients.	To reduce the risk of infecting the nursing staff.
4 The mortuary staff should be informed of the diagnosis.	
5 If the relatives want to view the body, they must be advised not to touch it.	To prevent contamination.

DISCHARGING THE PATIENT

Action	Rationale
1 The majority of precautions can cease.	Discharge normally implies the risk of cross-infection is no longer present.
2 The patient should be advised not to share razors, toothbrushes or similar personal property likely to be contaminated by blood.	To prevent cross-infection.
3 If bleeding occurs, the patient clears up the blood himself/herself and disposes safely of such items as contaminated tissues by burning, flushing down the toilet or sealing in a polythene bag for routine council rubbish collection. If regular persistent blood-stained waste is generated, the health authority must be requested to make special collections.	To prevent cross-infection.

4 If emergency treatment or dental care is required, the patient must inform the health care worker of the fact that he/she has a recent history of hepatitis B infection.

To allow the correct precautions to be taken.

ACQUIRED IMMUNE DEFICIENCY SYNDROME (AIDS)

Definition

AIDS is a state of immunosuppression caused by the human immunodeficiency virus (HIV). Because no overall description can be made for AIDS an internationally agreed case definition has been made (Centers for Disease Control, 1987).

REFERENCE MATERIAL

The human immunodeficiency virus has been isolated in the blood (Gallo *et al.*, 1984), semen (Zagury *et al.*, 1984), tears and saliva (Fujikawra *et al.*, 1985), breast milk (Thiry *et al.*, 1985), genital secretions of women (Wofsy *et al.*, 1986) and cerebrospinal fluid and the brain (Levy, 1985). Transmission of the virus between individuals most often occurs during sexual activity, by needle sharing in drug abusers, by the administration of contaminated blood and blood products and by vertical transmission from mother to baby.

When an individual is infected with HIV, antibodies to the virus can be demonstrated by using an antibody screening test. The limitations of this test are discussed by Adler (1987a).

The Department of Health and Social Security (1985) recommends that no patient should be tested for HIV antibodies without full informed consent and that counselling should be offered to the patient before and after the test. Miller (1987) discusses the information which should be included in the counselling sessions while Grimshaw (1987) suggests that time spent on counselling not only provides psychological and emotional support but also is a good basis for future communication.

Adler (1987b) reports that not all infected persons go on to develop AIDS and reports that some present with lymphadenopathy (PGL), with 10% eventually developing AIDS or AIDS-related complex (ARC) of whom 25% will then proceed to develop AIDS within 36 months. The mean survival of an AIDS patients is directly related to the presentation. Patients presenting with *Pneumocystis carinii* pneumonia have a mean survival time of 12.5 months, while those presenting with Kaposi's sarcoma have 21 months.

Up to the end of December 1987, 1,227 cases of AIDS had been reported to the Communicable Diseases Study Centre. Of these, 697 have been reported dead. In addition, 6,635 persons had been reported as HIV positive. No overall figures are available because AIDS is not a notifiable disease.

There is no effective treatment for AIDS and no prophylactic treatment can be given in the event of an inoculation accident involving an AIDS patient. Jeffries (1987) recommends that self-inoculation must be avoided and any broken skin covered with a waterproof dressing when caring for patients as all patients are a potential risk. In the event of gross contamination of intact skin, the affected area must be washed thoroughly with soap under hot running water. Scrubbing brushes which could cause skin damage should not be used. Splashes into the eyes or mouth should be diluted by washing and sterile eye wash bottles should be provided in areas where this is likely to occur, such as theatres or intravenous treatment rooms. Information about the action to take should a puncture wound or cut occur is found later in this section.

Mindel (1987) discusses the importance of confidentiality when dealing with any antibody-positive patient. This is supported by the United Kingdom Central Council for Nursing, Midwifery and Health Visitors (1986) and the Department of Health and Social Security (1986) which also states that health care workers dealing with known or suspected seropositive patients or specimens must be made fully aware of the risk.

The Public Health (Infections Diseases) Regulations 1985 make certain provisions to safeguard public health where a person is suffering from AIDS, stressing that these are only to be used in exceptional circumstances where transmission of HIV may occur.

References and further reading

Adler, M.N. (ed.) (1987a) *The ABC of AIDS*, British *Medical Journal* Publication, London.

Adler, M.N. (1987b) Range and natural history of infection, *British Medical Journal*, Vol. 294, pp. 1145–7.

Advisory Committee on Dangerous Pathogens (1986) *LAV/HTLF III – The Causitive Agent of AIDS and*

Related Conditions – Revised Guidelines, HMSO, London.

Centers for Disease Control (1987) Revision of CDC surveillance case definition for acquired immunodeficiency syndrome, *Morbidity and Mortality Weekly Report*, Vol. 36 (suppl. 1S), pp. 3S–15S.

Department of Health and Social Security (1986) *AIDS Booklet 3: Guidance for Surgeons, Anaesthetists, Dentists and Their Teams in Dealing with Patients Infected with HTLV III*, (CMO (86) 7), HMSO, London.

Department of Health and Social Security (1985) The Public Health (Infectious Diseases) Regulations 1985 (HC (85) 17) (LAC (85) 10), HMSO, London.

Elliott, J. (1987) Nursing care, *British Medical Journal*, Vol. 295, pp. 104–6.

Fujikawara, L.S. *et al.* (1985) Isolation of human T lymphotropic virus type III from tears of patients with AIDS, *Lancet*, Vol. II, pp. 529–30.

Gallo, R.C. *et al.* (1984) Frequent detection and continuous production of cytopathic retroviruses (HTLV III) from patients with AIDS and at risk for AIDS, *Science*, Vol. 224, pp. 497–500.

Grimshaw, J. (1987) Being HIV antibody positive, *British Medical Journal*, Vol. 295, pp. 256–7.

Jeffries, D. (1987) Control of Infection Policies, *British Medical Journal*, Vol. 295, pp. 33–5.

Levy, J.A. (1985) Isolation of AIDS associated retroviruses from cerebrospinal fluid and brain of patients with neurological symptoms, *Lancet*, Vol, ii, pp. 586–8.

Miller, D. *et al.* (eds.) (1986) *The Management of AIDS Patients*, Macmillan, London.

Miller, D. (1987) Counselling, *British Medical Journal*, Vol. 294, pp. 1670–4.

Mindel, A. (1987) Management of early HIV infection, *British Medical Journal*, Vol. 294, pp. 1145–7.

PHLS Communicable Disease Surveillance Centre (1986) *The Acquired Immune Deficiency Syndrome: 1985* (CDR 86/15).

PHLS Communicable Disease Surveillance Centre (1987) *HIV Exposure in Health Care Workers: a Prospective Study* (CDR 87/24).

Pratt, R.J. (1988) *AIDS – A Strategy for Nursing Care*, Edward Arnold, London.

Royal College of Nursing (1987) *Nursing Guidelines on the Management of Patients in Hospital and the Community Suffering from AIDS*, RCN, London.

Thiry, L. et al. (1985 Isolation of AIDS virus from cell free breast milk of three healthy virus carriers, *Lancet* Vol. i, pp. 891–2.

United Kingdom Central Council for Nursing, Midwifery and Health Visitors (1986) *Confidentiality – An Elaboration of Clause 9 of the Second Edition of the UKCC's Code of Professional Conduct*, UKCC, London.

Wofsy, C.B. *et al.* (1986) Isolation of AIDS associated retrovirus from genital secretions of women with antibodies to the virus, *Lancet*, Vol. i, pp. 527–9.

Zagury, D. *et al.* (1984) HTLV III cells culture from semen to two patients with AIDS, *Science*, Vol. 226, pp. 449–51.

GUIDELINES: ACQUIRED IMMUNE DEFICIENCY SYNDROME IN A GENERAL WARD

Procedure

Action	Rationale
1 It is not recommended that pregnant staff should nurse patients with AIDS or suspected AIDS.	AIDS patients may excrete high levels of cytomegalovirus which causes congenital deformities in babies.
2 Staff suffering from eczema should not nurse patients with AIDS or suspected AIDS.	Any break in staff members' skin should be covered with a waterproof dressing to prevent entry of HIV. This would be difficult to accomplish with eczema lesions and would exacerbate the eczema.
3 Immunodeficient-compromised staff, either through illness or therapy, should not nurse patients with AIDS or suspected AIDS.	AIDS patients who present with generalized infection could put this category of staff at risk.

4 All staff should read and be familiar with government guidelines on AIDS and their own hospital's codes of practice.	To ensure all staff are aware of, and take, the necessary precautions.
5 Hospital staff should cover any broken skin with a waterproof dressing.	To prevent the entry of infectious material.
6 Accidental inoculatins must be avoided at all cost.	There is no prophylactic treatment available.
7 In the event of gross contamination of intact skin the affected area must be washed thoroughly with soap under hot water. A scrubbing brush must not be used.	Intact skin is a natural barrier against infection. By thorough washing the infectious material can be removed. Scrubbing brushes can cause skin damage which allows infection to enter.
8 Puncture wounds or cuts must be made to bleed freely and washed under hot running water.	To flush out infectious material.
9 A waterproof dressing must be applied and medical advice sought for large wounds.	To prevent further infection.
10 An accident form must be filled in immediately and taken to bacteriology, the occupational health physician or other medical advisor as appropriate.	It is important to have accurate records of all accidents and incidents in order to monitor events.

LOW-RISK, HIV-POSITIVE INDIVIDUALS

Action	**Rationale**
1 If a low-risk, HIV-positive individual develops an infection, is undergoing invasive procedures or becomes incontinent, nursing care will commence as for high-risk, HIV-positive persons.	Incontinent, bleeding HIV antibody-positive patients have the potential risk of transmitting the HIV virus to others.

HIGH-RISK, HIV-POSITIVE INDIVIDUALS

Action	**Rationale**
1 Known or strongly suspected HIV antibody positive patients who are bleeding, incontinent infected with a contagious disease or receiving invasive procedures should be nursed in a single room with its own toilet and hand washing facilities.	To minimize the risk of transmitting infection to the patient from hospital pathogens and to protect other susceptible patients.

ENTERING THE ROOM

Action	**Rationale**
1 When the patient is not bleeding, coughing, incontinent or receiving procedures, protective clothing is not required. For prolonged close work such as making beds, a plastic apron is advisable.	Transmission of HIV is not possible from casual social contact. A plastic apron will prevent transmission of organism to or from the nurse's uniform.

Action	Rationale
2 When the patient is incontinent, bleeding or undergoing invasive procedures, disposable well-fitting gloves and a plastic apron are needed.	Transmission of HIV is possible from body fluids.
3 If there is a possibility of airborne contamination a correctly fitting theatre mask and safety spectacles should be worn.	Transmission of HIV is possible if contaminated material is allowed to contaminate mucous membrane.

LIQUID WASTE

Action	Rationale
1 All liquid waste from AIDS patients must be disposed of in a bedpan washer immediately, taking care to avoid splashing.	To prevent contamination of the environment.
2 Areas without bedpan washers will need to use the slop hopper. Great care must be taken to pour waste slowly and carefully down the hopper to avoid splashing. The hopper must be flushed twice.	To prevent contamination of the environment.

NON-DISPOSABLE EQUIPMENT

Action	Rationale
1 Cleaning of non-disposable equipment needs to be performed thoroughly and in a safe manner.	Careless cleaning, immersion, drying, etc. can increase contamination of the environment.
2 Gloves/aprons must be worn, together with masks/eye protection if appropriate.	To prevent self-contamination.
3 Prior to disinfection, equipment must be cleaned with soap and water, avoiding splashing.	Disinfectants cannot completely penetrate organic matter.
4 The equipment must then be dried carefully.	Wet objects would alter the disinfectant's strength and could inactivate the solution if soap and soiling were still present.
5 If equipment will not be damaged by immersion in freshly activated 2% glutaraldehyde for 30 minutes, this is the method of choice.	Glutaraldehyde's bacteriostatic action is completely effective against the AIDS retrovirus.
6 If the equipment will be damaged by immersion in the glutaraldehyde solution, or is too big to fit into the disinfection container, these items must be first washed thoroughly with soap and water and dried, followed by washing and drying with a hypochlorite 1% solution, i.e. Precept tablets.	Precept tablets have a non-corrosive action for delicate equipment and are less toxic to staff than glutaraldehyde.

7 If the equipment can be autoclaved it must be placed in a central sterile supplies department (CSSD) bag, taped shut with biohazard tape and marked with a biohazard label. The bag must then be taken to CSSD.

Autoclaving is the most effective sterilization method. Correct bagging and transportation of the equipment will prevent contamination of the environment.

8 Expensive, delicate items which have had prolonged close contact with the patient, i.e. a ventilator, will require ethylene oxide disinfection.

Ethylene oxide disinfection is the second process of choice after autoclaving.

9 Prior to the ethylene oxide disinfection process, these items must have all their disposable parts, filters, etc. removed and the whole item cleaned completely and thoroughly with hypochlorite 1% solution and dried carefully.

To prevent contamination of the environment.

10 The transportation and ethylene oxide process will take at least 1 week. Thought must be given beforehand to the use of this equipment for actively bleeding, incontinent patients.

Ethylene oxide disinfection involves lengthy airing of equipment after the process to ensure it is safe to re-use. During this time other patients may be deprived of the item.

OTHER HOSPITAL DEPARTMENTS

Action

Rationale

1 It is essential that all request cards for such items as specimens have the biohazard label attached.

To ensure all departments are informed that the sample is potentially dangerous.

2 All specimens must have the biohazard label attached and be double bagged in a specimen polythene biohazard bag with a biohazard label attached to the bag.

To ensure the laboratory is aware of potential risk and that the specimen is correctly contained to prevent cross-infection. (For further information on specimen collection see p. 335).

3 The specimen should be taken to the laboratory in a washable, covered container.

To prevent contamination of the environment.

4 A nurse should accompany an AIDS patient to other departments. If there is not a departmental nurse in the department, the ward nurse should remain with the patient.

To give help and advice.

5 The patient will normally be given the first or last appointment of the day.

The department will be less crowded and busy, thus allowing time for appropriate precautions to be taken.

DOMESTIC STAFF

Action

Rationale

1 The room must be prepared and cleaned. (For further information see pp. 13–17.)

To minimize the risk of cross-infection.

2 A nurse must check the patient's room to establish that it is suitable for the domestic staff to clean.

To ensure the room is not contaminated with blood or body fluids.

Action

Rationale

3   If contamination of the environment with blood or body fluids occurs it must be treated with a hypochlorite solution containing 10,000 ppm available chlorine.

To prevent cross-infection.

THERMAL CLEANING OF THE ROOM

Action

Rationale

1   The room must be cleared of all equipment before it is cleaned.

It is impossible to clean thoroughly if potentially contaminated items are in the room.

2   The carpet must be steamed if contamination by blood or excreta has occurred.

Organisms have been known to survive in carpets. Steam cleaning destroys these.

3   The walls should only be cleaned if contamination is known to have occurred.

HIV does not survive on intact walls.

4   The curtains must be changed if contamination has occurred.

Discretion and assessment need to be used. If the room has only been used for a short time for a patient who has not contaminated the environment, curtains would not need changing.

THE PATIENT

Action

Rationale

1   As soon as possible, the probable/known diagnosis must be discussed with the patient and the hospital policy explained.

It is essential that the patient understands fully the reason for these restrictions which, while protecting contacts, also protect the patient from further risks of infection.

2   Psychological support is essential.

Psychological dysfunction is likely and should be recognized and treated early to alleviate and contain the mental distress which an AIDS patient may experience.

3   It is necessary that all nurses caring for AIDS patients are familiar with treatment and care procedures.

To ensure appropriate nursing care is delivered.

4   Staff should adopt a non-judgemental approach in their dealings with AIDS patients.

It is the responsibility of all health professionals to care for patients not to pass moral judgements.

5   It may be appropriate to recommend voluntary agencies to AIDS patients.

Support groups have knowledge and experience which can help HIV antibody-positive individuals.

VISITING

Action

Rationale

1   There should be no restrictions on visiting.

2   The diagnosis of AIDS is confidential and should not be disclosed.

To maintain confidentiality.

DISCHARGING THE PATIENT

Action

1   Almost all patients with AIDS will require community services at some time during their illness.

2   If an AIDS patient requires community services, the patient must have given consent for HIV antibody-positive diagnosis to be given to the general practitioner and community care personnel.

Rationale

AIDS patients will need to be admitted to hospital for the treatment of clinical illness but when in remission will be encouraged to resume their normal activities.

Confidentiality must not be breached without the patient's consent. However, health care workers such as ambulancemen and district nurses will need to take precautions if bleeding, incontinence or infections are present.

DISPOSAL OF WASTE IN THE COMMUNITY

Action

1   Excreta, infected fluids and such items as sanitary towels can be discarded into the toilet in the normal manner.

2   Infected waste such as dressings, gloves and aprons, must be burned or placed in polythene bags and the local authority asked to collect them.

3   Sharps must be placed in a sharps box and stored in a safe place when full. They should then be placed in a yellow polythene bag and collected by the local health authority.

Rationale

To prevent contamination of the environment.

Yellow is the international colour for infected waste bags, and they are available on request from the local authority.

To prevent inoculation accidents.
Yellow is the international colour coding for clinical waste.

LAUNDRY IN THE COMMUNITY

Action

1   Clothes and linen which are heavily soiled or blood-stained should be washed separately, boiled before hand washing or machine washed at 95°C for 10 minutes. Wash as for above in a public launderette.

2   If the person is not fit enough, infected linen should be placed in red alginate plastic bags and the local authority asked to arrange collection and laundering.

Rationale

Heat is effective in destroying the HIV.

Red alginate plastic bags are the international colour coding for infected linen.

COOKERY AND CUTLERY

Action

1   Crockery and cutlery must be hand washed in hot soapy water or in a dishwasher.

Rationale

Heat is effective in destroying the HIV.

Action	Rationale
2 There is no need to keep a separate store of crockery and cutlery.	Crockery and cutlery present no risk of contamination.

PROTECTIVE CLOTHING IN THE COMMUNITY

Action	Rationale
1 Disposable apron and gloves need only be worn when blood or excreta are being handled.	There is no risk of acquiring infection from casual contact.
2 Disinfectants are only required if blood or excreta spillage has occurred. A strong hypochlorite solution (1 part household bleach to 10 parts water) is recommended.	Unnecessary use of disinfectants is expensive and may be potentially hazardous to staff and the environment.

VISITORS IN THE COMMUNITY

Action	Rationale
1 Visitors should be encouraged.	There is no risk of acquiring infection from casual contact.
2 The patient should be encouraged to resume social activities.	Social activities will help to contain any symptoms such as stress and depression.

PREVENTION OF FURTHER INFECTION

Action	Rationale
1 The patient should be encouraged to stay away from individuals with infections.	AIDS patients are susceptible to infections.
2 If the patient develops any signs and symptoms of ill health the general practitioner or hospital must be informed immediately.	Early treatment of symptoms will enhance the chances of containing the disease.

(For further details on discharge planning see p. 118.)

DEATH

Action	Rationale
1 The body should be laid out as described in the Procedure, Last Offices (p. 213). In addition the nurse should wear gloves and a plastic apron.	To prevent self-contamination.
2 All orifices must be packed.	The body continues to secrete fluids after death has occurred. Any leakage may contaminate the environment.

3 Any wounds, intravenous sites or skin breakages must be sealed with waterproof dressing.

To prevent leakage of contaminated fluids.

4 All documentation relating to this procedure must have a biohazard label attached.

To alert administration, portering and mortuary staff of the infection risks.

5 Once the body has been laid out and the room made presentable, family and friends may view the body.

Once the body has left the ward or home, viewing will be difficult, if the funeral director adheres strictly to infectious diseases regulations.

6 The body must be placed in a cadaver bag and sealed securely with biohazard tape.

The cadaver bag will prevent contamination of the environment and ensures infectious diseases regulations are complied with.

7 Porters must be given gloves and plastic aprons to wear when carrying the bag.

There is no infection risk when the body is sealed in a cadaver bag unless the bag becomes torn or damaged in transportation. Gloves and aprons will prevent contamination of the staff handling the body.

FUNERAL ARRANGEMENTS

Action

Rationale

1 Ideally the hospital administration should have a list of funeral directors who will attend to an AIDS patient.

It is important that the bereaved relatives are given every help and support to prevent unnecessary distress.

THE HERPES VIRUSES

The herpes viruses described in this section include herpes simplex (types 1 and 2) and varicella zoster virus (varicella and zoster).

REFERENCE MATERIAL
Herpes Simplex

Herpes simplex virus (HSV) infections are among the most common illnesses affecting humans; often annoying and troublesome, they are only life-threatening when afflicting immunosuppressed patients (Meyers *et al.*, 1980; Ramsey, 1982).

Nahmias *et al* (1970) showed that 80–100% of adults of a lower socioeconomic status in the USA possessed antibodies to HSV, compared to 30–50% of adults of higher socioeconomic groups, due to an increased frequency of both HSV1 and HSV2 infections in adults of lower socioeconomic status.

Herpes simplex virus can be subdivided into two groups: HSV1 – associated with oral, facial and neurological lesions; and HSV2 – associated with genital lesions (Corey *et al.*, 1983a, b). HSV2 has been impli-

cated in cervical cancer (Rawls *et al.*, 1977).

Herpes simplex virus may become latent within the sensory nerve ganglia, despite the presence of circulating antibodies. Relapses are common; a survey of over 6,000 persons with symptomatic recurrent genital herpes indicated the median number of yearly recurrences of genital herpes was between 5 and 8 (Knox *et al.*, 1982).

Transmission of HSV is by direct contact, particularly with oral and/or genital secretions. Prevention involves avoiding contact with infected lesions and therefore gloves are essential for all health care professionals who come into direct contact with lesions. The use of condoms to prevent genital spread during sexual intercourse is advisable (Corey *et al.*, 1983b). Caesarean section for mothers with clinically apparent cervical or genital infection will prevent the baby from acquiring the infection provided the mother implements good infection control practices when handling the baby (Corey *et al.*, 1983a).

The majority of infections resolve spontaneously, although antiviral drugs such as acyclovir are valuable for severe cases (Selby *et al.*, 1979).

NURSING CARE
For details on nursing care refer to pp. 13–17.

Varicella zoster virus (VZV)

Initial infection with VZV causes varicella (chicken pox). Following clinical recovery, the virus persists in a latent form in the dorsal root ganglia of nerves. Reactivation of the latent VZV causes zoster (shingles). Many years can elapse between varicella and zoster infections. It is probable that a person becomes infected with varicella only once apart from exceptional instances, such as bone marrow transplantation, when varicella can be contracted twice (Mandal, 1987).

Zoster appears more frequently as a debilitating disease in certain high-risk groups such as transplant recipients (Atkinson *et al.*, 1980; Hurley *et al.*, 1980), immunocompromised patients (Mazur *et al.*, 1978) and the elderly (Miller, 1980). Infection is directly related to the intensity of immunosuppression experienced by patients receiving combined radiotherapy and chemotherapy, who show a higher incidence than those receiving either radiotherapy or chemotherapy alone (Guinee *et al.*, 1985). Lesions often arise in the irradiated areas, and Mandal (1987) questions whether this implies some form of localized triggering influence. Zoster can recur, usually in the same site, more commonly in individuals with malignant disease.

Susceptible contacts can acquire varicella from individuals infected with varicella or zoster. There is little evidence, however, to support the view that zoster can be contracted by exposure to zoster or varicella (Dolin *et al.*, 1978).

The varicella incubation period is 11–21 days. The infected individual is infectious for 2 days before the rash appears and remains so until all the lesions have healed.

Neuralgia often proclaims the onset of zoster and can occur several days before the vesicles. The vesicles generally correspond in distribution to one or more sensory nerves, most commonly the thoracic and less commonly the cranial nerve.

Recovery from varicella in a fit person is usually spontaneous without sequelae, except for a very low incidence of complications including superinfection of skin, lung, encephalitis and arthritis (Gershon, 1980).

In the immunocompromised a much more serious presentation occurs. Fieldman *et al.* (1975) demonstrated a 7% mortality rate for children with cancer who develop varicella infection, although the mortality rate varies with the type of cancer and treatment given. Anti-varicella zoster immune globulin can be given to those who are in close contact with varicella. It produces immediate protection and has been shown to prevent illnesses in normal persons (Brunell *et al.*, 1969) and to prevent, or at least modify, the illness in high-risk persons (Brunell, 1972; Gershon *et al.*, 1974).

Treatment of varicella is normally only necessary for high-risk groups and involves the use of an antiviral agent such as acyclovir (Balfour *et al.*, 1983).

NURSING CARE

For details on nursing care refer to pp. 13–17. Ideally, children with varicella should be discharged home as varicella can quickly spread in hospital environments. Only staff who have had varicella should have contact with patients with varicella or zoster.

References and further reading

Atkinson, K. *et al.* (1980) Varicella Zoster virus infection after marrow transplantation for aplastic anaemia or leukaemia, *Transplantation*, Vol. 29, pp. 47–50.

Balfour, H.H. *et al.* (1983) Acyclovir halts progression of herpes zoster in immuno-compromised patients, *New England Journal of Medicine*, Vol. 308, pp. 1448–53.

Brunell, P.A. (1972) Prevention of varicella in high risk children – a collaborative study, *Paediatrics*, Vol. 50, pp. 718–21.

Brunell, P.A. *et al.* (1969) Prevention of varicella by zoster immune globulin, *New England Journal of Medicine*, Vol. 280, pp. 1191–4.

Corey, L. *et al.* (1983a) Genital herpes simplex virus infection – clinical manifestation, course and complications, *Annals of Internal Medicine*, Vol. 98, pp. 958–72.

Corey, L. *et al.* (1983b) Genital herpes simplex virus infections – current concepts in diagnosis, therapy and prevention, *Annals of Internal Medicine*, Vol. 98, pp. 973–83.

Dolin, R. *et al.* (1978) Herpes zoster–varicella infections in immuno-suppressed patients, *Annals of Internal Medicine*, Vol. 89, pp. 375–88.

Fieldman, S. *et al.* (1975) Varicella in children with cancer – 77 cases, *Paediatrics*, Vol. 56, pp. 388–97.

Gershon, A.A. (1980) Live attenuated varicella–zoster vaccine, *Review of Infectious Diseases*, Vol. 2, pp. 393–405.

Gershon, A.A. *et al.* (1974) Zoster immune globulin, *New England Journal of Medicine*, Vol. 290, pp. 243–5.

Guinee, V.F. *et al.* (1985) The incidence of herpes zoster in patients with Hodgkin's disease; an analysis of prognostic factors, *Cancer*, Vol. 56, pp. 642–8.

Hurley, J.K. *et al.* (1980) Varicella zoster infection in paediatrics renal transplant recipients, *Archives of Surgery*, Vol. 115, pp. 715–52.

Knox, S.R. *et al.* (1982) Historical findings in subjects from a high socio-economic group who have genital infections with herpes simplex virus, *Sexual Transmitted Diseases*, Vol. 9, pp. 15–20.

Mandal, B.K. (1987) Herpes zoster and the immuno-compromised, *Journal of Infection*, Vol. 14, pp. 1–5.

Mazur, M.H. *et al.* (1978) Herpes zoster at the NIH, a 20-year experience, *American Journal of Medicine*, Vol. 65, pp. 738–44.

Meyers, J.D. *et al.* (1980) Infections with herpes simplex virus and cell mediated immunity after marrow transplant, *Journal of Infectious Diseases*, Vol. 142, pp. 338–46.

Miller, A.E. (1980) Selective decline in cellular immune response to varicella-zoster in the elderly, *Neurology*, Vol. 30, pp. 582–7.

Nahmias, A.J. *et al.* (1970) Antibodies to herpes virus hominis types 1 and 2 in humans, *American Journal of Epidemiology*, Vol. 91, pp. 539–46.

Ramsey, P.G. (1982) Herpes simplex virus pneumonia – clinical presentation and pathogenesis, *Annals of Internal Medicine*, Vol. 97, pp. 813–20.

Rawls, W.E. *et al.* (1977) Relation of herpes simplex virus to human malignancies, *Current Topic Microbiology Immunology*, Vol. 87, p. 71.

Selby, P.J. *et al.* (1979) Parental acyclovir therapy for herpes virus infections in man, *Lancet*, Vol. ii, pp. 1267–70.

TUBERCULOSIS

Definition

Tuberculosis is a chronic, granulomatous infection caused by two species of mycobacteria – *Mycobacterium tuberculosis*, which can cause disease in almost every organ of the body but predominates in the lungs, and *Mycobacterium bovis*, which rarely causes human disease in the United Kingdom and involves the intestines and lymph nodes of the neck.

REFERENCE MATERIAL

There is an overall reduction in the number of new cases of human tuberculosis, with approximately 2,000 new cases being reported each year (Galbraith, 1981). About 10% of cases are fatal (Stanford, 1980; Department of Health and Social Security, 1987). With the increase in AIDS in the United Kingdom there may be an increase in tuberculosis, if the findings of a study in the USA, which demonstrated the rate of tuberculosis among AIDS patients was more than 100 times the incidence in the general public, are borne out (Morbidity and Mortality Weekly Report, 1987).

Certain conditions contribute to the development of tuberculosis including general physical debilitation, lowered resistance due to disease, immunosuppressive drugs and alcoholism, in addition to poor economic status, populations with little immunity such as Asians, and the very young and elderly (Galbraith, 1981).

The mode of spread for tuberculosis is principally inhalation and, less commonly, ingestion. It is thought that fairly prolonged close contact is required for cross-infection to occur. Transmission appears to be directly related to the presence and severity of a cough (Loudon *et al.*, 1969).

The Joint Tuberculosis Committee of the British Thoracic Society (1983) states that a patient with pulmonary tuberculosis who has smear-positive sputum suggests high infectivity and there is potential for cross-infection. All close contacts should be followed up and receive a chest X-ray six months after contact. If a patient is smear negative but culture positive, this indicates that the patient is not infectious and no follow-up is necessary.

The priorities for tuberculosis control are early detection of cases, barrier nursing, if appropriate, plus immunization with Bacillus Calmette–Guérin vaccine (BCG) of tubercle-negative persons (Galbraith, 1981).

Treatment until the 1960s included bed rest, diet, collapse therapy and isolation. Chemotherapy is now the preferred treatment.

Treatment in the initial stages involves the use of three drugs designed to reduce viable bacteria as rapidly as possible, to minimize the risk of ineffective treatment in those patients infected by drug-resistant bacteria (Cook, 1985). These antibiotics continue for at least eight weeks when they can be reduced to two drugs for 6–18 months (British Thoracic Association, 1980). Treatment failure occurs generally due to poor compliance by the patient plus improper supervision (Fox, 1983). A patient on combination chemotherapy is considered non-infectious after two weeks of treatment (Joint Tuberculosis Committee of the British Thoracic Society, 1983).

Tuberculosis is a notifiable disease under the Public Health Act 1985. It is the responsibility of the medical officer for environmental health to follow up all contacts of infected persons. Generally, hospital staff are followed up by the hospital infection control officer in liaison with the hospital occupational health unit (Thornbury, 1985).

Immunization involves vaccination with BCG to all contacts of known respiratory tuberculosis plus health service staff, school children between the ages of 10 and 13 years and students (Department of Health and Social Security, 1987).

Apart from newborn babies, testing for hypersensitivity to tuberculoprotein (tuberculin skin testing) is essential (Department of Health and Social Security,

1987) using the Mantoux, Heaf or tine test before BCG is administered.

Special attention must be given to equipment contaminated with Mycobacterium species. Autoclaving will steralize and is the method of choice. Certain equipment, such as endoscopes, are damaged by autoclaving and disinfection must be used instead. As greater resistance to glutaraldehyde solution is suspected, equipment should be totally immersed for 60 minutes in a freshly prepared glutaraldehyde solution (Department of Health and Social Security, 1986).

References and further reading

British Thoracic Association (1980) Short course chemotherapy in pulmonary tuberculosis, third report, *Lancet*, Vol. i, pp. 1182–83.

Joint Tuberculosis Committee of the British Thoracic Society (1983) Control and prevention of tuberculosis: a code of practice, *British Medical Journal*, Vol. 287, pp. 1118–21.

Cook, N.J. (1985) Treatment of tuberculosis, *British Medical Journal*, Vol. 291, pp. 497–8.

Department of Health and Social Security (1978) *Health Services Management, Control of Tuberculosis in NHS Employees*, HC (78):3.

Department of Health and Social Security (1986) *Safety Information Bulletin* 28, DHSS, London.

Department of Health and Social Security (1987) *Immunisation Against Infectious Diseases*, amended section, Tuberculosis and B.C.G. vaccination, DHSS, London.

Fox, W. (1983) Compliance of patients and physicians, experience and lessons from tuberculosis, *British Medical Journal*, Vol. 287, pp. 101–5.

Galbraith, N.S. (1981) Changing patterns of infectious diseases in the general population of England and Wales, in *Infection Control Nurses' Association Twelfth Annual Symposium*, pp. 61–5.

Joint Committee on Vaccination and Immunisation (1984) *Immunisation Against Infectious Disease*, HMSO, London.

Loudon, R.G. *et al*. (1969) Cough frequency and infectivity in patients with pulmonary tuberculosis, *American Review Respiratory Disease*, Vol. 99, pp. 109–11.

Morbidity and Mortality Weekly Report (1987) Tuberculosis and AIDS – Connecticut, *Journal of the American Medical Association*, Vol. 257, no. 13, pp. 1705–6.

Rouillon, A. *et al*. (1976) Transmission of tubercle bacilli, the effects of chemotherapy, *Tubercle*, Vol. 57, pp. 275–99.

Stanford, J.L. (1980) Protection of hospital staff from tuberculosis, *Journal of Hospital Infection*, Vol. 1, pp. 183–6.

Thornbury, G. (1985) TB or not TB, *Nursing Times*, Vol. 81, no. 32, pp. 43–4.

GUIDELINES: TUBERCULOSIS

PATIENTS WITH SMEAR-POSITIVE SPUTUM

Action	Rationale
1 The patient must be nursed in a well-ventilated single room.	Patients are infectious and segregation from susceptible patients is essential.
2 Strict barrier nursing is not necessary if the actions listed below are taken.	Prolonged close contact with a patient with a productive cough is required to cause cross-infection.
3 Wearing a plastice apron is advisable for prolonged close work, i.e. bed making.	Uniforms could become contaminated during prolonged close work.
4 The wearing of masks for staff is not necessary unless the patient has a very productive cough or when the patient is unable to cover mouth with his/her hand when coughing, i.e. unconscious patient being suctioned.	A mask will protect the wearer from inhaling organisms disseminated by the patient.

5	The patient is taught to cover his/her mouth when coughing and sneezing.	To prevent droplet transmission of organisms.
6	When leaving the room, the patient must wear a well-fitting mask.	A mask will prevent the dissemination of organisms from the nose and mouth of the patient during breathing, talking, sneezing and coughing.
7	The patient must be taught to expectorate into a sputum pot with a well-fitting lid which must be changed frequently, at least daily.	Sputum will initially contain viable tubercle bacilli which could cause cross-infection if not properly contained.
8	Filled sputum pots and tissues to be disposed of in a yellow waste bag.	Yellow is the international colour coding for clinical waste.
9	Vomit, which could also contain sputum, must be disposed of carefully into a heat disinfecting bedpan washer to prevent splashing of the environment.	To minimize the risk of cross-infection occurring.
10	Crockery and cutlery must be washed in a heat disinfecting dishwasher. In the absence of such a machine, disposable crockery and cutlery must be used.	Dishwashing machines should give a final rinse temperature of at least 80°C to ensure disinfection.
11	The bed linen to be treated as infected.	To prevent cross-infection.
12	The patient's room to be cleaned scrupulously daily, with equipment kept solely for this area.	Tubercle bacilli remain viable in dust and therefore must be removed immediately and prevented from being carried to other ward areas.
13	On discharge the patient's room to be stripped of all disposable items such as toilet paper, tissues, soap, and washable items.	To allow for complete cleaning.
14	The room to be terminally cleaned to include all areas and furniture, using detergent and hot water. If heavy contamination has occurred, a phenolic disinfectant, for example Hycolin 1%, should be used.	To minimize the risk of furniture harbouring organisms. Phenolic disinfectants have good bactericidal activity against tubercle bacilli.
15	All precautions can cease after 2 weeks' combination chemotherapy unless the patient has a resistant organism or the patient is extremely ill, e.g. an AIDS patient who may have a slower recovery.	The patient is considered non-infectious after 2 weeks, unless there are specific medical reasons present.

PATIENTS WITH SMEAR-NEGATIVE SPUTUM

	Action	**Rationale**
1	These patients may be nursed in a general ward.	They are not infectious. Routine infection control measures will be adequate while caring for this patient.
2	Safe disposal of sputum and used tissues into yellow clinical waste bags is advisable.	Sputum and tissues used for respirtory secretions should be handled with care at all times, regardless of the patient's diagnosis.

PATIENTS WITH NON-PULMONARY TUBERCULOSIS

Action	Rationale
1 These patients may be nursed in a general ward.	They are not infectious, providing drainage and dressings are handled with care.
2 Safe disposal of dressings immediately into a polythene bag which is then disposed of into a yellow clinical waste bag is essential.	To prevent contamination of the environment and therefore – cross infection. Yellow is the international colour coding for clinical waste.
3 Wound drainage to be disposed of into a disinfecting bedpan washer, with great care being taken to avoid splashing of the environment.	To prevent contamination of the environment which could cause cross-infection.
4 Drainage bottles to be sent to CSSD for disinfection and sterilization.	Autoclaving is the preferred means for achieving sterilization.

NURSING THE NEUTROPENIC PATIENT

Definition

Neutrophils are the circulating white blood cells essential for phagocytosis, which is the process in which micro-organisms are engulfed, destroyed and removed.

One of the major side-effects of cytotoxic chemotherapy and radiotherapy is neutropenia, which is the term used to denote a reduction in the number of neutrophils.

As the neutrophil count decreases the risk of infection increases. The longer the period of neutropenia the higher the risk of infection. Barrier nursing of a neutropenic patient is usually termed 'protective isolation' or 'reverse barrier nursing'.

Indications

Protective isolation provides a safe environment for patients who are susceptible to infection but can be an appropriate form of care for other patients, e.g. burns cases and children with immunodeficiency disease.

The procedure described below is intended to protect the patient whose period of neutropenia can reasonably be expected to be measured in days. It does not involve the special precautions of full protective isolation with protection from commensal infection in patients whose neutropenia is likely to be prolonged. Such patients should be nursed in a reverse barrier nursing unit. The present procedure should be used under the following circumstances:

1   following high-dose cytotoxic chemotherapy with autologous bone marrow 'rescue';
2   where there is idiosyncratic haematological sensitivity to cytotoxic agents, if the period of neutropenia is expected to be short.

REFERENCE MATERIAL

Bacterial, fungal and viral infections may all occur during a period of neutropenia.

Bacterial infections are commonly caused by Gram-negative organisms, such as Pseudomonas species, *Escherichia coli* and Klebsiella species, normally found in the gastrointestinal tract, and *Staphylococcus epidermidis*, usually a skin contaminant.

The commonest fungal infection is *Candida albicans*, most usually in the oral cavity, but which may affect the oesophagus, bowel or vagina, and cause systemic infection, pneumonia and septicaemia.

Herpetic lesions may result from the herpes simplex virus, and herpes zoster is more common in patients who are immunosuppressed or neutropenic.

The main route of infection transmission is by contact transmission from hands and clothes. Airborne infectious micro-organisms, notably staphylococci, may be inhaled or transferred to the patient through wounds, intravenous cannulae, etc. Patients may also infect themselves directly from their own micro-organisms.

Food chosen from the hospital menu is acceptable, but raw fruit, salads and uncooked vegetables should be avoided to reduce endogenous infection.

Early detection of infection is vital. Four-hourly recordings of temperature, pulse and blood pressure will facilitate this. The patient may carry out self-screening of the mouth, intravenous site and other areas of potential infection if able; otherwise a nurse should do this and report any evidence of infection to allow prompt treatment with intravenous antibiotics.

Blood product therapy may be required during the neutropenic period.

Opinions vary as to the degree of protective care required, and to the ideal method; controlled trials are difficult to organize and to evaluate, and results are often conflicting. It is generally accepted, however, that the neutropenic patient who is given some protection will have fewer infections, fewer days of fever, and reduced morbidity and mortality compared with the unprotected patient.

The system chosen will depend on local resources. The success of the system relies heavily on the education and attitude of hospital staff, the patient, his/her relatives and friends who may wish to visit.

References and further reading

Ayliffe, G.A.J. *et al.* (1979) A unit for source and protective isolation in a general hospital, *British Medical Journal*, Vol. 2, pp. 461–5.

Bagshawe, K.D. *et al.* (1978) Isolating patients in hospital to control infection. Part I. Sources and routes of infection, *British Medical Journal*, Vol. 2, pp. 609–12.

Bates, M. (1980) Factors related to infection in cancer patients and implications for care, in R. Tiffany (ed.) *Cancer Nursing Update*, Baillière Tindall, London.

Hann, I.M. and Prentice, H.G. (1984) Infection prophylaxis in the patient with bone marrow failure, *Clinics in Haematology*, Vol. 13, no. 3, pp. 523–47.

Hodges, D. and Griffiths, G. (1982) Prevention versus cure, *Nursing Mirror*, Vol. 154, no. 7, pp. 24–6.

Jenner, E.A. (1977) Intravenous infusion – a cause for concern? *Nursing Times*, Vol. 73, pp. 156–8.

Kominos, S.D. *et al.* (1972) Introduction to *Pseudomonas aeruginosa* into a hospital via vegetables, *Applied Microbiology*, Vol. 25, no. 4, pp. 567–70.

Lidwell, O.M. *et al.* (1974) Transfer of micro-organisms between nurses and patients in a clean air environment, *Journal of Applied Bacteriology*, Vol. 37 no. 4, pp. 649–56.

Pizzo, P.A. *et al.* (1982) Microbiological evaluation of food items, *Journal of the American Dietetic Association*, Vol. 81, pp. 272–9.

Remington J.S. and Schimpff, S.C. (1981) Please don't eat the salads, *New England Journal of Medicine*, Vol. 304, pp. 433–4.

Smith, B.J. (1983) The infection-prone child. 1. Aspects of microbiology, *Nursing Times*, Vol. 79, no. 25, pp. 56–60.

Smith, B.J. (1983) The infection-prone child. 3. Evaluation, *Nursing Times*, Vol. 79, no. 27, pp. 28–30.

Taylor, L.J. (1978) An evaluation of hand washing techniques, *Nursing Times*, Vol. 74, no. 2, pp. 54–5.

Whitby, J.L. and Rampling, A. (1972) *Pseudomonas aeruginosa* contamination in domestic and hospital environment, Lancet, Vol. i, pp. 15–17.

GUIDELINES: NURSING THE NEUTROPENIC PATIENT

Procedure

PREPARATION OF THE ROOM AND MAINTENANCE OF GENERAL CLEANLINESS

Action	Rationale
1 A single room should be used if possible.	To reduce airborne transfer of micro-organisms.
2 A toilet to be kept for the sole use of the patient.	To reduce the risk of cross-infection.
3 Area to be cleaned meticulously before the patient is admitted.	To reduce the risk of infection.
4 Equipment and supplies to be kept for the sole use of the patient. (This must also include any cleaning equipment used by domestic staff.)	To reduce the risk of cross-infection. Cleaning equipment can easily become colonized with micro-organisms which may cause cross-infection.
5 Surfaces and furniture to be damp dusted daily using disposable cleaning cloths and detergent solution.	Damp dusting and mopping removes micro-organisms without distributing them into the air.

Action	Rationale
6 Floor to be mopped daily using soap and water.	To reduce the risk of cross-infection.
7 Mop head to be laundered daily.	As above.
8 Bucket and mop handle to be cleaned and dried and stored in the isolation area.	As above.

NURSING PROCEDURE

Action	Rationale
1 Hands must be washed thoroughly with a bactericidal skin cleanser such as Hibiscrub.	Hands are regarded as the principle source of transfer of micro-organisms. (For further information on aseptic technique see pp. 7–8.)
2 A disposable plastic apron should be worn for all nursing procedures.	Staff clothing can easily become contaminated. A disposable plastic apron reduces the risk of transfer of organisms.
3 Door of room to be kept closed. Ideally the air in the room should be under slightly positive pressure. The air flow should be from the room into the corridor.	To reduce the risk of airborne transmission of infection by inhaling organisms from the rest of the ward when entering the protective isolation room.

VISITORS

Action	Rationale
1 The patient should be asked to nominate close relatives and friends who may then, after education, visit freely. The patient or his or her representative should inform casual acquaintances or non-essential visitors that they should avoid visiting during the period of neutropenia.	The incidence of infection increases in proportion to the number of people visiting. Large numbers of visitors are difficult to screen and educate. Unlimited visiting by close relatives and friends diminishes the sense of isolation that the patient may experience.
2 Any visitor with an infection or who has been in contact with infection should be excluded.	Neutropenic patients are susceptible to infection.
3 Children, unless very close relatives, should be discouraged.	Children are more likely to have been in contact with infectious diseases which can have serious consequences if transmitted to a neutropenic patient.

DIET

Action	Rationale
1 Educate the patient to choose only cooked food from the hospital menu and avoid raw fruit, salads and uncooked vegetables, whether on the menu or brought in by visitors.	Uncooked foods are often heavily colonized by micro-organisms, particularly from negative bacteria.

2 Food brought into the hospital by visitors must be:

   (a) obtained from well-known reliable firms;

   (b) in undamaged sealed tins and packets;

   (c) within expiry date.

Correctly processed and packaged foods are acceptable as they should not be unacceptably infected.

3 Water should be boiled and allowed to cool in a covered jug.

Tap water is perfectly safe to drink but can become colonized by organisms, particularly from negative organisms found in the plug hole of sinks or overflow outlet when the water is being filled.

4 Bottled concentrated fruit drinks made from whole fruit and containing sugar are invariably pathogen free.

Pathogens do not easily survive or multiply in a high sugar concentrate.

5 Sealed packets of fruit juice (long shelf-life varieties, particularly those rich in vitamins) are suitable. It should be poured directly into a clean jug and drunk the same day.

These juices have been pasteurized and remain pathogen-free until they are opened.

DISCHARGING THE PATIENT

Action

Rationale

1 Crowded areas, for example shops, cinemas, pubs and discos, should be avoided.

Although the patient's white cell count is usually high enough for discharge, the patient remains immunocompromised for some time.

2 Pets should not be allowed to lick the patient and new pets should not be obtained.

Pets are known carriers of infection.

3 Certain foods, for example take-away meals, should continue to be avoided.

Take-away meals are subject to handling by a large number of individuals and are stored for longer periods, both of which increase the likelihood of contamination.

4 Salads and fruit should be washed carefully, dried and, if possible, peeled.

To remove as many pathogens as possible.

5 Any sign or symptoms of infection should be reported to the patient's general practitioner or to the discharging hospital immediately.

Any infection may continue to have serious consequences if left unlocated.

4

Bladder Lavage and Irrigation

Definition
LAVAGE
Bladder lavage is the washing out of the bladder with sterile fluid.

IRRIGATION
Bladder irrigation is the continuous washing out of the bladder with sterile fluid.

Indications
Bladder lavage or irrigation is indicated for the following reasons:

LAVAGE
1 To clear an obstructed catheter.
2 To remove potential sources of obstruction, e.g. blood clots or sediment from infection.
3 To cleanse the bladder with urinary disinfectants when some types of urinary infections are present and to prevent the spread of such infection, e.g. to the kidney.

IRRIGATION
1 To prevent the formation and retention of blood clots, e.g. following prostatic surgery.
2 On rare occasions to remove heavily contaminated material from a diseased urinary bladder.

REFERENCE MATERIAL
Solutions used for lavage and irrigation
A number of solutions are available for cleansing the bladder and the selection of a particular solution will depend on its therapeutic properties in relation to the patient's needs. Recently studies have suggested that the use of bladder washout regimens to reduce, prevent or treat urinary tract infection (UTI) is ineffective (Warren et al., 1978; Dudley and Barriere, 1981; Stickler et al., 1981). The following conclusions were suggested by these studies:

1 regular bladder irrigation leads to infection with resistant organisms and may lead to higher rates of infection;
2 noxythiolin (Noxyflex) had no bactericidal effect unless in contact with infected urine for 2 hours;
3 chlorhexidine was found to lead to the selection of resistant bacterial species.

The use of bladder lavage, however, to reduce or prevent catheter obstruction may be beneficial with certain patients (Brocklehurst and Brocklehurst, 1978; Ferrie et al., 1979; Blannin and Hobden, 1980).

Normal saline is the agent most commonly recommended for lavage and irrigation and should be used in every case unless an alternative solution is prescribed. Normal saline is isotonic so it does not affect the body's fluid or electrolyte levels, therefore large volumes may be used as necessary. Three-litre bags of saline are available for irrigation purposes.

Studies of water and saline (Harper and Matz, 1975, 1976) showed them to be the least erosive irrigating solution when tested in rat bladders. Ferrie et al. (1979) and Blannin and Hobden (1980) recommend the use of tap water as a purely mechanical means of flushing out the catheter for patients at home. The use of large volumes of sterile water is not recommended, however, as its absorption through the bladder wall may increase the blood volume to unacceptable levels.

The use of chlorhexidine gluconate as a bladder washout is not recommended unless it is specifically prescribed. The 0.02% solution provided for intravesical use is a disinfectant which is effective against vegetative bacteria, especially Gram-positive organisms. Its activity is reduced, however, by blood and other organic matter (Martindale, 1982) and can cause haematuria and bladder erosion (Harper, 1981).

Noxythiolin (Noxyflex) is occasionally prescribed as a bladder installation solution and is reported to be a more effective antibacterial and antifungal agent than chlorhexidine gluconate. A solution of 1% Noxyflex was found to be as effective as a 2.5% solution and caused less haematuria (MacFayden, 1976). However, the significant amount of haematuria associated with the use of Noxyflex may restrict its use.

A number of other solutions have been recommended for use in specific circumstances but their effectiveness has not been established (Kennedy, 1984). They include citric acid (3.23%) to prevent and dissolve crystallization in the catheter or bladder; mandelic acid (1%) to prevent the growth of urease-producing bacteria by bladder acidification; and citric acid (6%) to dissolve persistent crystallization in the bladder or catheter.

Cytotoxic agents given intravesically

For details on the administration of cytotoxic agents, see pp. 111–13.

Catheters used for lavage and irrigation

A three-way urinary catheter must be used for irrigation in order that fluid may simultaneously be run into, and drained out from, the bladder. This catheter is routinely passed in theatre when irrigation is required, e.g. after prostatectomy. Occasionally bladder irrigation is started on the ward. If the patient has an ordinary catheter, this must be replaced with a three-way type (see Figure 4.1).

For bladder lavage it is not necessary to use a three-way catheter. There are three reasons for this:

1   obstruction is more likely to occur when the drainage lumen is small, as in the three-way type;
2   the catheter may not drain if there is an obstruction. Such an obstruction is most likely to have occurred within the drainage lumen, and lavage via the side-arm is unlikely to have much, if any, effect on the cause of the obstruction;
3   the risk of infection from the recatheterization with a three-way catheter is much greater than the risk of infection from disconnecting a closed drainage system, provided that aseptic techniques are strictly adhered to.

It is recommended, however, that a three-way catheter is passed if frequent intravescial installations of drugs or antiseptic solutions are prescribed and the risk of catheter obstruction is not considered to be very great. In such cases the most important factor is minimizing the risk of introducing infection and maintaining a closed urinary drainage system, for which the three-way catheter allows.

References and further reading

Blannin J. and Hobden, J. (1980) The catheter of choice, *Nursing Times*, Vol. 76, pp. 2092–3.

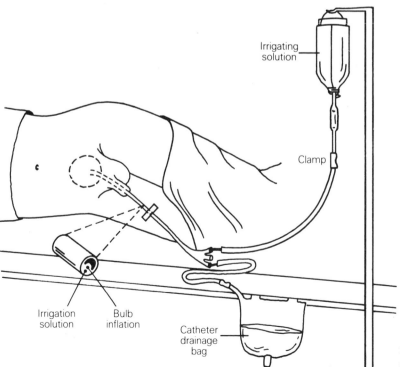

Irrigating solution

Clamp

Irrigation solution

Bulb inflation

Catheter drainage bag

Figure 4.1   Closed urinary drainage system with provision for intermittent or continuous irrigation.

Brocklehurst, J.C. and Brocklehurst, S. (1978) Management of indwelling catheters, *British Journal of Urology*, Vol. 50, pp. 102–5.

Datta, P.K. (1981) The post prostatectomy patient, *Nursing Times*, Vol. 77, pp. 1759–61.

Dudley, M.N. and Barriere, S.L. (1981) Antimicrobial irrigations in the prevention and treatment of catheter related urinary tract infections, *American Journal of Hospital Pharmacy*, Vol. 38, pp. 59–65.

Ferrie, B.G. *et al.* (1979) Long term urethral catheter drainage, *British Medical Journal*, Vol. 279, pp. 1046–7.

Harper, W. (1981) An appraisal of 12 solutions used for bladder irrigation or installation, *British Journal of Urology*, Vol. 53, pp. 433–8.

Harper, W. and Matz, L. (1975) The effect of chlorhexidine irrigation of the bladder in the rat, *British Journal of Urology*, Vol. 47, pp. 539–43.

Harper, W. and Matz, L. (1976) Further studies on effects of irrigating solutions on rat bladders, *British Journal of Urology*, Vol. 48, pp. 463–7.

Kennedy, A. (1984) Trial of new bladder washout system, *Nursing Times*, Vol. 80, pp. 48–51.

MacFayden, I.R. (1976) Comparison of noxythiolin 'Noxyflex' and chlorhexidine 'Hibitaine' installation after intermittent catheterisation, *Clinical Trials Journal*, Vol. 4, pp. 654–6.

Martindale. W. (1982) *The Extra Pharmacopoeia*, 28th edn, The Pharmaceutical Press, London.

Stickler, D.J. *et al.* (1981) Some observations on the activity of three antiseptics used as bladder irrigants in the treatment of UTI in patients with indwelling catheters, *Paraplegia*, Vol. 19, pp. 325–33.

Warren, J. *et al.* (1978) Antibiotic irrigation and catheter associated urinary tract infection, *New England Journal of Medicine*, Vol. 299, pp. 570–3.

GUIDELINES: BLADDER LAVAGE

Equipment

1 Sterile dressing pack
2 Bladder syringe, 60 ml
3 Sterile jug
4 Antiseptic solution, such as Savlodil
5 Alcohol-based hand wash solution, such as Hibisol
6 Sterile gloves
7 Clamp
8 New catheter bag (for Foley-type catheter) or sterile spigot (for three-way catheter)
9 Sterile receiver
10 Sterile solution for lavage.

Procedure

Action	Rationale
1 Explain the procedure to the patient.	To obtain the patient's consent and co-operation.
2 Screen the bed. Ensure that the patient is in a comfortable position allowing access to the catheter.	For the patient's privacy and to reduce the risk of cross-infection. Curtains are drawn at this stage so that dust and airborne organisms disturbed by the curtains do not settle on the sterile field.
3 Perform the procedure using an aseptic technique.	To prevent infection. (For further information on aseptic technique see pp. 5–8.)
4 Draw up solutions from vials, e.g. Noxyflex, using a 60-ml bladder syringe with needle adapter. Cap the syringe and place it in a sterile receiver.	It is easier to draw up solutions from vials in the clinical area than at the bedside.

5   Take the trolley to the bedside. Open the outer wrappings of packs and put them on the top shelf of the trolley.

6   Prepare the sterile field. Pour the lavage solution into the sterile jug.

7   Clean your hands with the appropriate antiseptic solution, such as Hibiscrub, and put on gloves.

To minimize the risk of infection.

8   Clamp the catheter. Place a sterile paper towel under the junction of the catheter and the tubing of the drainage bag and disconnect them.

To prevent leakage when the catheter is disconnected. When the patient has a three-way catheter the drainage bag will not need disconnecting as the washout fluid is injected through the side-arm of the catheter. This should be spigoted off after use and the fluid remaining in the bladder will drain into the catheter bag.

9   Clean gloved hands with an alcohol-based hand wash solution, such as Hibisol. Using an aseptic technique, clean around the end of the catheter with sterile cotton wool and an antiseptic solution, such as Savlodil.

To remove surface organisms from gloves and catheter and thus reduce the risk of introducing infection into the catheter.

10   Draw up the irrigating fluid into the bladder syringe and insert the nozzle into the end of the catheter.

11   Release the clamp on the catheter and gently inject the contents of the syringe into the bladder, trying not to inject air.

Rapid injection of fluid could be uncomfortable for the patient. Large volumes of air in the bladder cause distension and discomfort.

12   Remove the syringe and allow the bladder contents to drain by gravity into a receiver placed on a sterile towel.

13   Repeat steps 11 and 12 of the procedure until the washout is complete or the returning fluid is clear.

14   If the fluid does not return naturally, aspirate gently with the syringe.

Gentle suction is sometimes required to remove obstructive material from the catheter.

15   Connect a new catheter bag or sterile pigot if a three-way catheter is in place, and allow the remaining fluid to drain out.

A closed drainage system must be re-established as soon as possible to reduce the risk of bacterial invasion through the catheter.

16   If the solution is to remain in the bladder, the catheter should be clamped when all the fluid has been injected and the clamp released after the desired period.

17   Measure the volume of washout fluid returned and compare it with the volume of fluid injected. Record any discrepancies of volume in the appropriate documents.

To keep an accurate record of urinary output and to observe for catheter obstruction.

18   Make the patient comfortable, remove equipment and clean the trolley.

19   Wash hands.

To prevent cross-infection.

As an alternative to the use of bladder syringe and irrigating solution a pre-packed filled reservoir with sterile catheter adaptor called Uro-tainer is now available. Kennedy (1984) found that the use of Uro-tainer compared with traditional saline washout procedure produced a reduced incidence of urinary tract infection.

GUIDELINES: CONTINUOUS BLADDER IRRIGATION

Equipment

1 Sterile dressing pack
2 Antiseptic solution, such as Savlodil
3 Alcohol-based hand wash solution, such as Hibisol
4 Sterile gloves
5 Clamp
6 Sterile irrigation fluid
7 Disposable irrigation set
8 Infusion stand
9 Sterile jug

Procedure

COMMENCING BLADDER IRRIGATION

Action	Rationale
1 Explain the procedure to the patient.	To obtain the patient's consent and co-operation.
2 Screen the patient and ensure that he or she is in a comfortable position allowing access to the catheter.	For the patient's privacy and to reduce the risk of cross-infection. Curtains are drawn at this stage so that dust and airborne organisms disturbed by the curtains do not settle on the sterile trolley.
3 Perform the procedure using an aseptic technique.	To prevent infection. (For further information on aseptic technique, see pp. 5–8.)
4 Open the outer wrappings of the pack and put it on the top shelf of the trolley.	
5 Insert the end of the irrigation giving set into the fluid bag and hand the bag on the infusion stand. Allow fluid to run through the tubing so that air is expelled.	To prime the irrigation set so that is is ready for use. Air is expelled in order to prevent discomfort from air in the patient's bladder.
6 Clamp the catheter.	
7 Prepare the sterile field.	
8 Clean hands with an antiseptic solution, such as Hibiscrub. Put on gloves.	To minimize the risk of cross-infection.
9 Place a sterile paper towel under the irrigation inlet of the catheter and remove the spigot.	To prevent leakage of urine through the irrigation arm when the spigot is removed.
10 Discard the spigot.	

11	Clean gloved hands with an alcohol-based hand wash solution, such as Hibisol. Using an aseptic technique, clean around the end of the irrigation arm with sterile cotton wool and an antiseptic solution such as Salvodil.	To remove surface organisms from gloves and catheter and to reduce the risk of introducing infection into the catheter.
12	Attach the irrigation giving set to the irrigation arm of the catheter. Keep the clamp of the irrigation giving set closed.	To prevent over-distension of the bladder, which can occur if fluid is run into the bladder before the drainage tube has been unclamped.
13	Release the clamp on the catheter tube and allow any accumulated urine to drain into the catheter bag. Empty the urine from the catheter bag into a sterile jug.	Urine drainage should be measured before commencing irrigation so that the fluid balance may be monitored more accurately.
14	Discard the gloves.	These will be contaminated, having handled the catheter bag.
15	Set irrigation at the required rate and ensure that fluid is draining into the catheter bag.	To check that the drainage system is patent and to prevent fluid accumulating in the bladder.
16	Make the patient comfortable, remove unnecessary equipment and clean the trolley.	
17	Wash hands.	To prevent cross-infection.

CARE OF THE PATIENT DURING IRRIGATION

	Action	**Rationale**
1	Adjust the rate of infusion according to the degree of haematuria. This will be greatest in the first 12 hours following surgery (average fluid input is 6–9 litres during the first 12 hours, falling to 3–6 litres during the next 12 hours). The aim is to obtain a drainage fluid which is rosé in colour.	To remove blood from the bladder before it clots and to minimize the risk of catheter obstruction and clot retention.
2	Check the volume in the drainage bag frequently when infusion is in progress, e.g. half-hourly or hourly.	To ensure that fluid is draining from the bladder and to detect blockages as soon as possible; also to prevent over-distension of the bladder and patient discomfort. Frequent checking means, in addition, that full catheter bags are noticed and can be emptied before they reach capacity.
3	Using rubber-tipped 'milking' tongs, 'milk' the catheter and drainage tube regularly, as required.	To remove unseen clots from within the drainage system and to maintain an efficient outlet.
4	Record the fluid balance chart accurately. The fluid balance of all patients having bladder irrigation must be monitored.	So that urine output is known and any related problems, e.g. renal dysfunction, may be detected quickly and easily.

(A) Date and time	(B) Volume put up	(C) Volume run in	(D) Total volume	(E) Urine	(F) Urine running total

Figure 4.2 Bladder irrigation recording chart.

BLADDER IRRIGATION RECORDING CHART

The bladder irrigation recording chart (Figure 4.2) is designed to provide an accurate record of the patient's urinary output during the period of irrigation.

PROCEDURE FOR THE USE OF THE CHART

Record the time (column A) and the fluid volume in each bag of irrigating solution (column B) as it is put up.

When the irrigating fluid has all run from the first bag into the bladder, record the original volume in the bag in column C. Record the corresponding time in column A. Do not attempt to estimate the fluid volume run in while a bag is in progress as this will cause inaccuracies. If, however, a bag is discontinued, the volume run in can be calculated by measuring the volume left in the bag and deducting this from the original volume. This should be recorded in column C.

The catheter bag should be emptied as often as is necessary, the volume being recorded in column D and the corresponding time in column A. The catheter bag must also be emptied whenever the bag of irrigating fluid is empty, and the volume recorded in column D.

When each bag of fluid has run through, add up the total volume drained by the catheter in column D, and write this in red. Subtract from this the total volume run in (column C) to find the urine output. Write this in column E. Draw a line across the page to indicate that this calculation is complete and continue underneath for the next bag.

NURSING CARE PLAN

Problem	Cause	Suggested action
Fluid retained in the bladder when the catheter is in position.	Fault in drainage apparatus, e.g.:	
	Blocked catheter.	'Milk' the tubing. Wash out the bladder with normal saline.
	Kinked tubing.	Straighten the tubing.
	Overfull drainage bag.	Empty the drainage bag.
	Catheter clamped off.	Unclamp the catheter.
Distended abdomen related to an overfull bladder during the irrigation procedure.	Irrigation fluid is infused at too rapid a rate.	Slow down the infusion rate
	Fault in drainage apparatus.	Check the patency of the drainage apparatus.
Leakage of fluid from around the catheter.	Catheter slipping out of the bladder.	Insert the catheter further in and inflate the balloon more.
	Catheter too large or unsuitable for the patient's anatomy.	If leakage is profuse or unacceptable for the patient's comfort, replace the catheter with one of smaller size.
Patient experiences pain during the lavage or irrigation procedure.	Volume of fluid in the bladder is too great for comfort.	Reduce the fluid volume within the bladder.
	Solution is painful to raw areas in the bladder.	Inform the doctor. Administer analgesia as prescribed.
Retention of fluid with or without distended abdomen with or without pain.	Perforated bladder.	Stop irrigation. Call medical assistance. Monitor vital signs. Monitor patient for pain, tense abdomen.

5

Bone Marrow Aspiration

Definition

Bone marrow aspiration is the aspiration of sufficient bone marrow from the iliac crest or sternum, using a special needle, to enable laboratory testing.

Indications

Bone marrow aspiration is a procedure performed by trained medical staff to evaluate haematopoiesis and so establish a diagnosis in certain haematological disorders, e.g. anaemia, leukaemia, myeloma, metastatic carcinoma. It is also performed to monitor both the course of the patient's disease and his/her response to therapy.

Contraindications

This procedure is contraindicated in those patients who are unable to co-operate, or who have a coagulation defect.

REFERENCE MATERIAL

Bone marrow aspiration was first introduced in Naples in 1909 by Pianese. By 1933 Custer had developed it into a routine technique. It is a quick and relatively simple method of obtaining a marrow specimen and can be performed either in the hospital ward or in an outpatient clinic.

Anatomy and physiology

The bone contains two types of marrow:
1 yellow marrow, which is a mainly fatty substance;
2 red marrow, which is responsible for the production of red and white blood cells.

In certain diseases, such as leukaemia, the immature cells of the red marrow may proliferate and replace the yellow marrow.

Red marrow is found in the cavities of all bones during the first years of life. In adults it is found mainly in the flat bones, e.g. skull, vertebrae, clavicles, scapulae, sternum and iliac crests.

The preferred sites for marrow aspiration, in an adult, are the iliac crests and the sternum (see Figure 5.1). The iliac crests are often used for patients requiring frequent marrow aspirations as the use of the right and left crests can be alternated, both anterior and posterior surfaces may be used and there are no vital organs nearby that may be punctured during the procedure. The posterior iliac crest is often preferred as the procedure can then be performed outside the patient's field of vision, thus reducing his/her anxiety.

The actual aspiration of marrow from the bone cavity is painful despite the local anaesthetic which dulls the pain of the passage of the biopsy needle through the skin, subcutaneous layer and, to a large extent, the periosteum. To enable the patient to cope with the pain he/she should be warned about its inevitability beforehand but it should be emphasized that the pain will only be of short duration.

Very anxious patients and children may be prescribed a mild sedative, such as diazepam, to be given before the procedure begins. In some units the procedure is carried out under a light general anaesthetic.

Complications

Complications are extremely rare but include the following:
1 *cardiac tamponade*, which can occur following sternal puncture;
2 *haemorrhage*, which occurs almost exclusively in those patients suffering from thrombocytopenia. It may be avoided by applying adequate pressure to the puncture site for a few minutes following aspiration.

References and further reading

Abrahams, P. and Webb, P. (1975) *Clinical Anatomy of Practical Procedures*, Pitman Medical, London.

Bevan, J. (1978) *A Pictorial Handbook of Anatomy and*

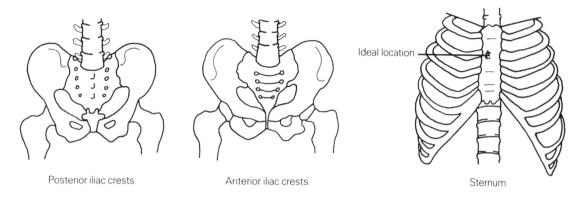

Posterior iliac crests   Anterior iliac crests   Sternum

Ideal location

Figure 5.1   Common sites for bone marrow examination, arranged in order of preference. Normally only aspirations, not biopsies, are done on the sternum because of its small size and proximity to vital organs.

Physiotherapy, Mitchell Beazley, London.

Booth, J.A. (1983) *Handbook of Investigations*, Harper & Row, London.

Brunner, L.S. and Suddarth, D.S. (1982) *The Lippincott Manual of Medical–Surgical Nursing*, Vol. 2, Harper & Row, London.

Frazer, I. and Gough, K.R. (1968) Bone marrow biopsy, in A.E. Read (ed.) *Biopsy Procedures in Clinical Medicine*, John Wright, Bristol.

Markus, S. (1981) Taking the fear out of bone marrow examinations, *Nursing* (US), Vol. 11, no. 4, pp. 64–7.

Navarett, D. (1981) Assisting with bone marrow aspiration, in J. Hirsch and J. Hancock (eds.) *Mosby's Manual of Clinical Nursing Procedures*, C.V. Mosby, St Louis.

Pagnana, K.D. and Pagnana, T.J. (1986) *Diagnostic Testing and Nursing Implications*, 2nd edn, C.V. Mosby, St Louis.

Skydell, B. and Crowder, A. (1975) *Diagnostic Procedures – A Reference for Health Practitioners and a Guide for Patient Counselling*, Little, Brown, Boston.

GUIDELINES: BONE MARROW ASPIRATION

Equipment
1   Antiseptic skin cleansing agent
2   Sterile dressing pack
3   Selection of syringes and needles
4   Local anaesthetic
5   Sterile gloves
6   Marrow aspiration needle and guard, e.g. Salah needle
7   Microscope slides and coverslips
8   Specimen bottles (plain and with heparin)
9   Plastic dressing or plastic dressing spray.

Procedure

Action

1   Explain the procedure to the patient.

Rationale

To reinforce what the doctor has told him/her and thus ensure his/her co-operation.

Action	**Rationale**
2 Give medication as ordered, allowing sufficient time for it to have effect.	Usually this is only necessary for very anxious patients.
3 Help the patient into the correct position: (a) Supine (b) Prone or on side.	For sternal puncture. For anterior or posterior iliac crest puncture.
4 Continue to observe the patient throughout the procedure. Assist the doctor as required. Reassure the conscious patient. Follow the appropriate procedure if the patient is anaesthetized.	
5 Procedure is performed by a doctor: (a) Skin is cleansed with antiseptic solution (b) Local anaesthetic is injected intradermally and through the various layers until the periosteum is infiltrated. (c) Once the local anaesthetic has taken effect the doctor inserts the marrow needle, with the guard on, into the anaesthetized area. (d) If the patient has not been anaesthetized, the doctor warns the patient that he/she will feel a brief episode of sharp pain as the marrow is withdrawn. The needle is advanced into the bone marrow and the required amount of marrow is withdrawn. (e) The needle is removed from the puncture site.	To maintain asepsis throughout the procedure and thus minimize the risk of infection. To minimize pain during the procedure and to ensure the maximum degree of co-operation of the patient. Transitory pain will be felt both as the periosteum is punctured and when the marrow is aspirated. The needle guard ensures the correct positioning of the needle in the marrow cavity and diminishes the risk, particularly in the sternal puncture, of inadvertently puncturing vital organs. To allay anxiety and to ensure the patient's maximum co-operation.
6 Once the doctor has removed the needle, apply pressure over the puncture site using a sterile topical swab until the bleeding stops.	To minimize bruising and to prevent haematoma formation. Prolonged pressure, 5–10 minutes, is required if the patient has a low platelet count (thrombocytopenia).
7 Once bleeding stops, cover the site with plaster or a plastic dressing. Ask the patient not to bathe or wash the area for 24 hours.	
8 Make the patient comfortable. He/she may be mobile, as desired, depending on the level of sedation.	Some patients will have this procedure performed in the outpatient department and will be asked to wait in the clinic for a further 30 minutes to ensure that no further bleeding occurs.
9 Remove and dispose of equipment.	To prevent spread of infection.
10 Record necessary information in the appropriate documents and ensure that specimens are sent to the appropriate laboratory department, correctly labelled and with the necessary forms.	

NURSING CARE PLAN

Problem	Cause	Suggested action
Pain experienced over the puncture site for 1–2 days following the procedure.	Bruising of the tissues at the time of puncture or haematoma formation due to inadequate pressure on the puncture site following the procedure.	Administer a mild analgesic as ordered by the doctor.
Haemorrhage from the puncture site following the procedure.	Low platelet count or inadequate pressure on the puncture site following the procedure.	Ensure that pressure is applied for a minimum of five minutes on the puncture site. Report excessive, uncontrollable bleeding to the appropriate personnel.
Haematoma formation over the puncture site.	Haemorrhage following the procedure.	Administer analgesics as ordered. If the haematoma is severe, report this to the doctor as aspiration may be required.

6

Bowel Care

GENERAL INTRODUCTION

It should be borne in mind that many patients are too embarrassed to talk about bowel function and will often delay reporting the problem until it has been present for a few days. Generally complaints will be either that the patient has diarrhoea or that he/she is constipated. Both diarrhoea and constipation should be seen as symptoms of some underlying disease or malfunction and managed accordingly.

The nurse's priority in either case is immediate resolution of the problem and re-education of the patient to avoid such problems in the future. In the management of diarrhoea, the nurse can ensure that the patient's diet is altered. Foods having a high fibre content can be avoided and fluid intake can be increased. Such measures as the provision of soft toilet paper, easy access to toilet facilities and a suitable barrier cream to prevent anal excoriation can be implemented and will be much appreciated by the patient. Constipation, however, demands the use of more elaborate nursing skills.

REFERENCE MATERIAL
Anatomy and physiology

From the ileocaecal sphincter to the anus the colon is approximately 1.5 m in length. Its main function is to eliminate the waste products of digestion by the propulsion of faeces towards the anus. In addition, it produces mucus to lubricate the faecal mass, thus aiding its expulsion. Other functions include the absorption of fluid and electrolytes, the storage of faeces and the synthesis of vitamins B and K by bacterial flora.

Faeces consist of any unabsorbed end products of digestion, bile pigments, cellulose, bacteria, epithelial cells, mucus and some inorganic material. They are semisolid in consistency and contain about 70% water.

The colon absorbs about 2 litres of water in 24 hours. If faeces are not expelled they will, therefore, gradually become hard due to dehydration and will be difficult to expel. If there is insufficient roughage (fibre) in the faeces, colonic stasis will lead to continued water absorption and the faeces will harden even further.

The movement of faeces through the colon towards the anus is by peristaltic action.

Faeces normally remain in the sigmoid colon until the stimulus to defaecate occurs. This stimulus varies in individuals according to habit. The stimulus can be controlled by conscious effort. After a few minutes the stimulus disappears and does not return for several hours. If these natural reflexes are inhibited on a regular basis they are eventually suppressed and reflex defaecation is inhibited. The result is that the individual becomes severely constipated. If the stimulus is responded to then faeces will move into the rectum.

The rectum is very sensitive to rises in pressure, even of 2–3 mm Hg, and distension will cause a perineal sensation with a consequent desire to defaecate.

A co-ordinated reflex empties the bowel from mid-transverse colon to the anus. During this phase the diaphragm, abdominal and levator ani muscles contract and the glottis closes. Waves of peristalsis occur in the distal colon and the anal sphincter relaxes, allowing the evacuation of faeces.

Constipation

Constipation is a symptom. Its management depends on its cause. Definitions and classifications differ but for most patients it means irregular, infrequent defaecation associated with the passage of hard faeces (see Figure 6.1). The patient usually complains of difficulty in defaecating with accompanying discomfort or pain.

Traditionally, the treatment of constipation has been left to the nurse (Milton-Thompson, 1971). As the patient often presents in hospital with an acute problem of constipation, nurses will need to formulate a short-term plan to evacuate the bowel as completely and as quickly as possible. For this reason enemas, suppositories and laxatives have remained the treatments of choice. Very often little thought is given either to the

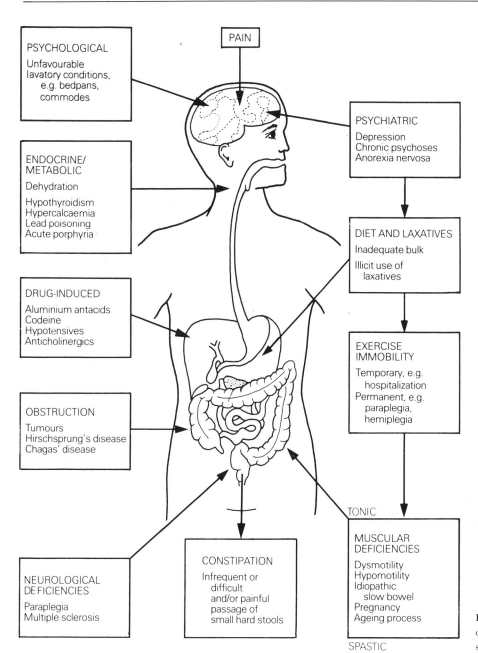

PAIN

PSYCHOLOGICAL

Unfavourable
lavatory conditions,
e.g. bedpans,
commodes

ENDOCRINE/
METABOLIC

Dehydration

Hypothyroidism
Hypercalcaemia
Lead poisoning
Acute porphyria

DRUG-INDUCED

Aluminium antacids
Codeine
Hypotensives
Anticholinergics

OBSTRUCTION

Tumours
Hirschsprung's disease
Chagas' disease

NEUROLOGICAL
DEFICIENCIES

Paraplegia
Multiple sclerosis

PSYCHIATRIC

Depression
Chronic psychoses
Anorexia nervosa

DIET AND LAXATIVES

Inadequate bulk

Illicit use of
laxatives

EXERCISE
IMMOBILITY

Temporary, e.g.
hospitalization
Permanent, e.g.
paraplegia,
hemiplegia

TONIC

MUSCULAR
DEFICIENCIES

Dysmotility
Hypomotility
Idiopathic
slow bowel
Pregnancy
Ageing process

SPASTIC

CONSTIPATION

Infrequent or
difficult
and/or painful
passage of
small hard stools

Figure 6.1 Classification of constipation – combined sources.

cause of the problem or to a more long-term plan. Duffin *et al.* (1981) have shown that a total of 3,428 enemas were given on the geriatric wards of a district general hospital over a 6-month period. There were 1,120 admissions in this period which gave an overall average of three enemas per patient. The same study found that although enemas frequently produced a good bowel evacuation, they also embarrassed the patient and produced symptoms ranging from nausea and abdominal pain to faecal incontinence. Hurst (1970) felt that enemas were prob-

ably only of use where there was a mechanical delay between the splenic flexure and anus. Dorgu (1971) felt that the main benefit of enemas was that they acted within minutes of their administration and were useful in acute conditions of impaction before drug therapy could be effective.

Assessment of the problem

The myth of daily bowel evacuation being essential to healthy living has persisted through the centuries. This myth has resulted in laxative abuse becoming one of the commonest type of drug abuse in the Western world.

On the use and abuse of purgatives Hurst (1970) showed that £10 million was expended in 1921 on patent medicines, the majority of which contained purgatives. In the 1960s, a survey of Londoners showed that over 30% were treating themselves with laxatives (Rutter and Maxwell, 1976).

However, the indications for the use of laxatives are fairly limited. The nurse should always stress the importance of diet and exercise to the patient before recommending other ways of evacuating the bowel.

Defining constipation is undoubtedly a problem while the notion of essential daily evacuations persists. The first objective should be for the nurse to assess what is 'normal' for that patient. A bowel action every third day may be quite adequate for some people; for others three times a day will be the norm. This does not mean that the first person is constipated or that the second has diarrhoea.

Many factors may affect normal bowel functioning. Among those pertinent to hospital admission are the following:
1 change in diet;
2 lack of exercise;
3 X-ray investigation of the bowel involving the use of barium;
4 the use of drugs, particularly analgesics.
Purgatives are often required to overcome these effects.

The nurse should always make a rectal examination to establish whether the patient is constipated and to what degree. Wilson and Muir (1975) in their trial on geriatric faecal incontinence found that there was little correlation between a nurse's subjective assessment of whether a patient was constipated and the actual evidence gained from a rectal examination.

Wherever possible the most natural means of bowel evacuation should be employed. This will mean, after initial solution of the problem by the use of purgatives, re-educating the patient about dieting and exercise.

The use of the bedpan should always be avoided if possible. If the patient can get out of bed, a commode is preferable as the amount of energy expended is considerably less than that required for balancing on a bedpan. Lewin (1976) quoted from research by an American team investigating the straining forces of bowel evacuation by objective methods. They showed that straining was increased three to six times when a patient used the bedpan and that its use requires a 50% greater consumption of oxygen than a commode by the bedside.

In all cases manual evacuation of the rectum should be avoided. It is a distressing, often painful and potentially dangerous procedure for the patient. It may be necessary to sedate the patient before carrying out the procedure. It is recommended by Pirrie (1980) that it should only be performed by medical staff.

Laxatives

The use of purgatives should be avoided and certainly they ought not to be used unless prescribed by a doctor. Purgatives alter the natural functioning of the alimentary tract and often a period of no bowel evacuations will follow their use. This usually causes the patient to take more laxatives and a cycle of dependence ensues (Mortimer, 1970).

Stool softeners lower the surface tension of the faeces and allow penetration by water. They act within 24–48 hours. Liquid paraffin is a stool softener as well as a lubricant, but its use should be avoided as droplets of oil may be accidentally inhaled, especially by the very young or the elderly, and cause lipoid pneumonia or even pulmonary tumours which may imitate carcinoma (Milton-Thompson, 1971). Repetitive use of liquid paraffin and the mineral oils also interferes with the absorption of fat-soluble vitamins and may increase the risks of alimentary tract malignancies (Janes, 1979).

Osmotic agents retain water in the small bowel and increase the flow of fluid into the colon. This increased volume will cause peristalsis and consequent expulsion of faeces. Osmotic agents work within 3–6 hours. Magnesium salts are contraindicated for patients suffering from chronic renal failure as magnesium poisoning may result (Milton-Thompson, 1971). Sodium-containing laxatives should not be used for patients with cardiac problems or inflammatory bowel disease (Corman et al., 1975).

Chemical stimulants cause irritation of mucosa, nerves or smooth muscle. Most of the stimulants act within 2–8 hours. The amount of abdominal cramping produced and the time taken for them to work vary from drug to drug. These drugs can produce electrolyte imbalance, histological changes (melanosis coli) and damage to the mysenteric plexi. Eventually permanent damage to the motility of the colon can occur, leading the patient to take increasing doses of the drug (Rutter and Maxwell, 1976).

Recently more favour has been shown towards the bulk laxatives, particularly those, such as bran, which can be incorporated into the diet, e.g. in bran cereals and high-fibre bread. Bulk laxatives work by increasing the mass of the faeces. They do this by attracting water. This in turn promotes peristalsis and reduces the time taken by the faeces to move through the colon. An increased fluid intake is required when bulk laxatives are used, particularly in the elderly, to prevent intestinal obstruction occurring. Another problem initially is that bulk laxatives tend to distend the abdomen, often making the

Table 6.1 Types of Laxatives

Type of laxative	Example	Brand names and sources
Bulk producers	Dietary fibre	Bran, wholemeal bread
	Mucilaginous polysaccharides	Metamucil, Isogel, Normacol
	Methylcellulose	Celevac
Stool softeners	Synthetic surface active agents	Dioctyl
Lubricants	Liquid paraffin	Agarol, Petrolager
	Mineral oil, hydrocarbon mixtures	
Osmotic agents	Sodium, potassium and magnesium salts	Magnesium sulphate, Epsom salts, milk of magnesia
Chemical stimulants	Anthracene compounds	Senna, Senokot
	Polyphenolic compounds	Bisacodyl, Dulcolax
	Castor oil	
	Bile salts	Cholic acid, Taxol, Veracolate

patient feel full and uncomfortable. Sometimes this leads to temporary anorexia. Harris (1980) discussed fully the merits of introducing bran into the diet, especially of the elderly, and the consequent drastic reduction in the number of enemas administered. She also showed that the cost of using bran compared to other laxatives, even other bulk laxatives, was very much lower. It is often forgotten that bran also reduces glucose absorption from the small intestine and increases the time taken for the blood sugar level to reach its maximum. This could be beneficial when treating patients with maturity onset diabetes, although caution is needed if they are receiving oral hypoglycaemica.

ENEMAS

Definition
An enema is the introduction into the rectum or lower colon of a stream of fluid for the purpose of producing a bowel action or instilling medication.

Indications
Enemas may be prescribed for the following reasons:

1 to clean the lower bowel prior to surgery or childbirth, prior to X-ray examination of the bowel using contrast medium, prior to endoscopy examination or in cases of severe constipation;
2 to introduce medication into the system;
3 to soothe and treat irritated bowel mucosa;
4 to decrease body temperature (due to contact with the proximal vascular system);
5 to stop local haemorrhage;
6 to reduce hyperkalaemia (calcium resonium);
7 to reduce portal systemic encephalopathy (phosphate enema).

Contraindications
Enemas are contraindicated under the following circumstances:
1 cases of paralytic ileus;
2 cases of colonic obstruction;
3 the administration of tap water or soap and water enemas which may cause circulatory overload, water intoxication, mucosal damage and necrosis, hyperkalaemia and cardiac arrhythmias;
4 the administration of large amounts of fluid high into the colon which may cause perforation and haemorrhage;
5 following gastrointestinal or gynaecological surgery, where suture lines may be ruptured (unless medical consent has been given).

REFERENCE MATERIAL
Types of enemas
EVACUANT ENEMAS

An evacuant enema is a solution introduced into the rectum or lower colon with the intention of its being expelled, along with faecal matter and flatus, within a few minutes. The following solutions are commonly used:

1　phosphate enemas with standard or long rectal tubes in single-dose disposable packs;
2　dioctyl sodium sulphosuccinate 0.1%, sorbitol 25% in single-dose disposable packs;
3　sodium citrate 450 mg, sodium alkysulphoacetate 45 mg, sorbic acid 5 mg in single-dose disposable packs;
4　sodium citrate 450 mg, sodium laurylsulphoacetate 45 mg, glycerol 625 mg with citric acid, potassium sorbate and sorbitol in single-dose disposable packs;
5　sodium citrate 450 mg, sodium laurylsulphate 75 mg, sorbic acid 5 mg, in a viscous solution in single-dose disposable packs;
6　oxyphensiatin (Veripaque) in powder for reconstitution;
7　tap water.

Enemas containing dioctyl sodium sulphosuccinate lubricate and soften impacted faeces. Phosphate enemas are useful in bowel clearance prior to X-ray examination and surgery.

Tap water may be dangerous when administered as an enema to a child or to those with poor cardiac function as excessive absorption could lead to circulatory overload (Milton-Thompson, 1971).

Green soap was formerly very popular as an evacuant enema, especially prior to childbirth. Its use has now, however, fallen into disfavour due to numerous adverse reports of mucosal damage, necrosis, extensive sloughing of mucosa, sever haemorrhage, anaphylactic shock and death (Lewis, 1965; Smith, 1967; Pike *et al.*, 1971; Edgell and Johnson, 1973). The limiting factors in soap are alkalis, potash and phenol. In Hirschsprung's disease, deaths following soap enema have occurred when a potassium-based soap was used. Hyperkalaemia resulted, causing cardiac dysrhythmias (Lewin, 1976). Soap is probably a simple irritant; the higher the concentration the greater the mucosal inflammation.

RETENTION ENEMAS

A retention enema is a solution introduced into the rectum or lower colon with the intention of its being retained for a specified period of time. Three types of retention enema are in common use:

1　arachis oil (may be obtained in a single-dose disposable pack);
2　olive oil;
3　prednisolone.

Enemas containing olive oil will soften and lubricate impacted faeces. Retention enemas given to administer medications will be prescribed by the doctor. The product must be checked with the prescription before its administration.

SUPPOSITORIES

Definition

A suppository is a solid or semisolid pellet introduced into the anal canal for medicinal purposes.

Indications

The use of suppositories is indicated under the following circumstances:

1　to empty the bowel prior to certain types of surgery;
2　to empty the bowel to relieve acute constipation or when other treatments for constipation have failed;
3　to empty the bowel prior to endoscopic examination;
4　to introduce medication into the system;
5　to soothe and treat haemorrhoids or anal pruritus.

Contraindications

The use of suppositories is contraindicated when one or more of the following pertain:

1　chronic constipation, which would require repetitive use;
2　cases of paralytic ileus;
3　cases of colonic obstruction;
4　following gastrointestinal or gynaecological operations, unless on the specific instructions of the doctor.

REFERENCE MATERIAL

Many elderly people find repeated enemas both unpleasant and uncomfortable and in cases of severe stasis and impaction whole gut irrigation or colonic lavage may be preferable (Currie, 1979). Hunt (1974) states that the advantages of colonic lavage are that it clears the colon more effectively when visual observation of the interior of the colon is necessary and in cases of disordered action with constipation. However, the disadvantages include the risk of bowel perforation and the inadvertent washing away of the protective mucus which the bowel secretes. Its use is contraindicated in cases of diverticular disease and colitis.

Suppositories may be favoured as they are both easier to administer (see Figure 6.2) and generally cause the patient less discomfort.

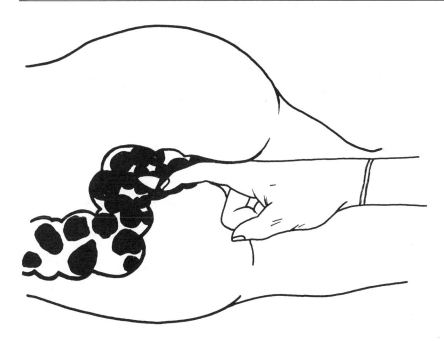

Figure 6.2 Administration of suppositories.

ADMINISTRATION OF SUPPOSITORIES
The use of suppositories dates back to about 460 BC. Hippocrates recommended the use of cylindrical suppositories of honey smeared with ox gall (see Hurst, 1970). Several types are now commercially available.

Lubricant suppositories, e.g. glycerine, should be inserted directly into the faeces and allowed to dissolve to enable softening of the faecal mass (see Figure 6.2). However, stimulant types, such as bisacodyl, must come into contact with the mucous membrane of the rectum if they are to be effective. Other types, such as sodium bicarbonate and anhydrous sodium acid phosphate (Beogex), exert their influence by releasing carbon dioxide, causing rectal distension when they contact water or mucous membrane.

Walker (1982) has shown that if a suppository is being used to obtain a systemic action it should be inserted blunt end forward to minimize rectal discomfort or irritation and maximize the retention period. For local action to promote defaecation it should be inserted in the conventional manner (Figure 6.3).

RECTAL LAVAGE

Definition
Rectal lavage is the washing out of the rectum using large volumes of non-sterile fluid.

Indications
Rectal lavage is performed for the following purposes:
1   to clear the lower bowel prior to investigation by barium enema and thus enable good images to be obtained;
2   to assist in clearing the lower bowel prior to major abdominal surgery and thus decrease the risk of infection and aid satisfactory healing;
3   to clear the lower bowel of residual faecal matter following previous surgery, e.g. formation of colostomy.

Contraindications
Rectal lavage is contraindicated in patients who have a history of any one of the following:
1   severe or prolapsed haemorrhoids;
2   anal fissure;
3   inflammatory bowel disease;
4   large tumour in the rectum or sigmoid colon;
5   post-radiation proctitis;
6   internal fistulae;
7   previous extensive deep X-ray therapy to the pelvis;
8   recent bowel surgery;
9   congestive cardiac failure;
10   impaired renal function.

In 1–8 of the contraindications listed above, the reason for employing caution is because of the damage that could be inflicted by the mechanical aspects of

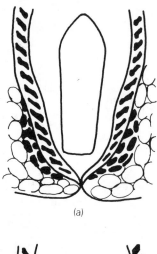

(a)

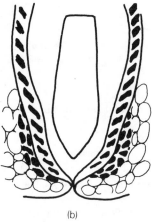

(b)

Figure 6.3   *a*, A suppository administered in the conventional manner to have a local action and promote defaecation. *b*, A suppository administered blunt end forward to minimize local discomfort and maximize systemic therapy.

rectal lavage. When the bowel has already been traumatized there is a greater potential risk of causing irritation or, in extreme cases, perforation, while inserting the catheter and running large volumes of fluid in and out of the rectum.

With the last two contraindications the potential risk lies with the possibility of large amounts of fluid and/or electrolytes becoming absorbed through the bowel. (Generally speaking, with the amounts and type of fluid used and the relatively short time that it stays in the bowel, it should not present a major problem.)

REFERENCE MATERIAL
Choice of fluid

Several solutions can be used to clear the bowel.

SOAP SOLUTIONS

Soap solutions can be made from either 'hard' soap, i.e. from olive oil and sodium hydroxide, or 'soft' soap, which is a combination of potassium and vegetable products. Soft soaps are more irritating than hard soaps and the usual dilution is 5 ml of soap in 1000 ml or more of water. Soap solutions stimulate peristalsis by chemical irritation and intestinal distension. However, they can also cause a whole range of symptoms, which extends from simple hyperaemia to gangrene and the occasional fatality. Lewis (1965) in his survey of five Seattle hospitals reported 'definite undesirable and unnecessary morbidity' related to the use of soap solutions. He further reported that the strengths of solutions used were arbitrary and haphazard, often far exceeding the recommended concentration.

Soap solutions are unsuitable for use prior to bowel surgery or rectal examination because of their effect on the mucosa, and Lewis' investigations leave much doubt as to whether they are of any real value (see Enemas, pp. 59–60).

HYPERTONIC SOLUTIONS

Hypertonic solutions, e.g. sodium phosphate and sodium biphosphate in solution, act by drawing water from the intestinal cells by osmosis. This increases the fluid in the faecal mass, causing first distension then contraction and defaecation.

For patients who have a large amount of faecal matter to evacuate, small volumes of these solutions are very effective. Hypertonic solutions should not be given to patients whose capacity to utilize sodium is affected as some sodium may be absorbed. These are available as commercially prepared enemas but are not suitable for administration in large volumes.

TAP WATER

Rectal lavage is a procedure that is normally used in combination with other methods of clearing the bowel, e.g. oral aperients and dietary restrictions. In this situation, it can be anticipated that there will be very little residue remaining in the lower bowel. What is needed, therefore, is a simple, non-sterile solution that can be used with relative safety in large volumes to wash out the residual faecal matter. The solution which fulfils these criteria ideally is tap water.

Rectal lavage using tap water is not without risk as large volumes of this hypotonic solution can upset the patient's electrolyte balance. Water is drawn by osmosis into the intestinal cells and water intoxication can result with symptoms of weakness, sweating, pallor, vomiting, coughing and dizziness. However, this is a relatively rare complication and generally tap water is very well tolerated.

The other advantages of tap water are as follows:
1   it is cheap and easily available;
2   it can be easily warmed to the correct temperature;
3   it is non-irritant to the bowel mucosa;
4   it does not cause excessive peristalsis with resulting cramps and colic.

Caution should be exercised when giving tap water lavage to infants or patients with altered kidneys or cardiac reserve, but otherwise tap water is the solution of choice.

ISOTONIC SALINE

For patients with compromised electrolyte status an isotonic saline solution can be substituted. This is prepared by adding two teaspoonsful of salt to 1 litre of plain water. Its effect on the bowel is similar to that of water in that it stimulates peristaltic action by distending the intestinal walls. With isotonic saline, however, there is less danger of electrolyte imbalance.

Choice of catheter

Several manufacturers produce rectal catheters. The criteria for selection should be as follows:
1   the catheter should be of an adequate length. Most are approximately 30 cm;
2   the lumen should be large enough to allow the free drainage of particulate matter, i.e. a minimum Charrière gauge of 24;
3   the tip of the catheter should be open ended or have large opposed eyelets to minimize the possibility of blockage;
4   the catheter should be made from a soft flexible material; rubber or plastic is suitable.

References and further reading

British Medical Association Pharmaceutical Society of Great Britain (1988) *British National Formulary*, BMA, London.

Cooper, P. (1976) The treatment of constipation, *Midwife, Health Visitor and Community Nurse*, Vol. 12, p. 165.

Corman, M. *et al.* (1975) Cathartics, *American Journal of Nursing*, Vol. 75, pp. 273–9.

Currie, J.E.J (1979) Whole gut irrigation, *Nursing Times*, Vol. 75, pp. 1570–1.

Dorgu, R.E.O. (1971) *Bowel Function – Disorders and Management*, Butterworth, London.

Duffin, H.M. *et al.* (1981) Are enemas necessary? *Nursing Times*, Vol. 77, pp. 1940–1.

Edgell, R.W. and Johnson, W.D. (1973) Postpartum hypotension and erythema: an adverse reaction to soap enema, *American Journal of Obstetrics and Gynecology*, Vol. 117, pp. 1146–7.

Harris, W. (1980) Bran or aperients? *Nursing Times*, Vol. 76, pp. 811–13.

Hunt, T. (1974) Colonic irrigation, *Nursing Mirror*, Vol. 139, no. 1, pp. 76–7.

Hurst, Sir A. (1970) *Selected Writings of Sir Arthur Hurst (1879–1944)*, Spottiswoode, Ballantyne.

Janes, E. (1979) Constipation: keeping a true perspective, *Nursing Mirror*, Vol. 149, no.13, Supplement, p.x.

Lewin, D. (1976) Care of the constipated patient, *Nursing Times*, Vol. 72, pp. 444–6.

Lewis, A.E. (1965) Dangers inherent in soap enemas, *Pacific Medicine and Surgery*, Vol. 73, pp. 131–3.

Milton-Thompson, G.J. (1971) Constipation, *Nursing Mirror*, Vol. 132, pp. 30–3.

Mortimer, P.M. (1970) A worrying problem – constipation, *Health Visitor*, Vol. 43, pp. 47–8.

Pike, B.F. *et al.* (1971) Soap colitis, *New England Journal of Medicine*, Vol. 285, no. 4, pp. 217–18.

Pirrie, J. (1980) Constipation in the elderly, *Nursing* (1st series), no. 17, pp. 753–4.

Rutter, K. and Maxwell, D. (1976) Constipation and laxative abuse, *British Medical Journal*, Vol. 2, pp. 997–1000.

Smith, D. (1967) Severe anaphylactic reaction after a soap enema, *British Medical Journal*, Vol. 215, no. 4, p. 215.

Smith, S. (1987) Drugs and the gastrointestinal tract, *Nursing Times* Vol. 83, no. 26, pp. 50–2.

Thompson, M. and Bottomley, H. (1980) Normal and abnormal bowel function, *Nursing* (1st series), no. 17, pp. 721–2.

Walker, R. (1982) Suppository insertion, *World Medicine*, Vol. 18, p. 58.

Wieck, L. *et al.* (1986) *Illustrated Manual of Nursing Techniques*, 3rd edn, J.B. Lippincott, Philadelphia.

Wilson, A. and Muir, T. (1975) Geriatric faecal incontinence, *Nursing Mirror*, Vol. 140, no. 16, pp. 50–2.

GUIDELINES: ADMINISTRATION OF ENEMAS

Equipment

1 Disposable incontinence pad
2 Disposable gloves
3 Topical swabs
4 Lubricating jelly
5 Rectal tube and funnel (if not using a commercially prepared pack)
6 Solution required or commercially prepared enema pack (check prescription with another nurse before administering a medicinal enema, e.g. Predsol retention enema)
7 Bath thermometer.

Procedure

Action	Rationale
1 Explain the procedure to the patient.	To obtain the patient's consent and co-operation.
2 Ensure privacy.	To avoid unnecessary embarrassment to the patient.
3 Ensure that a bedpan, commode or toilet is readily available.	In case the patient feels the need to expel the enema before the procedure is completed.
4 Warm the enema to the required temperature, testing with a bath thermometer. A temperature of 40.5–43.3 °C is recommended for adults. Oil retention enemas should be warmed to 37.8 °C.	Heat is an effective stimulant of the nerve plexi in the intestinal mucosa. An enema temperature of body temperature or just above will not damage the intestinal mucosa. The temperature of the environment, the rate of fluid administration and the length of the tubing will all have an effect on the temperature of the fluid on reaching the rectum.
5 Assist the patient to lie in the required position, i.e. on the left side, with knees well flexed, the upper higher than the lower one, and with the buttocks near the edge of the bed.	This allows ease of passage into the rectum by following the natural anatomy of the colon. In this position gravity will aid the flow of the solution into the colon. Flexing the knees ensures a more comfortable passage of the enema nozzle or rectal tube.
6 Place a disposable incontinence pad beneath the patient's hips and buttocks.	To reduce potential infection caused by soiled linen. To avoid embarrassing the patient if the fluid is ejected prematurely following administration.
7 Wash hands and put on disposable gloves.	To reduce cross-infection.
8 Place some lubricating jelly on a topical swab and lubricate the nozzle of the enema or the rectal tube.	To prevent trauma to the anal and rectal mucosa by reducing surface friction.
9 Expel excessive air and introduce the nozzle or tube slowly into the anal canal while separating the buttocks. (A small amount of air may be introduced if bowel evacuation is desired.)	The introduction of air into the colon causes distension of its walls, resulting in unnecessary discomfort to the patient and increases peristalsis. The slow introduction of the lubricated tube will minimize spasm of the intestinal wall. (Evacuation will be more effectively induced due to the increased peristalsis.)
10 Slowly introduce the tube or nozzle to a depth of 10–12.5 cm.	This will bypass the anal canal (2.5–4 cm in length) and ensure that the tube or nozzle is in the rectum.

11 If a retention enema is used, introduce the fluid slowly and leave the patient in bed with the foot of the bed elevated by 45° for as long as prescribed.

To avoid peristalsis. The slower the rate at which the fluid is introduced the less pressure is exerted on the intestinal wall. Elevating the foot of the bed aids in retention of the enema by force of gravity.

12 If an evacuant enema is used, introduce the fluid slowly until the pack is empty or the solution is completely finished.

The faster the rate of flow of the fluid the greater the pressure on the rectal walls. Distension and irritation of the bowel wall will produce a strong persistalsis which is sufficient to empty the lower bowel.

13 If using a funnel and rectal tube, adjust the height of the funnel according to the rate of flow desired.

The forces of gravity will cause the solution to flow from the funnel into the rectum. The greater the elevation of the funnel, the faster the flow of the fluid.

14 Clamp the tubing before all the fluid has run in.

To avoid air entering the rectum and causing further discomfort.

15 Slowly withdraw the tube or nozzle.

To avoid reflex emptying of the rectum.

16 Dry the patient's perineal area with a gauze swab.

To promote patient comfort and avoid excoriation and infection.

17 Ask the patient to retain the enema for 10–15 minutes before evacuating the bowel.

To enhance the evacuant effect.

18 Ensure that the patient has access to the nurse call system, is near to the bedpan, commode or toilet, and has adequate toilet paper.

19 Remove and dispose of equipment.

To avoid infection.

20 Wash hands.

21 Record in the appropriate documents that the enema has been given, its effects on the patient and its results (colour, consistency, content and amount of faeces produced).

To monitor the patient's bowel function.

NURSING CARE PLAN

Problem	Cause	Suggested action
Unable to insert the nozzle of enema pack or rectal tube into the anal canal.	Tube not adequately lubricated.	Apply more lubricating jelly.
	Patient in an incorrect position.	Ask the patient to draw his/her knees up further towards his/her chest.
	Patient apprehensive and embarrassed about the situation.	Ensure adequate privacy and give frequent explanations to the patient about the procedure.

Problem	Cause	Suggested action
	Patient unable to relax his/her anal sphincter	Ask the patient to take deep breaths and 'bear down' as if defaecating.
Unable to advance the tube or nozzle into the anal canal.	Spasm of the canal walls.	Insert the tube or nozzle more slowly, thus minimizing spasm.
Unable to advance the tube or nozzle into the rectum.	Blockage by faeces.	Allow a little solution to flow and then insert the tube further.
	Blockage by tumour	If resistance is still met, stop the procedure and inform a doctor.
Patient complains of cramping or the desire to evacuate the enema before the end of the procedure.	Distension and irritation of the intestinal wall, which produce a strong peristalsis sufficient to empty the lower bowel.	Temporarily stop the insertion of fluid by clamping the tubing or lowering the funnel until the patient says the feeling has subsided.
Patient unable to open his/her bowels after an evacuant enema and the fluid has not returned.	Reduced neuromuscular response in the bowel wall.	Insert a rectal tube and try to siphon the fluid off. Measure and record the amount. If this is not successful, perform rectal lavage. (For further information on rectal lavage see pp. 61–3.) Measure and record the amount returned.

GUIDELINES: ADMINISTRATION OF SUPPOSITORIES

Equipment
1 Disposable incontinence pad
2 Disposable glove
3 Topical swabs or tissues
4 Lubricating jelly
5 Suppository(ies) as required (check the prescription before administering a medicinal suppository, e.g. aminophylline).

Procedure

Action	Rationale
1 Explain the procedure to the patient.	To obtain the patient's consent and co-operation.
If you are administering a medicated suppository, it is best to do so after the patient has emptied his/her bowels.	To ensure that the active ingredients are not impeded from being absorbed by the rectal mucosa or that the suppository is not expelled before its active ingredients have been released.
2 Ensure privacy.	To avoid unnecessary embarrassment to the patient.
3 Ensure that a bedpan, commode or the toilet is readily available.	In case of premature ejection of the suppositories or rapid bowel evacuation following their administration.

4   Assist the patient to lie in the required position, i.e. on the left side, with his/her knees flexed, the upper higher than the lower one, with the buttocks near the edge of the bed.

This allows ease of passage of the suppository into the rectum by following the natural anatomy of the colon. Flexing the knees will reduce discomfort as the suppository is passed through the anal sphincter.

5   Place a disposable incontinence pad beneath the patient's hips and buttocks.

To avoid unncessary soiling of linen, leading to potential infection and embarrassment to the patient if the suppositories are prematurely ejected or there is rapid bowel evacuation following their administration.

6   Wash hands and put on gloves.

To reduce cross-infection.

7   Place some lubricating jelly on the topical swab and lubricate the *blunt* end of the suppository if it is being used to obtain systemic action. Separate the patient's buttocks and insert the suppository, blunt end first, advancing it for about 2–4 cm. Repeat this procedure if a second suppository is to be inserted.

Lubricating reduces surface friction and thus eases insertion of the suppository and avoids anal mucosal trauma. Research has shown that the suppository is more readily retained if inserted blunt end first. (For further information see pp. 60–1.) The anal canal is approximately 2–4 cm long. Inserting the suppository beyond this ensures that it will be retained.

8   Once suppository(ies) has been inserted, clean any excess lubricating jelly from the patient's perineal area.

To ensure the patient's comfort and avoid anal excoriation that may then lead to infection.

9   Ask the patient to retain the suppository(ies) if it is of an evacuant type. If it is medicated, ask the patient to retain the suppository for 20 minutes, or until he/she is no longer able to do so.

This will allow the suppository to melt and release its active ingredients.

10   Remove and dispose of equipment.

To avoid infection.

11   Record that the suppository(ies) has been given, the effect on the patient and the result (amount, colour, consistency and content) in the appropriate documents.

To monitor the patient's bowel function.

GUIDELINES: ADMINISTRATION OF RECTAL LAVAGE

Equipment
1   Rectal lavage pack containing a large funnel, rubber tubing, a straight connector, a 1 litre jug and a rectal catheter (Charrière gauge 24)
2   Non-sterile topical swabs
3   Lubricating jelly
4   Disposable gloves
5   Disposable incontinence pad
6   Plastic sheet and draw sheet
7   Large non-sterile jug
8   Bucket
9   Gate clip or clamp
10   Toilet paper or tissues
11   Disposable plastic apron
12   Large disposable bag
13   Measured volume of warm tap water (37–40 °C).

Procedure

Action	Rationale
1 Explain the procedure to the patient.	To obtain the patient's consent and co-operation.
2 Prepare the area where lavage is to be performed, i.e. the patient's bed or a couch in the room where rectal lavage is to take place. Protect the bed or couch with a plastic sheet and draw sheet. Place a disposable incontinence pad on the floor.	To prevent non-disposable equipment becoming contaminated with faecal matter, thus minimizing the risk of cross-infection.
3 Wash and dry hands, clean the trolley and prepare the equipment for the procedure by opening the pack and laying out the contents on the top of the shelf.	Although this is not an aseptic procedure, care must be taken to avoid unnecessary contamination.
4 Attach a large disposable bag to the trolley.	To provide a suitable receptacle for safe disposal of potentially large amounts of contaminated waste.
5 Fill a large non-sterile jug with a measured volume of warm (37–40 °C) tap water. Check the temperature with a lotion thermometer. Place the filled jug on the lower shelf of the trolley. Put a bucket for receiving effluent by the side of the bed or couch.	As the bowel is not sterile, there is no need to use sterile fluid. A large volume needs to be available for use, although the total amount used will vary with each patient. If the solution is too warm, the intestinal mucosa may be damaged; if too cold, unnecessary cramping may occur.
6 Assist the patient to lie in the required position, i.e. on the left side, with his/her knees well flexed, the upper higher than the lower one, and with the buttocks near the edge of the bed. Tilt the bed slightly if possible.	This position allows ease of access for insertion of the catheter into the rectum, follows the natural anatomy of the colon and aids gravity in promoting the flow of fluid into the sigmoid and descending colon. Tilting the bed also aids the flow.
7 Check that the patient's clothing is tucked out of the way and that both the patient and the bed are adequately protected. Ensure that the patient is as comfortable as possible before continuing with the procedure.	As the procedure can be lengthy and is potentially messy, the patient needs to be as relaxed and well protected as possible to aid successful completion.
8 Wash hands and put on disposable gloves and a disposable plastic apron.	To reduce cross-infection.
9 Connect up the funnel, tubing and rectal catheter, using a straight connector between the latter two items. Fix a gate clamp or clip in position approximately 15 cm from the end of the rectal catheter.	To allow the tubing and the catheter to be primed and filled with fluid, thus preventing the entry into the rectum and discomfort to the patient.
10 Using non-sterile topical swab lubricate the last 15 cm of the rectal catheter with a generous amount of jelly.	To aid insertion and minimize patient discomfort and trauma to the rectal mucosa.
11 Fill a small jug with 1 litre from the measured volume of warm tap water.	A small jug is more manageable and allows measurement of the amount of fluid used each time.
12 Prime the catheter and tubing.	
13 Gently insert 7.5–10 cm of the catheter into the rectum.	The rectum is approximately 12.5 cm long and the anal canal 2.5 cm. Inserting the catheter 7.5–10 cm ensures that the rectum will be adequately filled with the minimum trauma to the patient.

14   Encourage the patient to take deep breaths.

Deep breathing relaxes the anal sphincter.

15   Check that the patient is comfortable.

16   Fill the funnel with approximately 400 ml of fluid from the jug.

The rectum will hold 200–400 ml without causing trauma.

17   Hold the funnel about 30 cm above the rectum, release the clamp and allow the fluid to run into the rectum, holding the catheter in position.

Aqueous solution exerts pressure of 0.225 kgf for every 30 cm of elevation. The pressure should not exceed 0.45 kgf as this may cause cramping or even rupture of the intestinal wall.

18   Ask the patient to rock gently from side to side.

To ensure efficient lavage of the bowel lumen.

19   Before the funnel is completely empty, invert it over the bucket to allow the lavage fluid and faecal material to drain out.

To prevent unnecessary amounts of air entering the rectum and causing the patient discomfort.

20   Refill the funnel with another measure of fluid, keeping the tubing pinched or clamped and the funnel at patient level until it is filled.

21   Repeat the last two procedures until
   (a)   The effluent runs clear.
   (b)   A maximum volume of 6 litres has been used.

If the bowel is not clear after this volume, other methods need to be employed.

22   Note how much fluid was used during the procedure.

To ensure that not more than 6 litres are used.

23   At the end of the procedure
   (a)   Measure the amount of effluent obtained and compare it with the volume run in.
   (b)   Clear away and dispose of equipment.
   (c)   Ensure that the patient is clean and dry.

To ensure that the patient has not absorbed fluid in such a quantity that will carry the risk of fluid overload.
To avoid infection.

23   Settle the patient into bed, on an incontinence pad and with a bedpan or commode at hand.

To reduce potential infection caused by soiled linen.

NURSING CARE PLAN

Problem	Cause	Suggested action
Fluid will not run in freely.	Catheter is pressed against the bowel wall.	Gently manoeuvre the catheter around in the rectum.
	Catheter is blocked with faecal material.	Remove the catheter and unblock. Reinsert and recommence procedure.
	Insufficient gravity flow.	Raise the funnel slightly, but never over 60 cm above the mattress.
Leakage of fluid around the catheter.	Poor positioning of the catheter or displacement following insertion.	Check that the catheter is 7–10 cm into the rectum. Hold it gently in position.
	Poor tone of the anal sphincter muscles.	Ask the patient to try and tighten muscles as fluid is run in. Elevate the foot of the bed to aid flow.

Problem	Cause	Suggested action
Discomfort and/or cramping when the fluid is run in.	Fluid is too cold.	Check the temperature of the fluid and warm it if necessary.
	Pressure of the fluid entering the rectum is too high.	Lower the funnel to stop fluid from running until the spasm passes, but leave the catheter in to relieve distension.
	Extreme tension and anxiety.	When the spasm has passed, gradually raise the funnel and allow fluid to enter very slowly. Encourage deep breathing through the mouth to relax the abdominal muscles and decrease colonic pressures.
	Perforation of the rectum.	Stop the procedure immediately.
Severe pain accompanied by perspiration, pallor and tachycardia.	Perforation of the gut around the site of a large tumour due to increased peristalsis.	Check the patient's vital signs. Inform a doctor. Do not allow the patient to eat or drink until seen by a doctor.
Blood is returned in the effluent.	Insertion of the catheter has caused internal haemorrhoids to bleed.	Stop the procedure and inform a doctor. Record the appropriate amount of blood that has been passed and observe further bowel motions.
	Trauma to rectal mucosa.	
Large discrepancy between the amount of fluid run in and the effluent obtained.	Excessive leakage on to pads during the procedure.	Try to estimate the amount of fluid on pads, etc.
	Patient has retained a certain amount of fluid that may be passed later.	Measure carefully all subsequent bowel actions.
	Patient has absorbed the excess fluid.	Check the patient's vital signs. Record further intake and output carefully. Inform a doctor.
Sudden onset of pallor, perspiration, vomiting, coughing and dizziness.	Water intoxication due to excessive absorption of water from the rectum.	Stop the procedure immediately. Inform a doctor. Check the patient's vital signs.

7

Cardiopulmonary Resuscitation

Definition
Cardiac arrest may be defined as the abrupt cessation of cardiac function which is potentially reversible. The heart may be in one of two states during cardiac arrest, either asystole or ventricular fibrillation.

Indications
Indications of cardiac arrest, are as follows:
1   sudden loss of consciousness;
2   absence of radial, femoral and carotid pulses;
3   cessation of respirations;
4   dilatation of the pupils;
5   marked cyanosis.

REFERENCE MATERIAL
Principles
The primary objectives of cardiopulmonary resuscitation are twofold:
1   to restore effective circulation and ventilation;
2   to prevent irreversible cerebral damage due to anoxia. When the heart fails to maintain the cerebral circulation for approximately 4 minutes, the brain may suffer irreversible damage.

Resuscitation consists of meeting the following needs (ABC sequence):
1   A(irway) is met by maintaining an open, clear airway;
2   B(reathing) is met by maintaining artificial ventilation;
3   C(irculation) is met by maintaining external cardiac massage.

Causes
1   *Cerebral:* cerebral causes are due to depression of the respiratory centre, e.g. overdose of depressant drugs, hypothermia, trauma, hypotension, lesions of the central nervous system.
2   *Respiratory:* respiratory causes are due to respiratory obstruction, e.g. foreign bodies, pulmonary embolism, pneumothorax, haemothorax, drowning.
3   *Cardiac:* cardiac causes are due to coronary occlusion, pericardial tamponade, cardiac myopathy and electrocution.
4   *Hepatic:* liver disfunction may cause electrolyte imbalance, e.g. hyper-or hypokalaemia.

Treatment
Treatment of cardiac arrest is carried out in three stages:
1   cardiopulmonary resuscitation;
2   correction of acid–base balance;
3   assessment and correction of electrolyte balance.

Drugs
A range of drugs is used in the treatment of cardiac arrest:

Atropine sulphate: to increase the heart rate by blocking the slowing effect of vagal activity.

Adrenaline 1:10,000: to increase excitability and tone of the myocardium.

Lignocaine: to lower the excessive excitability of cardiac contraction.

Sodium bicarbonate 8.4%: to correct acidosis associated with cardiopulmonary arrest.

Calcium chloride 10%: to increase the contractability of the myocardial muscle.

Isoprenaline 0.002%: to maintain cardiac output by stimulating the ventricles to contract with greater power.

Aminophylline: to reduce pulmonary oedema, left ventricular fibrillation and bronchospasm. To a lesser extent it causes coronary artery dilatation, increases urinary output and the rate and power of cardiac contraction.

Frusemide: to increase diuresis and reduce pulmonary oedema.

The way in which these drugs are used in relation to defibrillation is set out by the Resuscitation Council (1984).

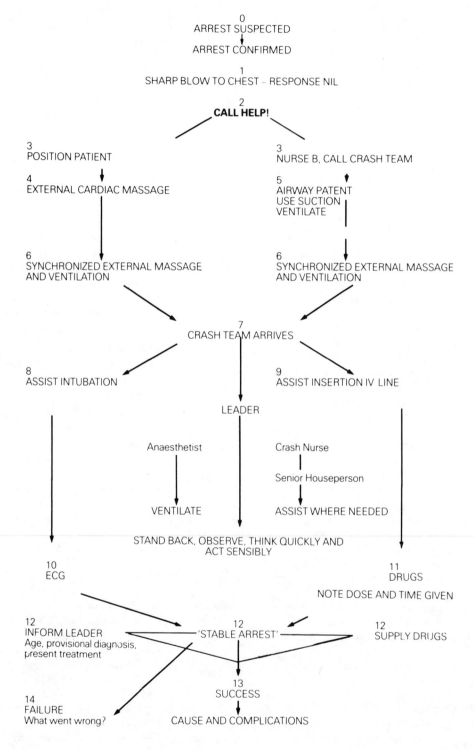

Figure 7.1 Flow chart to illustrate the management of cardiopulmonary resuscitation.

Aftercare

1 Monitor pulse, blood pressure and urinary output.
2 Connect up oscilloscope.
3 Give oxygen therapy.
4 Transfer to special units (coronary care).

Intravenous infusion and intubation

If the procedure is performed by a doctor, the nurse's responsibilities are as follows:

1 to check what equipment the doctor needs to use and to prepare it for use;
2 to assist as required;
3 to clear away equipment.

Defibrillation

The carrying out of defibrillation by nurses is more common in the United States than it is in the United Kingdom, although those nurses working in special units in the UK are accepting responsibility for this procedure. A useful outline of the principles and the equipment may be found in Matheny (1981).

It is recommended that nurses receive proper training before taking on this extended role.

The resuscitation team

Wilson and Aarvold (1975) recommend that four or five personnel are adequate:

1 a senior physician to diagnose and direct the treatment;
2 an anaesthetist, anaesthetic nurse or a nurse trained to perform endotracheal intubation;
3 one or two nurses to perform external cardiac massage;
4 one nurse to administer prescribed drugs and intravenous infusion.

These authors also warn of the dangers engendered when personnel not directly involved gather around the area where the arrest has occurred.

Statistics

It has been estimated by Thompson (1982) that 80–90% survival can be anticipated on the coronary care unit in patients with primary ventricular fibrillation. Survival rates on the ward are approximately 20% lower. Surviv-al rates in the community are nil. Peatfield *et al.* (1977), in a study based on the Central Middlesex Hospital, found that of 1,063 arrests in the hospital over a 10-year period, 345 patients were successfully resuscitated but 252 of these died later in hospital, giving 93 survivors. The number of cardiac arrest calls varied between 77 and 134 per year and the percentage surviving to discharge varied from 4 to 13.8%. Survival rates for males and females were equal. (The study was based on arrests in the general areas of the hospital, excluding the coronary and intensive care units.)

Ethics

The criteria used to assess the suitability of a patient for resuscitation are controversial. Factors that need to be considered are the patient's age, the nature and extent of the principal and/or secondary diseases, the quality of life experienced by the patient prior to admission and that to be expected after discharge. All personnel in the clinical team must be aware of the resuscitation status of each individual patient.

References and further reading

Brunner, L.S. and Suddarth, D.S. (1982) *The Lippincott Manual of Medical–Surgical Nursing*, Vol. 2, Harper & Row, London.

Cochrane, G.M. (1978) Saving life after cardiac arrest, *Nursing Mirror*, Vol. 147, no. 2, pp. 17–20.

Evans, T.R. (ed.) (1986) *ABC of resuscitation*, British *Medical Journal* Publication, London.

Matheny, L.G. (1981) Defibrillation: when and how to use it, *Nursing* (US), Vol. 11, no. 6, pp. 69–72.

Newbold, D. (1987) External chest compression – the new skills, *Nursing Times*, Vol. 83, pp. 41–3.

Peatfield, R.C. *et al.* (1977) Survival after cardiac arrest in hospital, *Lancet*, Vol. i, pp. 1223–5.

Resuscitation Council (1984) *Cardiopulmonary Resuscitation*, Laerdal Medical, Norway.

Thompson, D.R. (1982) *Cardiac Surgery*, Baillière-Tindall, London.

Wilson, P. and Aarvold, J.A. (1975) The organization and operational nursing management of cardiac arrest, *International Journal of Nursing Studies*, Vol. 12, pp. 23–32.

GUIDELINES: CARDIOPULMONARY RESUSCITATION

Equipment

All items should be kept together and a checklist of these items should be drawn up. The list should be checked at least once a week and immediately after use.

1   Airway
2   Ambu bag with valve and mask
3   Oxygen tubing
4   Tongue forceps
5   Mouth gag
6   High capacity clearance catheters for aspirating the buccal cavity
7   Laryngoscope with spare bulbs and batteries
8   Intubating forceps
9   Endotracheal tubes
10 Topical swabs
11 Lubricating jelly
12 Syringe
13 Artery forceps
14 Endotracheal suction catheters
15 Hypo-allergenic tape
16 Scissors
17 Catheter mount and swivel connector
18 Plaster
19 Tracheostomy set
20 Tracheostomy tubes
21 Emergency cardiac drugs
22 Intravenous infusion giving sets
23 Intravenous infusion cannulae
24 Syringes and needles
25 Swabs saturated with isopropyl alcohol 70%
26 Intravenous infusion stands
27 Cardiac needle
28 Oscilloscope
29 Electrode pads
30 Defibrillator
31 Lubricating jelly suitable for defibrillation paddles.

Procedure

Action	Rationale
1 Note the time of the arrest, if witnessed.	Lack of cerebral circulation for approximately 3–5 minutes will result in irreversible brain damage.
2 Give the patient a short, sharp blow to the chest.	This may restore a cardiac rhythm which will give an adequate cardiac output.
3 Summon help. If a second nurse is available, he/she should call the emergency resuscitation team, bring equipment needed for cardiopulmonary resuscitation, prepare the environment and screen off the area.	Cardiopulmonary resuscitation is more effective when carried out by two people. Two nurses carrying out efficient cardiac massage and assisted ventilation can support the patient for 20 minutes plus. Medical intervention is required immediately.
4 Lie the patient in a supine position on a firm, non-metallic surface.	To allow for effective compression of the sternum against the spine during cardiac massage and to safeguard patients and personnel if defibrillation is required.

5   Remove the head of the bed if the patient is in bed.

To allow easy access to the patient's head. To assist in the intubation procedure.

6   Ensure a clear airway by removing debris, secretions, vomit and prostheses from the buccal cavity. Hyperextend the neck by tilting the chin upwards and backwards.

Maintains a clear airway by moving the tongue away from the pharyngeal wall.

7   Insert the airway.

8   Place the mask of the Ambu bag over the patient's mouth and nose.

To inflate the lungs. To ensure an airtight seal.

9   Compress the lower third of the sternum with the heel of one hand. Place the palm of the other hand over the back of this hand. Keep your arms straight and elbows locked.

The heart is situated between this area of the sternum and the spine. Pressure will massage the heart and maintain circulation. The brain is more susceptible to ischaemia than anoxia and external cardiac massage should commence prior to ventilation, if both cannot be instituted simultaneously.

10   Depress the bag in a rhythmical fashion.

To ensure a constant, steady supply of oxygen.

11   Attach the Ambu bag or rebreathing bag (open valve a half turn when using rebreathing circuit) to an oxygen source as soon as possible. A minimum of 4 litres per minute at 100% should be delivered.

Brain damage begins to occur once the blood's small store of oxygen is used up. There is a lack of sufficient oxygen in atmospheric air (approximately 21%).

12   Inflate the lungs and compress the heart in the ratio 1:5 or 2:15 if one person only. Cardiac massage must continue until the patient is able to maintain his/her own blood pressure.

To maintain circulation and oxygenation at an acceptable rate (a pulse of 60 beats per minute and respirations of 15 per minute).

13   When the resuscitation team arrives, one nurse should be responsible for recording information in the appropriate documents.

To ensure accurate information about the nature and course of the emergency.

At this stage the resuscitation team becomes responsible for the management of the emergency. All other personnel not directly involved should return to their duties.

INTUBATION

Action

Rationale

14   Continue to ventilate and oxygenate the patient before intubation begins.

Cardiac dysrhythmias due to hypoxia are decreased.

15   Attach the patient to an oscilloscope by applying electrode pads, check switches, connections and gain.

Accurate recording of cardiac rhythms will enable appropriate treatment to be initiated.

16   Before handing equipment to the medical staff check that:
    (a) The suction equipment is operational.
    (b) The endotracheal tube is lubricated.
    (c) The endotracheal tube cuff inflates and deflates.
    (d) The catheter mount and the swivel connector are attached.

Action	Rationale
17 Recommence ventilation and oxygenation immediately intubation is completed.	

INTRAVENOUS LINE

Action	Rationale

Such a line will allow for the resoration of acid base and electrolyte imbalance, the administration of drugs and the replacement of body fluids.

Action	Rationale
18 Asepsis must be maintained throughout.	To prevent local and/or systemic infection.
19 The correct rate of infusion is required.	To ensure maximum drug and/or solution effectiveness.
20 Accurate recording of the administration of solutions infused and drugs added is essential.	To provide a point of reference in the event of any queries.

DEFIBRILLATION

Used to terminate ventricular fibrillation.

NURSING CARE PLAN

Problem	Action	Rationale
Only one nurse available immediately.	Shout for help and keep shouting. Inflate the lungs and compress the heart in the ratio 2:15.	To make it obvious that help is needed. This will give a pulse of 80 beats per minute.
Absence of chest expansion.	Check that the airway is clear and that the head is in the correct position.	To provide and maintain a clear airway so that forceful ventillation may occur.
	If an Ambu bag is used, check that the valve is working, i.e. that the flaps open and close.	
	Check that the mouthpiece of the Ambu bag is covering the nose and the mouth.	To provide an airtight seal.
	Check endotracheal tube cuff is inflated.	
	Inform medical staff.	Possibility of oesophageal intubation, intubation of right bronchus or stiff non-compliant lungs. Pneumothorax.

Patient is a child.	Omit precordial thump. Use only two fingers over the lower sternum to compress the heart.	Undue pressure will fracture a child's ribs, with potential rupture of the lungs leading to haemopneumothorox.
	An increased rate of compression is also necessary.	Children normally have a pulse rate of 20–40 beats per minute more than an adult.
	Ensure that appropriate equipment of paediatric size is available, e.g. airway and Ambu bag.	Adult-size equipment would cause trauma and be inadequate for this purpose.
	If equipment is unavailable, use mouth to mouth–nose method, i.e. cover child's mouth and nose and inflate lungs.	To ensure an airtight seal and adequate oxygenation.
Patient has a radioactive source implanted.	See the procedures for Iodine 131 (p. 205), and Sealed Radioactive Sources (p. 318).	

8

Central Venous Catheterization

Definition

Placement of an indwelling catheter within the superior or inferior vena cava or right atrium, or a large vein leading to these vessels.

Indications

This procedure is indicated in the following circumstances:

1 to monitor central venous pressure in seriously ill patients;
2 for the administration of large amounts of intravenous fluid or blood, e.g. in cases of shock or major surgery;
3 to provide long-term access for:
    (a) hydration or electrolyte maintenance;
    (b) repeated administration of drugs, such as cytotoxic and antibiotic therapy;
    (c) repeated transfusion of blood or blood products;
    (d) repeated specimen collection.
4 for total parenteral nutrition.

REFERENCE MATERIAL
The catheter

In the past decade there have been numerous developments in both catheter design and materials, resulting in a greater range of devices. This has had a beneficial effect on patient care due to improvements in insertion techniques and nursing management.

Table 8.1 lists examples of available catheters. This is not intended to be a comprehensive list as recent progress has been rapid, with many new products entering clinical use. Double- and triple-lumen catheters have provided solutions to the problems of multiple access and the inclusion of extra features such as 'on/off' switches has simplified nursing practice.

INSERTION OF THE CATHETER

The catheter may be inserted at any of the sites shown in Figure 8.1. If the site chosen is the antecubital fossa, a 'long line' will be used as the catheter has to pass a substantial distance through the venous system.

The catheter may be inserted directly into the vein or it may be tunnelled subcutaneously for a short distance prior to entry (see Figure 8.1). Skin tunnelling is usually performed if the catheter is intended to provide long-term access over a number of months, during which the patient may be discharged and readmitted. The purpose of the tunnel is to remove the entry site into the vein from the exit site on the skin, so providing a barrier to infection. Catheters specifically designed for skin tunnelling frequently have a Dacron cuff sited part way along their length. This cuff is positioned in the subcutaneous tunnel and tissue granulates around it so reinforcing the barrier to invading organisms and providing security. Local site infection can be observed and treated, the incidence of septicaemia is reduced and removal of the catheter due to contamination is not always necessary. An example of this type of catheter is the Hickman.

A recent development aimed at further reducing infectious complications is an implantable drug delivery system, consisting of a portal attached to a silicone catheter (Figure 8.2). The portal is placed under the skin and sutured to the chest wall. The catheter is tunnelled as previously described and the tip rests in a major vein. The re-formation of the skin barrier prevents the entry of micro-organisms and strict aseptic technique should result in a minimal contamination rate.

The portal is accessed using a special Huber point needle when therapy is required and this may remain in place for up to one week. During this time, management is as for a central venous catheter.

The hazards associated with the insertion of a central venous catheter are substantial (Table 8.2) and for this reason the procedure should be performed in a controlled environment. The operating theatre or anaesthetic room is preferred. When this is not possible, a quiet environment with a minimum of activity is desirable.

Table 8.1 Examples of Common Catheter Materials

Catheter material	Recommended indwelling life	Common site(s) of insertion	Capacity for skin tunnelling
Teflon	5–7 days	Jugular	No
Polyethylene	8–10 days	Jugular Subclavian Antecubital fossa	No
Silicone	Indefinite	Cephalic Axillary Subclavian Antecubital fossa	Yes (may be connected to an implanted port)
Polyurethane	Indefinite	Subclavian	No

A general anaesthetic may be necessary for some insertions, but often the procedure is performed under heavy sedation or using local anaesthesia. The doctor inserts the catheter with the nurse assisting. The nurse's responsibilities are as follows:

1   to provide the patient with a full explanation of the procedure and to teach the patient techniques which may be required during insertion, for example the Valsalva manoeuvre (see p. 80);
2   to ensure that any specific preoperative instructions have been carried out;
3   to explain the postoperative procedures and the appearance/function of the catheter or device;
4   to assemble the equipment requested;
5   to prepare fluids with which to test the patency of the catheter, and to prime the administration set and extension set;
6   to prepare local anaesthesia and dressing materials;
7   to ensure the correct positioning of the patient during insertion, that is, in the supine or Trendelenburg position with the head down and a roll of towel along the spinal column;
8   to attend to the physical and psychological comfort of the patient during and immediately following the procedure;
9   to ensure that no fluid or medication is infused before the correct position of the catheter is confirmed.

Prevention of the afore-mentioned complications and distress to the patient may be achieved by careful insertion techniques, strict asepsis, correct positioning and radiological confirmation of the catheter placement. The catheter should be heparinized or normal saline infused very slowly, 10–20 ml/h, until X-ray results are available.

Table 8.2 Hazards of Catheter Insertion

Sepsis	Brachial plexus injury
Air embolism	Thoracic duct trauma
Pneumothorax	Misdirection or kinking
Hydrothorax	Catheter embolism
Haemorrhage	Thrombosis
Haemothorax	

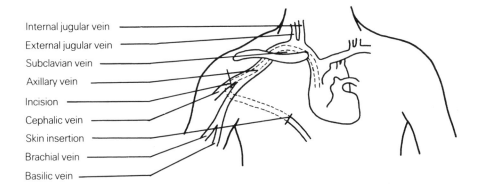

Internal jugular vein
External jugular vein
Subclavian vein
Axillary vein
Incision
Cephalic vein
Skin insertion
Brachial vein
Basilic vein

Figure 8.1 The ideal position and site for a long-term indwelling catheter.

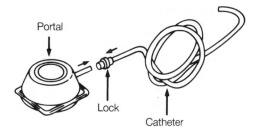

Figure 8.2 Components of the Port-a-Cath® implantable delivery system.

The Valsalva manoeuvre

This may be performed by conscious patients to aid the insertion of the catheter. The patient is placed in the supine or Trendelenburg position which increases venous filling. He/she is asked to breathe in and then try to force the air out with mouth and nose closed. This increases the intrathoracic pressure so that the return of blood to the heart is momentarily reduced and the veins in the neck region become engorged. A distension of the vein up to 2.5 cm can be achieved in this way.

Principles of catheter care
PREVENTION OF INFECTION

Strict aseptic technique and compliance with recommendations for equipment and dressing changes are essential if microbial contamination is to be prevented.

Sterile gloves should be worn whenever the insertion site is exposed or the closed system is broken. The insertion site should be regularly checked postoperatively and the dressing renewed if there is haemoserous discharge. When a skin-tunnelled catheter has been inserted there may be local swelling and drainage from the tunnel. A pressure dressing or the application of ice may reduce the severity of these problems. The sterile dressing over the insertion site may be renewed weekly if it is intact and not soiled. A complaint of soreness from the patient or an unexplained pyrexia is also a reason for earlier renewal (for further details see the guidelines: for changing the dressing, pp. 89–91).

At the time the dressing is changed the site should be observed for inflammation and/or discharge, and the conditions of the skin noted. Alternatives must be considered in situations where the skin is delicate and a conventional semi-occlusive dressing could traumatize it, for example in bone marrow transplant patients and children. For these patients a dry, sterile gauze dressing secured with a minimum of tape may be more suitable. This should be changed daily.

Following the healing of the skin tunnel and removal of the sutures from a Hickman-type catheter, at 14 days, no dressing is necessary unless the patient requests it.

Meticulous hand washing may replace the use of sterile gloves.

Manipulations of the catheter and intravenous pathway must be kept to a minimum, and changes of dressing, extension set, administration set or procedures such as blood sampling should be co-ordinated to reduce handling. The giving set must be changed every 24 hours but the extension set may be regarded as an integral part of the catheter and changed weekly.

MAINTENANCE OF A CLOSED SYSTEM

If equipment becomes disconnected, air embolism or profuse blood loss may occur, dependent on the condition and position of the patient at the time. Luer locks provide a more secure connection and all equipment should have these fittings, i.e. giving sets, extension sets, injection caps, syringes. Care should be taken to clamp the line firmly when changing equipment, or to use the switch provided on some catheters. Connections must be double checked and precautions should be taken to prevent the introduction of air into the system when making additions to, or taking blood from, the central line.

Data extrapolated from studies with animals suggests that 20cc of air per second is required to produce symptoms of air embolism and between 75 and 150 cc/sec to produce a fatality.

MAINTENANCE OF A PATENT CATHETER

Occlusion of the catheter is usually the result of one of the following:

1 an infusion running too slowly;
2 an administration set or mechanical aid turned off accidentally and left for a prolonged period;
3 infrequent flushing of the catheter when not in use.

In all these instances a clot will form in the catheter. Occasionally, a blockage may be the result of precipitate formation due to inadequate flushing between incompatible medications.

Meticulous intravenous technique and management will prevent the majority of these problems. However, little definitive research exists regarding the technique of heparinization. The amount of heparin required and the frequency at which flushing is performed are based on empiricism. The injection technique using positive pressure to ensure fluid is retained in the catheter does appear to be important.

When used for intermittent therapy, the catheter should be flushed after each use with a solution of heparinized saline, containing 10 units/ml. The volume injected must be between 2.5 and 5 ml. Commercial preparations of this strength are available.

Catheters made of polyurethane and silicone are often *in situ* for prolonged periods of time and may not be used frequently, especially if the patient is discharged. In this situation it is recommended that heparinization with the afore-mentioned solution is performed twice weekly.

If occlusion does occur, gentle aspiration may dislodge the clot and a flush with normal saline may be all that is required to restore patency. Gentle pressure and suction may need to be repeated if the catheter has been left for a long time and a larger thrombus has formed. Silicone catheters expand on pressure and allow fluid around a clot facilitating its dislodgement. Use of heparin solution may also be tried.

The enzymes urokinase and streptokinase have both been used to dissolve thrombi and restore catheter patency. Although effective, these are potentially dangerous substances and their use must be approved by the medical staff and prescribed accordingly.

When using implanted drug delivery systems, the manufacturer's literature should be consulted with reference to heparinization. The most widely stated recommendation is a flush with 500 units of heparin monthly.

PREVENTING DAMAGE OF THE CATHETER AND PERFORMING A REPAIR

Silicone catheters are prone to cracking or splitting if handled incorrectly but fortunately both temporary and permanent repairs can be performed. However, prevention of this occurrence is preferred.

Artery forceps, scissors or sharp-edged clamps should not be used on or near the catheter. A smooth clamp should be placed on the reinforced section of the catheter provided for this purpose. If this is not present, one can be created by placing a tape tab over part of the catheter. A second alternative is to move the clamp up or down the catheter at regular intervals.

Accidents do occur, however, and the nurse must be familiar with the action to be taken. Immediate clamping of the catheter proximal to the fracture or split is essential to prevent blood loss or air embolism. The split area should be covered with an alcohol swab and emergency repair equipment collected, together with sterile gloves to ensure that all manipulations are aseptic. Figure 8.3 illustrates the steps to be followed.

A permanent repair should be performed as soon as possible using the specific kit provided by the manufacturer. This should be done by a member of the medical staff or other designated personnel.

Total parenteral nutrition

Total parenteral nutrition (TPN) is the direct infusion, into a vein, of solutions containing the essential nutrients in quantities sufficient to meet all the daily needs of the patient.

The decision to commence TPN should be an elective one and should be used only if alternative enteral

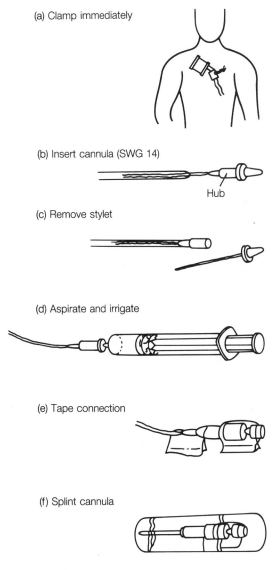

Figure 8.3 Temporary repair of a damaged silicone catheter (adapted from Ford, 1986).

methods are considered inappropriate or unsatisfactory. Total parenteral nutrition is indicated in any disease or circumstance when the digestive and absorptive functions of the small intestine are seriously impaired (see Table 8.3)

TPN SOLUTIONS

The nutrients for TPN are provided by an amino acid solution, a glucose solution, a solution containing an emulsion of lipids and solutions containing essential vitamins and minerals. The amount and concentration of solutions used can be varied in order to construct a

Table 8.3   Indications for Total Parenteral Nutrition (TPN)

Inflammatory bowel disease
Enterocutaneous fistulae
Short bowel syndrome
Severe burns
Bowel obstruction
Infants of very low birth weight
Major abdominal/thoracic surgery

regimen to suit the patient's needs. These solutions may be administered in one of three ways:

1 two solutions are infused concurrently with the third given separately;
2 the amino acids, glucose, vitamins and minerals are prepared either commercially or by pharmacy in a 2–3-litre bag and administered over 12–16 hours. The fat emulsion is then run in over 4–6 hours;
3 all solutions are prepared together in a 3-litre bag and administered over 16–24 hours.

Methods (2) and (3) are in use at The Royal Marsden Hospital and three standard regimens are in operation (see Table 8.4). Three days of feed may be ordered at any one time.

MONITORING OF TPN

During TPN regular observations are required. The following measurements are suggested:

Daily

Sodium mmol/l   Potassium mmol/l
Chloride mmol/l   Bicarbonate mmol/l
Urea mmol/l   Creatinine umol/l
Glucose mmol/l
Fluid balance

Twice weekly

Albumin g/l   Total protein g/l
Magnesium mmol/l   Calcium mmol/l
Phosphate mmol/l
Bilirubin µmol/l
Aspartate amino transferase (AST) i.u./l
Alkaline phosphatase (ALP) i.u./l
Haemoglobin g/dl
WBC $\times 10^9$/l
PCV %

Table 8.4   An Example of a TPN Regimen for Patients of Body Weight 60–75 kg

Components	Quantity
Vamin glucose	1500 ml (N_2 14.1 g, Zn 50 µmol)
Dextrose 10%	1000 ml (CHO 250 g, Fe 50 µmol)
Addiphos	15 ml (Fat 100 g, F 50 µmol)
Potassium chloride 15%	15 ml (Na 98 mmol, Mn 40 µmol)
Addamel	10 ml (K 82 mmol, Cu 5 µmol)
Zinc sulphate 50 µmol/ml	0.6 ml (Ca 8.8 mmol, I 1 µmol)
Magnesium sulphate 50%	1 ml (Mg 5.8 mmol)
Intralipid 20%	500 ml (PO_4 37.5 mmol)
Vitlipid adult	10 ml (Cl 126 mmol)
Solivito	1 vial

Non-protein Kcal/N_2 ratio 142:1
Total volume: 3,052 ml
Total Kcal: 2,000

DELIVERY OF TPN AND RECOMMENDATIONS FOR INTRAVENOUS MANAGEMENT

The major hazard associated with delivery of TPN is infection and the following detailed recommendations are designed to prevent this. They reflect the current policy of The Royal Marsden Hospital, compiled by a multidisciplinary team and is regularly reviewed.

1 catheter insertion must take place in theatre using full aseptic technique;
2 a skin-tunnelled silicone catheter is the catheter of choice for long-term nutrition;
3 a separate peripheral cannula may be required for insulin infusion via a syringe pump;
4 peripheral venous access should be assessed prior to catheter placement; if the veins available are considered inadequate to support the patient for the duration of therapy a double-lumen catheter should be inserted.
5 in the event of peripheral access deteriorating during the course of parenteral nutrition, and adaptor for dual access to the nutrition catheter should be used. The adaptor should be streamlined and possess Luer lock fittings.

DRESSING OF THE INSERTION SITE

A sterile semi-occlusive transparent dressing will be applied to the insertion site while the patient is in theatre. This should not be touched, but the site should be inspected daily. Exceptions to this are:

1 if the site is inflamed or sore;
2 if the dressing is not adequately secured, or torn.

The dressing must be performed in accord with the hospital procedure for the dressing of central venous lines. The entry site is cleaned with 0.5% chlorhexidine in 70% spirit, sprayed with povidone-iodine spray, then Opsite spray is also applied before the appropriate dressing.

If the site is inflamed a swab must be sent to bacteriology for culture and sensitivity and the medical staff notified.

ADMINISTRATION SETS

Administration sets must be changed every 24 hours, as directed by hospital policy, using sterile gloves and aseptic technique. Administration sets must have a Luer lock fitting.

Infusion containers will be prepared under aseptic conditions in the pharmacy and may be delivered to the ward with administration sets attached. In this instance, the nurse is required to prime the tubing and connect it to the catheter.

The inside and outside of the hub of the catheter and end of the administration set must be sprayed with isopropyl alcohol 70%, and allowed to dry before the connection is made. The hub will be set in an iodine-impregnated foam pad.

All connections must be checked.

Existing injection sites on the administration set should *never* be used for the giving of additional medications. They will be labelled accordingly.

Containers and administration sets should be scheduled for changing in daylight hours, even if this means discarding an incompletely used bag at a time specified on prescription sheet.

ADMINISTRATION OF MEDICATIONS

No additional medications or blood products should be given via a parenteral nutrition catheter. It should not be used for central venous pressure (CVP) measurements or blood sampling. The procedure detailed under catheter insertion should be followed, i.e. a peripheral line should be established (see pp. 78–9).

CONTROL OF INFUSION RATE

Total parenteral nutrition infusions must be closely monitored at all times. An infusion pump, drip rate or volumetric, must always be used, especially when TPN is given via a 3 litre bag.

No adjustment greater than 4 drops per minute every 15 minutes should be made to an infusion rate. *Never* attempt to 'catch up' rapidly if fluid is running slowly.

PYREXIA OF UNKNOWN ORIGIN

In the event of the patient developing a persistent pyrexia/tachycardia, contamination of the catheter should be suspected. However, the catheter should not be removed until infection has been confirmed, unless clinical condition dictates otherwise.

The following investigations must be performed:

1 blood cultures:
   (a) from the catheter;
   (b) from a peripheral vein;
2 a full blood count;
3 midstream specimen of urine for microscopy, culture and sensitivity;
4 chest X-ray;
5 other tests to eliminate other sources of infection, as appropriate, e.g. wound swabs, throat swabs, etc.

SEPTICAEMIA

If the patient has a suspected septicaemia, antibiotic cover should be initiated but no further action taken with reference to the catheter until positive blood culture results are received and further decisions made by medical staff concerned. The line should be heparinized and TPN infusion stopped.

Removal of the catheter

ELECTIVE

The catheter must be removed if blood cultures taken from the line are positive to micro-organisms, and the patient is symptomatic or has a pyrexia, after consultation with the medical staff.

A leaking or damaged catheter should be removed after consultation with the medical staff. The catheter must be removed carefully using aseptic technique and the tip sent for bacteriological examination.

Termination of therapy

Total parenteral nutrition should not be terminated (except for the above reasons) until oral or nasogastric feeding is well established. This will be discussed by the medical and surgical staff and dietitian.

At the end of parenteral nutrition, the catheter need not be removed immediately. It may continue to be used for access or fluids.

When the catheter is removed, aseptic technique must be used and the catheter tip sent to bacteriology. A sterile airtight dressing should be placed on the exit site and left in place for at least 24 hours.

HEPARINIZATION

Occasionally, certain investigations, e.g. computerized tomography, may require that the infusion be discontinued and the catheter heparinized. Simultaneous insulin infusions must also be discontinued. Partly used infusion containers should *never* be re-used but should be discarded and a fresh one requested, if necessary, from the pharmacy.

Problems should be referred to the appropriate member of medical, anaesthetic, pharmacy or nursing staff.

Reading central venous pressure

Central venous pressure (CVP) is the pressure within the superior vena cava or within the right atrium. Measurements of CVP reflect the relationship between the blood volume and cardiac competence (Figure 8.4).

PURPOSE OF CVP READINGS

1 To serve as a guide to fluid balance in seriously ill patients.
2 To estimate blood volume deficits.
3 To assist in monitoring circulatory failure.

MEASURING CVP

The CVP measurement should be taken from a site in line with the right atrium. Either of the sites indicated in Figure 8.5 may be used, but it should be established at the outset of the readings which point is to be used as there is a pressure difference of about 5 cm water between them. It is useful to mark the chosen site for future readings and to note this site both on the CVP recording chart and in the care plan for the patient.

The normal values for CVP readings are: 0–5 cm water at the sternal angle and 5–10 cm water at the mid-axilla.

Current models of some volumetric infusion pumps have electronic central venous pressure monitoring facilities. These are accurate, easy to use and remove many of the variables which lead to discrepancies in CVP readings, especially those related to the nurse. Examples of these are differences in the exact site used and problems of positioning the patient in an identical manner.

Discharging patients with a central catheter *in situ*

Patients with skin-tunnelled catheters or implanted devices may be discharged home with their line *in situ*. No

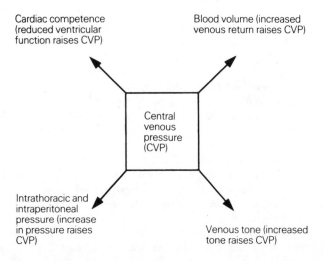

Figure 8.4   Determinants of central venous pressure.

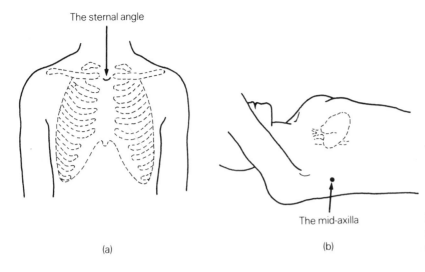

The sternal angle

The mid-axilla

(a)   (b)

Figure 8.5 Measuring central venous pressure. *a*, The sternal angle. *b*, The mid-axilla.

special instructions are required for implanted ports as the catheter will be heparinized and the needle removed before the patient leaves hospital. Reheparinization is not necessary for one month.

However, patients with Hickman-type catheters must be instructed and supervised in the care of their lines before discharge. Aspects to be covered with the patient, relatives and/or friends include:

1 care of the exit site;
2 heparinization techniques;
3 the amount and type of activity permitted.

At the time of discharge the catheter should be well established and the Dacron cuff covered with fibrous tissue, thus sealing off the catheter insertion site from the skin. In this instance, no dressing is needed unless the patient requests it. If this is so, sterile gauze swabs and hypo-allergenic tape may be supplied.

If the individual is discharged prior to suture removal, the site should be dressed according to hospital policy and arrangements made for this to be renewed weekly. The only other time when a dressing may be required is if the patient participates in water sports. In this instance, the whole catheter and exit site should be completely covered with an occlusive dressing one hour prior to the activity and removed immediately afterwards. The area should then be carefully dried. Such precautions are not necessary for daily showers or baths but it must be pointed out to the patient that the sponge/cloth used for general body washing should not come into contact with the exit site. Sterile wool balls should be supplied and the technique of cleansing with tap water demonstrated to the patient.

Prior to discharge the patient should observe the heparinization technique and perform it with and without supervision. Relatives and friends should be in-

volved in this procedure. Sufficient equipment must be supplied to enable the patient to care for the catheter from the time of discharge until the next outpatient appointment or admission. A kit has been assembled containing the following:

1 spare Luer lock caps with an injection site;
2 a spare smooth-edged clamp;
3 a supply of heparinized saline, 50 i.u. in 5 ml, for example Hepsal or Heplok;
4 isopropyl alcohol 70% swabs to clean the injection site on the cap;
5 a supply of sterile 5-ml syringes;
6 19G needles (white) to draw up heparinized saline;
7 25G needles (orange) to inject through the intermittent injection cap;
8 instruction booklet to provide the patient with a point of reference if in doubt about procedures when at home.

The patient's technique and confidence when caring for the catheter should be assessed prior to discharge and the importance of asepsis during all handling procedures stressed.

There are few restrictions with reference to activity. Modifications of dressing technique to permit swimming, etc. have already been mentioned. The psychological impact of an indwelling catheter on body image should not be overlooked, especially when patients are sexually active. Additionally, normal activities may be affected, for example driving may become uncomfortable due to pressure from a seat belt on the catheter/clamp/exit site.

Removal of the catheter
NON-SKIN TUNNELLED CATHETERS
If a catheter is not tunnelled through the skin it may be removed by nursing staff. The nurse should be familiar

with the procedure and confident about performing it. Aseptic technique must be adhered to and the site cleaned prior to removal to prevent a false positive when the catheter tip is sent for bacteriological examination. Major vessels usually heal quickly but pressure must be applied until lack of bleeding confirms this. A sterile dressing is applied and should remain in place for at least 24 hours.

SKIN-TUNNELLED CATHETERS

Removal techniques for skin-tunnelled catheters vary but the procedure is normally performed by a doctor due to the risk of the catheter breaking and subsequent catheter embolism. This has been reported in a number of studies.

It is recommended that the patient is placed in the same position as for insertion and that aseptic technique is used throughout. Sedation may be required by the patient to relieve anxiety. The exit site should be cleaned to prevent a false-positive tip culture being obtained. The catheter should be gripped firmly and constant traction applied. It may take a few minutes for the catheter and cuff to become loosened and slide free. Continued steady pressure will remove the complete line. This should be checked immediately after removal before the tip is cut and sent for microbiological examination. The catheter and cuff may be pulled through together, resulting in a slight bleeding from the exit site and complaints of a burning sensation from the patient. However, the cuff may remain attached to tissue. This is of no significance and it may be left in place. If the patient or medical staff wish it, the cuff may be surgically excised. Difficulty with removal or a break in the catheter will require surgical intervention. Major vessels usually heal quickly but a dressing may be needed on the exit site for 24 hours.

Note: intravenous management and administration of drugs may be undertaken via peripheral or central venous pathways. Therefore, only nurses in possession of a certificate of competence, or nurses supervised by a suitably qualified nurse should perform these procedures.

References and further reading

Anderson, M.A. *et al.* (1982) The double-lumen Hickman catheter, *American Journal of Nursing*, Vol. 82, no. 2, pp. 272–7.

Bjeletich, J. (1982) Repairing the Hickman catheter, *American Journal of Nursing*, Vol. 82, no. 2, p. 274.

Bjeletich, J. and Hickman, R.O. (1980) The Hickman indwelling catheter, *American Journal of Nursing*, Vol. 80, no. 1, pp. 62–5.

Brunner, L.S. and Suddarth, D.S. (1986) *The Lippincott Manual of Nursing Practice*, 4th edn, J.B. Lippincott, Philadelphia.

Dewar, B.J. (1986) Total parenteral nutrition at home, *Nursing Times*, Vol. 82, no. 28, pp. 35–8.

Flannigan, M. (1982) Intravenous feeding 1/2, *Nursing Mirror*, Vol. 154, no. 16, pp. 44–6; no. 17, pp. 48–52.

Ford, R. (1986) History and organisation of the Seattle-area Hickman catheter committee, Journal of the Canadian Intravenous Nurses Association, Vol. 2, no. 2, pp. 4–13.

Goodman, M.S. and Wickham, R. (1984) Venous access devices: an overview, *Oncology Nurses Forum*, Vol. 11, no. 5, pp. 16–23.

Gyves, J. *et al.* (1982) Totally implanted system for intravenous chemotherapy in patients with cancer, *American Journal of Medicine*, Vol. 73, pp. 841–5.

Hollingsworth, S. (1987) Getting on line, *Nursing Times*, Vol. 83, no. 29, pp. 61–2.

Hurtibise, M.R. *et al.* (1980) Restoring patency of occluded central venous catheters, *Archives of Surgery*, Vol. 115, pp. 212–13.

Keohane, P.P. *et al.* (1983) Effects of catheter tunnelling and a nutrition nurse on catheter sepsis during parenteral nutrition, *Lancet*, Vol. ii, no. 17, pp. 1388–90.

Lawson, M. *et al.* (1979) Long term I.V. therapy: a new approach, *American Journal of Nursing*, Vol. 79, no. 6, pp. 1100–3.

Lawson, M. *et al.* (1982) The use of urokinase to restore the patency of occluded central venous catheters, *American Journal of I.V. Therapy and Clinical Nutrition*, Vol. 9, no. 9, pp. 29–32.

Mann, R.L. *et al.* (1981) Comparison of electronic and manometric central venous pressure: influence of access routes, *Critical Care Medicine*, Vol. 2, pp. 98–100.

Mehtar, S. and Taylor, P. (1982) Bacteriological survey of patients undergoing TPN and an I.V. policy's effects, *British Journal of Intravenous Therapy*, Vol. 3, no. 8, pp. 3–11.

Ostrow, L.S. (1981) Air embolism and central venous lines, *American Journal of Nursing*, Vol. 81, no. 11, pp. 2036–9.

Sellu, D. (1985) Long-term intravenous therapy, *Nursing Times*, Vol. 81, no. 21, pp. 40–2.

Strong, A. (1983) Monitoring central venous pressure, *Nursing 83*, Vol. 10, pp, 8–10.

Wood, S. (1982) Parenteral nutrition, *Nursing*, Vol. 2, no. 4, pp. 105–7.

GUIDELINES: READING CENTRAL VENOUS PRESSURE

Equipment for the electronic measurement of central venous pressure is now available and should be used whenever possible as readings have been shown to reflect more accurately the physiological condition of the patient. This is in part due to the elimination of nursing error related to the location of the external reference point, construction of equipment or incorrect sighting of the scale, for example.

In the absence of an infusion pump with this facility the procedure outlined below should be carefully followed.

Equipment
1   Spirit level
2   Manometer
3   Central venous pressure monitoring intravenous administration set.

Procedure

Action	**Rationale**
1 Explain the procedure to the patient.	To obtain the patient's consent and co-operation.
2 Ascertain the point of CVP reading, i.e. sternal angle or mid-axilla. If the patient agrees, this point should be marked on the patient and noted in the care plan chart for future reference.	CVP must always be read from the same point because the sternal angle reading is about 5 cm water higher than the mid-axilla reading.
3 Assist the patient to get into a recumbent or semirecumbent position to a maximum angle of 45°.	The position of the patient must allow the baseline of the manometer to be level with the patient's right atrium. If the patient is upright or is lying on his/her side, the right atrium will not be in line with the sternal angle or the mid-axilla.
4 Position the manometer so that the baseline is level with the right atrium.	To obtain an accurate CVP reading the baseline and the right atrium must be level.
5 Loosen the securing screw and slide the scale up or down until the baseline figure lies next to the arm of the spirit level (Figure 8.6a) This figure may be 0 but is usually taken as +10 if the CVP reading is more than 2 cm below zero (Figure 8.6b).	Most scales do not extend below 2 cm, therefore the height of the scale must be altered to obtain a reading.

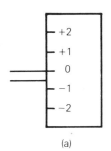

(a)

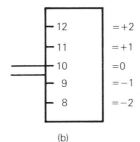

(b)

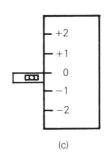

(c)

Figure 8.6   *a,b,* Setting the baseline, *c,* Checking the baseline.

Action

Rationale

6 Check that the baseline and right atrium are level by extending the arm of the spirit level to the sternal angle or to the mid-axilla. Move the manometer until the bubble is between the parallel lines of the spirit level (Figure 8.6c).

To ensure the patency of the line and to check for leaks, kinks, blockages, etc.

7 Flush the line well by allowing the intravenous fluid to run through into the patient.

To allow the intravenous fluid to run into the manometer.
To avoid:
  Bubbles, which cause inaccurate readings.
  Overfilling of, and spillage from, the manometer that would put the patient at risk from infection.

8 Turn off the three-way tap to the patient. Allow the manometer to fill slowly (Figure 8.7).

9 Turn off the three-way tap to the intravenous fluid (Figure 8.8).

To allow fluid from the manometer to enter the patient's right atrium.

10 When the level of fluid in the manometer ceases to drop, and rises and falls with the patient's respirations, this is the CVP reading.

The pressure of the column of water in the manometer now equals the pressure in the right atrium.

11 Turn off the three-way tap to the manometer (Figure 8.9).

To restore the intravenous line.

12 Readjust the infusion rate.

13 Record the CVP measurement on the appropriate chart. Compare this measurement with the patient's acceptable CVP limits as stated by the doctor or anaesthetist.

Acceptable CVP values vary with the patient and his/her overall condition. Deviations from these limits may require urgent medical intervention.

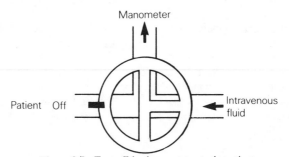

Figure 8.7   Turn off the three-way tap to the patient.

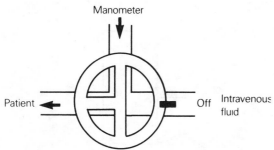

Figure 8.8   Turn off the three-way tap to intravenous fluid.

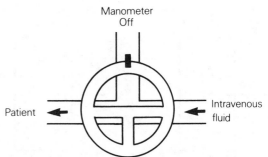

Figure 8.9   Turn off the three-way tap to manometer.

GUIDELINES: CHANGING THE DRESSING ON A CENTRAL VENOUS CATHETER INSERTION SITE

Before commencing the procedure it is important to check whether there is a variation to standard technique for individual patients, e.g. those receiving TPN, children, etc.

Equipment

1 Sterile dressing pack
2 Clamp for the catheter, if necessary
3 Alcohol-based hand scrub, e.g. Hibisol
4 Alcohol-based skin cleansing preparation, e.g. chlorhexidine 0.5% in 70% spirit
5 Topical skin disinfectant, e.g. povidone-iodine dry spray
6 Topical spray dressing, e.g. Opsite spray
7 Intravenous administration set and extension set primed with infusion fluid, if prescribed
   or
   Intermittent injection cap
8 Sterile padded dressing, e.g. Steripad
9 Hypo-allergenic tape
10 Bacteriological swab
11 Sterile gloves

Procedure

Action	Rationale
1 Explain the procedure to the patient.	To obtain the patient's consent and co-operation.
2 Perform the dressing using an aseptic technique.	To prevent infection. (For further information on asepsis, see the procedure on aseptic technique, pp. 5–8.)
3 Screen the bed. Assist the patient into supine position, if possible.	To allow dust and airborne organisms to settle before the wound and the sterile field are exposed. To help prevent embolus.
4 Wash hands with an appropriate solution, such as soap and water or Hibiscrub. Place all equipment required for the dressing on the bottom shelf of a clean dressing trolley.	
5 Prime the giving set, keeping the Luer lock sterile.	So that the infusion is ready for use when the current giving set is discontinued.
6 Take the trolley to the patient's bedside, disturbing the screens as little as possible.	To minimize airborne contamination.
7 Open the outer cover of the sterile dressing pack and slide the contents onto the top shelf of the trolley.	
8 Open the sterile field using the corners of the paper only. Using the forceps in the pack, arrange the sterile field with the handles of the instruments in one corner.	So that areas of potential contamination are kept to a minimum.

Action	**Rationale**
9 Attach a plastic disposal bag to the side of the trolley below the level of the top shelf.	So that contaminated material is below the level of the sterile field.
10 Open the other sterile packs, tipping their contents gently onto the centre of the sterile field. Pour lotions into gallipots or an indented plastic tray.	
11 Clean hands with an alcohol-based hand wash solution, such as Hibisol.	Hands may have become contaminated by handling the outer packs, etc.
12 Loosen the old dressing gently, touching only the tape, etc securing it.	So that the dressing can be lifted off easily with the forceps.
13 Using forceps, remove the old dressing and discard it together with the forceps into the plastic bag.	
14 If the site is red or discharging, take a swab for bacteriological investigation. *Note:* Routine samples should be taken weekly for all patients, including those having TPN, and twice weekly for susceptible patients.	For identification of pathogens. To predict colonization of the site.
15 Clean hands with an alcohol-based hand wash solution, such as Hibisol. Put on sterile gloves.	To minimize the risk of introducing infection.
16 Clean the wound as necessary, working from the inside to the outside of the area and dealing with the cleanest parts of the wound first.	To minimize the risk of infection spread from a 'dirty' to a 'clean' area.
17 Spray the site with a skin disinfectant solution, i.e. povidone-iodine.	
18 Apply a thin adhesive polyurethane film, such as Opsite spray.	To provide an airtight seal over the insertion site and to prevent the entry of bacteria.
19 Discontinue the infusion in progress. Clamp the catheter using a smooth clamp if the catheter is of silicone, or artery forceps over sterile topical swabs if it is of plastic, or move catheter 'on/off' switch to 'off'.	To prevent entry of air or leakage of blood when the catheter is disconnected. Swabs prevent cracking of a plastic catheter by artery forceps.
20 Clean gloved hands with an alcohol-based hand wash solution, such as Hibisol.	To minimize the risk of introducing infection into the catheter after handling unsterile parts of the system.
21 Ask the patient to perform the Valsalva manoeuvre. Disconnect the catheter from the old giving set and extension set and connect the prepared new set. Check that no air bubbles are present in the system. Unclamp the catheter and continue infusion.	To reduce the risk of air embolism.
22 Apply a sterile padded dressing, moulding it into place so that there are no folds or creases.	

23	Tape the extension set into a position comfortable for the patient, and attend to his/her general comfort.	To ensure the patient's comfort and to minimize the risk of accidental dislodging of the catheter.
24	Ensure that the drip rate is satisfactory.	
25	Alternatively, attach a Luer lock intermittent injection cap and heparinize the catheter, and extension set, if continuous infusion is not required (see p. 84).	To maintain a patent catheter for intermittent use.
26	Fold up the sterile field, place it in the plastic disposal bag and seal the bag before moving the trolley. Draw back the curtains. Dispose of waste in appropriate containers.	To prevent environmental contamination.

GUIDELINES: HEPARINIZATION OF A CENTRAL VENOUS CATHETER

This is a simple procedure which may be performed after each use or twice weekly when no therapy is necessary.

Equipment
1 Heparinized saline 50 i.u. 5 ml ready prepared in a syringe, with 25G (orange) needle attached, in clinically clean container
2 Isopropyl alcohol 70% swabs.

Procedure

Action	Rationale
1 Explain the procedure to the patient.	To gain the patient's consent and co-operation.
2 Wash hands thoroughly or use an alcohol-based hand scrub.	To avoid microbiological contamination.
3 Swab the injection cap with 70% alcohol and allow to dry.	To avoid microbiological contamination.
4 Insert the needle, unclamp the catheter and inject contents of the syringe.	To flush the line thoroughly.
5 Clamp the catheter while injecting the final 0.5 ml of solution.	To maintain positive pressure and prevent backflow of blood into the catheter, and possible clot formation.
6 Remove needle from cap and dispose of equipment safely.	To prevent injury.
7 Follow procedure meticulously.	To ensure the patient is aware of each step, and the need for good hand washing/drying techniques, etc. as he/she may be performing this procedure on discharge.

GUIDELINES: TAKING BLOOD SAMPLES FROM A CENTRAL VENOUS CATHETER

Equipment

1 Sterile dressing pack
2 Clamp for catheter, if necessary
3 Sterile gloves
4 Alcohol-based hand wash solution
5 Sterile 10-ml syringe or extra 10-ml blood bottle without heparin.
6 Sterile syringe of appropriate size for sample required
   or
   Vacuum system container holder (shell)
   Vacuum system adaptor
   Appropriate vacuumed blood bottles
7 Intermittent injection cap, if necessary
8 Heparinized saline, as per policy for flushing.

Procedure

Action	Rationale
1 Explain the procedure to the patient.	To obtain the patient's consent and co-operation.
2 Perform procedure using an aseptic technique.	To prevent infection. (For further information on asepsis see pp. 5–8.)
3 Wash hands with an appropriate solution, such as soap and water or Hibiscrub.	
4 Prepare a tray or trolley and take it to the bedside. Cleanse hands as above. Open sterile pack and prepare equipment.	
5 If intravenous fluid infusion is in progress, discontinue it.	
6 Clamp the catheter with a smooth clamp if the catheter is of silicone or with artery forceps over sterile topical swabs if is of plastic, or move catheter 'on/off' switch to 'off'.	To prevent entry of air or leakage of blood via the catheter. Swabs prevent the artery forceps from cracking a plastic catheter.
7 Clean hands with an alcohol-based hand wash solution, such as Hibisol. Put on sterile gloves.	To minimize the risk of introducing infection into the catheter.
8 Disconnect the giving set from the catheter and cover the end of the set with the syringe cover or remove the injection cap and discard.	To reduce the risk of contaminating the end of the giving set.
9 For syringe sampling:	
(a) Attach a 10-ml syringe to the catheter. Release the clamp and withdraw 5–10 ml of blood.	
(b) Reclamp the catheter and discard the sample and syringe.	To remove blood, heparin and intravenous fluids from the 'dead space' of the catheter. Samples from this 'dead space' are likely to cause inaccuracies in blood tests.
(c) Attach a new syringe of appropriate size. Release the clamp and withdraw the required amount of blood.	To obtain the sample. To prevent blood loss or air embolism.

(d) Reclamp the catheter and detach the syringe.

10 For vacuum sampling:
   (a) Attach vacuum container holder and release clamp. Withdraw 10 ml of blood into spare sample bottle.
   (b) Attach sample bottles for required specimens.
   (c) Reclamp catheter and detach vacuum container holder.

To remove blood, heparin and intravenous fluids from the 'dead space' of the catheter. Samples from this 'dead space' are likely to cause inaccuracies in blood tests.
To obtain sample. It is not necessary to clamp the catheter when changing collection bottles, as the system is not broken.

11 Reconnect the giving set, unclamp the catheter and recommence infusion *or* attach new intermittent injection cap, release clamp and heparinize catheter.

To continue therapy.
To prevent the catheter clotting in between uses.

12 Ensure that blood samples have been placed in the correct containers and agitated as necessary to prevent clotting. Label them with patient's name, number, etc. and send to the laboratory with the appropriate forms.

To make certain that the specimens, correctly presented and identified, are delivered to the laboratory, enabling the requested tests to be performed and the results returned to the correct patient's records.

Difficulty may be encountered when taking blood samples. This is particularly true when the central catheter is made of silicone and has been in place for a period of time. The main cause is that the tip of the soft catheter lays against the wall of the vessel and the suction required to draw blood brings this into close contact so leading to temporary occlusion.

Measures to try to dislodge the tip include asking the patient to:
1 cough and breathe deeply;
2 roll from side to side;
3 raise his/her arms;
4 perform the Valsalva manoeuvre, if possible;
5 increase general activity, e.g. walk up and down stairs.

If these are unsuccessful, irrigation of the catheter with normal saline or a dilute solution of heparin may be helpful. However, it may be necessary to take blood from a peripheral vein (see pp. 405–11).

GUIDELINES: REMOVAL OF A NON-SKIN TUNNELLED CENTRAL CATHETER

Equipment
As for a change of dressing for a central venous catheter insertion site (nos. 1–11, p. 89) plus:
12 Sterile scissors
13 Small sterile specimen container
14 Stitch cutter
15 Additional sterile gauze swab.
(A new administration set, etc. is not required.)

Procedure
Proceed as for a dressing procedure, steps 1–15 (pp. 89–90) then continue as follows:

Action

Rationale

16 Clean the insertion site.

To prevent contamination of the catheter on removal, and a false-positive culture result.

Action	Rationale
17 Spray the site with a skin disinfectant, i.e. povidone-iodine.	
18 Discontinue the infusion, if in progress. Clamp the catheter as previously described or move the catheter 'on/off' switch to 'off'.	To prevent entry of air or leakage of blood when the catheter is disconnected.
19 Clean gloved hands with an alcohol-based hand wash solution.	To minimize the risk of infection after handling unsterile parts of the system.
20 Cut and remove any skin sutures securing the catheter.	To facilitate removal.
21 Disconnect the catheter from the remainder of the infusion system.	To ease handling and removal.
22 Ask the patient to perform the Valsalva manoeuvre.	To reduce the risk of air embolus.
23 Cover the insertion site with a thick pad of several sterile topical swabs.	Swabs are used to discourage the entry of organisms into the insertion site and to absorb any leakage of blood.
24 Hold the catheter with one hand near the point of insertion and pull firmly and gently. As the catheter begins to move, press firmly down on the site with the swabs. Maintain pressure on the swabs for about 5 minutes after the catheter has been removed.	Pressure is applied to prevent haemorrhage and to encourage resealing of the vein wall. It also prevents the entry of air into the vein. Continued pressure is necessary to allow time for the puncture in the vein to close.
25 When bleeding has stopped (approximately 5 minutes), spray the insertion site with topical plastic spray dressing, e.g. Opsite, and cover with padded dressing.	To provide an airtight seal over the site and prevent the entry of bacteria.
26 Carefully cut off the tip (approx. 5 cm) of the catheter using sterile scissors and place it in a sterile container for microbiological investigation.	To detect any infection related to the catheter, and thus provide necessary treatment.
27 Fold up the sterile field, place it in the plastic disposal bag and seal the bag before moving the trolley. Dispose of the equipment in the appropriate containers.	To prevent environmental contamination.
28 Make the patient comfortable.	

This procedure may be adapted for removal of a skin-tunnelled line.

NURSING CARE PLAN

Problem	Cause	Suggested action
Dyspnoea, chest pain or cyanosis (may be slow in onset).	Hydrothorax, pneumothorax or haemothorax due to insertion technique.	Inform a doctor. Arrange for a chest X-ray. Assist with chest drainage, if necessary.

Change in pulse rate and rhythm after insertion of catheter.	Cardiac irritability or cardiac rupture due to insertion technique.	Inform a doctor.
Dyspnoea, chest pain, tachypnoea, disorientation, cyanosis, raised CVP, coma, cardiac arrest.	Air embolism due to air entering circulation during the insertion procedure or via the catheter.	Observe the patient closely. If signs/symptoms develop, clamp the catheter to prevent further air entry. Lay the patient on his/her left side in Trendelenburg position. Inform a doctor. Give oxygen or external cardiac compression.
Tingling in fingers, shooting pain down arm, paralysis.	Injury to brachial plexus during insertion.	Inform a doctor. Treatment is symptomatic. Physiotherapy may be necessary.
Oedema of the arm on the side of the catheter insertion, may be associated with pain or limb discolouration.	Thoracic duct injury at insertion, resulting in alterations in lymph flow. Thrombosis in major vessel due to irritation by foreign body (catheter).	Inform a doctor. Removal is usually necessary. Inform a doctor. Removal is usually necessary.
Pyrexia, tachycardia, rigors indicating systemic infection.	Poor aseptic technique. Careless use and handling of equipment, e.g. stopcocks, over-flooding of manometer.	Culture of the patient's blood is required. Take a swab of the infusion site, employing strict asepsis and minimum handling of the equipment. Administer antimicrobials as prescribed. Observe the patient closely.
Unable to draw back blood.	Catheter tip occluded by the vein wall.	Position the patient on his/her side where the catheter is inserted, and ask him/her to perform the Valsalva manoeuvre.
	Catheter blocked by blood clots due to i. Infusion being too slow or switched off ii. Heparinization not having been carried out previously.	Inject 1000 i.u./ml heparin (1 ml) and 1 ml normal saline into the catheter. Clamp and leave for 15 minutes. Attempt to aspirate with a 5- or 10-ml syringe to remove the clots. Irrigate with 5 ml heparinized saline. Repeat if necessary.
Leakage of fluid onto the dressing.	Loose connection in the system. Cracking of catheter or hub.	Check and tighten connections. Report to the intravenous nursing staff and/or medical staff.
Catheter required for many functions, e.g. blood sampling and extra drug administration.	Limited routes of access available to satisfy the patient's requirements.	Simple regimens and methods of administration. Use adaptors and administration sets available for this purpose. Consider multi-lumen catheter prior to insertion.
Fluid overload resulting in dyspnoea, oedema, raised pulse rate and blood pressure.	Infusion is too fast. Inaccurate fluid monitoring.	Use flow control devices. Keep accurate records of the patient's fluid balance and weight. Revise the patient's fluid intake regimen. Inform a doctor.

Problem	Cause	Suggested action
Inaccurate CVP readings.	Patient in a position different from that in which the initial reading was taken. Reference point on the patient not observed.	Position should be documented in the patient's records. Zero of the manometer must be level with the patient's right atrium at the point marked on the patient, i.e. mid-axilla or sternal angle.
	Faulty pressure reading technique.	If the CVP reading is outside the limits deemed acceptable for that patient and it is considered to be an accurate reading, recheck it after 15 or 30 minutes and inform a doctor if unchanged.
Elevated CVP.	Increased intrathoracic pressure caused by coughing, increased movement or pain. Lower extremities elevated.	Encourage coughing before taking the reading. Ensure that the patient is comfortable and pain free. Position the patient so that he/she is lying in a supine position. Give sedation as necessary to enable him/her to maintain this position.
	Patient having intermittent positive-pressure ventilation.	Read the CVP at the end expiratory level (lowest point of fluctuation). This will always be higher than the 'normal' reading.
	Anxiety and/or restlessness.	Verify the cause of the anxiety/restlessness.
	Blood in progress via the CVP line.	Flush the line well with normal saline and read again.
	Shivering and/or muscular spasm, e.g. post-anaesthetic reaction.	Assess the patient's general condition, e.g. pulse, blood pressure, temperature. Check that the patient is warm enough. Inform a doctor.
Low CVP reading.	Leak in the system or equipment adjusted inaccurately.	Check and readjust the system.
	Changing of the patient's position from recumbent to semirecumbent.	Reread with the patient in the original position.
Potential pulmonary embolus due to catheter tip embolus. Symptoms include chest pain, cool clammy skin, haemoptysis, tachycardia, hypotension.	Occasionally occurs after the removal of the catheter, especially the skin-tunnelled type.	All skin-tunnelled catheters must be removed by medical staff. Notify a doctor immediately if the patient develops any of the related symptoms.
Bleeding at the insertion site following removal of the catheter.	Opening in the vein wall.	Apply pressure over the site with sterile topical swabs. Cover the site with topical plastic spray and an occlusive dressing when the bleeding has stopped. Patients prescribed warfarin or heparin will require a longer period of pressure to compensate for the prolonged clotting time.

In addition, the care plan associated with intravenous management (p. 144) may contain useful and relevant information.

9

Cytotoxic Drugs: Handling and Administration

REFERENCE MATERIAL

In recent years there has been increasing concern about the occupational hazards associated with the handling of cancer chemotherapeutic agents. On the basis of the evidence available at the present time, risks to personnel involved in the reconstitution and administration of cytotoxic drugs fall into two categories:

1. The proven local effects caused by direct contact with the skin, eyes and mucous membranes. These include:
   (a) dermatitis;
   (b) inflammation of mucous membranes;
   (c) excessive lacrimation;
   (d) pigmentation;
   (e) blistering, associated with mustine;
   (f) other, miscellaneous, allergic reactions.

   These hazards have been recognized for a number of years, and protection using goggles and latex/PVC gloves is advised. The thickness of the gloves has been shown to be the most important consideration.

2. The potentially harmful short- or long-term systemic effects due to inhalation or ingestion of cytotoxic drugs during preparation. Many of these drugs have been shown to be mutagenic, and several are suspected of being teratogenic and/or carcinogenic when given at the therapeutic levels to animals and humans. With the majority of compounds there is little or no absorption through intact skin, the exceptions being those which are lipid soluble. Systemic complaints from handlers include:
   (a) lightheadedness;
   (b) dizziness;
   (c) nausea;
   (d) headache;
   (e) alopecia;
   (f) coughing;
   (g) pruritus;
   (h) general malaise.

   The working conditions in which these complaints were experienced were not desirable, i.e. a small unventilated medicine closet. No formal collection of data was performed and the author readily admits to gathering information on an anecdotal basis.

In a number of studies the urine of cytotoxic drug handlers, including nurses, has been collected and screened for mutagenic activity using an accepted test (Ames *et al.*, 1975). Although alterations in cell structure have been detected in many of the published works, they appear to be transient and of a low level. It has yet to be demonstrated whether these changes in cell structure are harmful and if this level of mutagenesis can be equated with more serious consequences. Inconclusive or contradictory data, together with doubts about the validity of this test, mean that hazards have yet to be quantified.

In summary, localized toxicity due to accidental contact with cytotoxic drugs is well documented and it is, therefore, only sensible to take precautions to minimize the risks. While long-term hazards remain largely undefined, the suggestion that some compounds may carry the insidious risk of teratogenicity or carcinogenicity is sufficiently strong that the only responsible course of action is that which minimizes exposure. This is best achieved through locally agreed policies based on the available national guidelines. In hospitals where cytotoxics are used frequently the most satisfactory procedure is for all doses to be prepared in the pharmacy department by trained staff working in a specially equipped area.

Whatever the situation, written guidelines should be available to cover:

1. preparation of compounds – environment, staff training, staff protection, techniques, equipment;
2. administration of drugs – staff training, staff protection, technique, equipment;
3. disposal – of drugs, equipment, waste and excreta;
4. accidents – spillage and contamination of nurse, doctor or patient;

5   a system for monitoring and recording any effects on hospital staff.

Note: Qualified nursing staff are increasingly given responsibility for the administration of intravenous medications, including cytotoxic drugs. For further information regarding these procedures see pp. 179–204.

References and further reading

Ames, B.N. *et al.* (1975) Methods for detecting carcinogens and mutagens with the salmonella/mammalian microsome mutagenicity tese, *Mutation Research*, Vol. 31, pp. 347–64.

Anderson, M. *et al.* (1983) Development and operation of a pharmacy-based intravenous cytotoxic reconstitution service, *British Medical Journal*, Vol. 286, pp. 32–6.

Anderson, R. *et al.* (1982) Risk of handling injectable antineoplastic agents, *American Journal of Hospital Pharmacy*, Vol. 39, pp. 1881–7.

Bauman, B. and Duvall, E. (1980) An unusual accident during the administration of chemotherapy, *Cancer Nursing*, Vol. 3, no. 4, pp. 305–6.

Calvert, A.H. (1981) The long term sequelae of cytotoxic therapy, *Cancer Topics*, Vol. 3, no. 7, pp. 77–9.

Colls, B.M. (1985) Safety of handling cytotoxic agents: a cause for concern by pharmaceutical companies, *British Medical Journal*, Vol. 291, pp. 318–19.

Cooke, J. *et al.* (1987) Environmental monitoring of personnel who handle cytotoxic drugs, *Pharmaceutical Journal*, Vol. 239, 6452 suppl. R2.

Crudi, C.B. (1980) A compounding dilemma: I've kept the drug sterile but have I contaminated myself? *National Intravenous Therapy Assocation*, Vol. 3.

Darbyshire, P. (1986) Handle with care, *Nursing Times*, Vol. 82, no. 40, pp. 37–8.

Department of Health and Social Security (1985) *Guidelines for the Safe Handling of Cytotoxic Drugs*, DHSS, London.

Earnshaw, M. *et al.* (1983) Introduction of a cytotoxic reconstitution service, *Hospital Pharmacy and the Patient*, MTP Lancaster.

Falck, K. *et al.* (1979) Mutagenicity in urine of nurses handling cytotoxic agents, *Lancet*, Vol. i, p. 1250.

Harris, J. and Dodds, L. (1985) Handling waste from patients receiving cytotoxic drugs, *Pharmaceutical Journal*, Vol. 235, no. 6345, pp. 289–91.

Health and Safety Executive (1983) *Precautions for the Safe Handling of Cytotoxic Drugs*, Medical Series HMSO 123, HMSO, London.

Knowles, R.S. and Virden, J.E. (1980) Handling of injectable antineoplastic agents, *British Medical Journal*, Vol. 2, pp. 589–91.

Laidlaw, J.L. *et al.* (1984) Permeability of latex and polyvinyl chloride gloves to 20 antineoplastic drugs, *American Journal of Hospital Pharmacy*, Vol. 41, pp. 2018–23.

New England Journal of Medicine, Correspondence related to Selevan, S.G. (1986) *New England Journal of Medicine*, Vol. 16, pp. 1048–51.

Nguyen, T.V. *et al.* (1982) Exposure of pharmacy personnel to mutagenic antineoplastic drugs, *Cancer Research*, Vol. 42, pp. 4792–6.

Oakley, P. and Reeves, E. (1984) Setting up a reconstitution service, Pharmaceutical Journal, Vol. 232, no. 6282, pp. 739–40.

Oncology Nursing Society (1984) *Cancer Chemotherapy Guidelines and Recommendations for Nursing Education and Practice*, Oncology, Nursing Society, Pittsburgh, USA.

Richardson, M.L. and Bowron, J.M. (1985) The fate of pharmaceutical chemicals in the aquatic environment, *Journal of Pharmaceutical Pharmacology*, Vol. 37, pp. 1–12.

Royal College of Nursing of the United Kingdom (1982) *Cytotoxic Drugs and Their Handling*, RCN, London.

Selevan, S.G. *et al.* (1985) A study of occupational exposure to antineoplastic drugs and fetal loss in nurses, *New England Journal of Medicine*, Vol. 19, pp. 1173–8.

Speechley, V. (1982) Better safe than sorry, *Nursing Mirror*, Vol. 154, no. 15, p. 11.

Stevin, M.L. *et al.* (1984) The efficiency of protective gloves used in the handling of cytotoxic drugs, *Cancer Chemotherapy* Pharmacol. Vol. 12, pp. 151–3.

Stoikes, M. *et al.* (1987) Permeability of latex and polyvinyl chloride gloves to fluorouracil and methotrexate, *American Journal of Hospital Pharmacy*, Vol. 44, pp. 1341–6.

Stuart, M. (1981) Sequence of administering vesicant cytotoxic drugs Part A, *Oncology Nursing Forum*, Vol. 9, no. 1, pp. 53–4.

Vennit, S. *et al.* (1983) Monitoring exposure of nursing and pharmacy personnel to cytotoxic drugs: urinary mutation assays and urinary platinum as markers of absorption, *Lancet*, Vol. i, pp. 74–6.

Working Party of the Pharmaceutical Society of Great Britain on the Handling of Cytotoxic Drugs (1983) Guidelines for the handling of cytotoxic drugs, *Pharmaceutical Journal*, Vol. 230, no. 6215, pp. 230–1.

GUIDELINES: PROTECTION OF THE ENVIRONMENT

MANAGEMENT OF SPILLAGE

Action	Rationale
1 Act immediately.	Any spillage may become a health hazard.
2 Collect spillage kit.	It contains all necessary equipment.
3 Put on latex/PVC gloves and disposable plastic apron/tabard.	To provide personal protection.
4 If there is visible powder spill, put on a good-quality surgical face mask.	To prevent inhalation of powder.
5 If spillage is on a hard floor, put on overshoes.	For protection and to minimize the spread of contamination.
6 Wipe up powder spillage quickly with well-dampened paper towels and dispose of them as 'high-risk' waste.	To prevent dispersal of powder. To protect others and ensure safe disposal by incineration.
7 Mop up liquids which have been spilled on a hard surface with paper towels and dispose of them as 'high-risk' waste.	To protect others and ensure safe disposal by incineration.
8 Wash hard surfaces well with copious amounts of cold soapy water and dry with paper towels.	To remove residual contamination.
9 If spillage is on clothing, remove it as soon as possible and treat as 'soiled linen'.	To decontaminate clothing without hazard to laundry staff.
10 If spillage has penetrated clothing, wash contaminated skin liberally with soap and cold water.	To decontaminate skin and prevent drug absorption.
11 If spillage is on bedlinen, change it immediately and treat as 'soiled linen'.	To protect the patient. To protect the laundry staff.
12 *Any* accident or spillage involving direct skin contact with a cytotoxic drug *must* be reported to the occupational health department (see following guideline, protection of nursing staff when handling cytotoxic drugs).	To ensure that details of accidental contact are entered in the nurse's health record, and appropriate follow-up initiated.

DISPOSAL OF WASTE

Action	Rationale
1 'Sharps' should be placed in the special container provided.	To ensure incineration and to prevent laceration and/or inoculation during transit and disposal.
2 Dry waste, intravenous administration sets and other contaminated material should be placed in 'high-risk' waste disposal bags.	To ensure careful handling and disposal by incineration.

Action	Rationale
3 Excess drug solutions should be flushed into the drainage system using copious amounts of cold water.	To ensure adequate dilution of any cytotoxic drugs.
4 Re-usable trays and other equipment should be washed with copious amounts of water followed by the usual procedure for disinfection.	To prevent cross-contamination and cross-infection.
5 Unused doses of cytotoxics should be returned, unopened, to the pharmacy.	To enable them to be relabelled and reissued, stability permitting, or to be safely destroyed.
6 Any unwanted doses in containers which have been opened should be carefully flushed into the drainage system using copious amounts of cold water.	To avoid the risks of transporting an unsealed dose container to the pharmacy.

DISPOSAL OF EXCRETA FROM PATIENTS RECEIVING CYTOTOXIC DRUGS

Few cytotoxic agents are excreted as unchanged drug or active metabolites in urine or faeces. Normal procedures and standards of personal hygiene, properly applied, should ensure that there is no direct contact with patients' excreta. The wearing of gloves is desirable for the handling of linen from patients who are incontinent during and immediately following a course of chemotherapy. These simple measures should ensure that risks to nursing staff in these circumstances are minimized.

GUIDELINES: PROTECTION OF NURSING STAFF WHEN HANDLING CYTOTOXIC DRUGS

Nursing staff should not be involved in routine reconstitution of cytotoxic drugs, as this is the function of the pharmacy unit. However, there may be emergency situations when the nurse is requested to prepare chemotherapy and it is essential that this is performed safely. The following procedure should be used for guidance.

Action	Rationale
1 Reconstitution of cytotoxic drugs should take place in a well-ventilated room. Doors and windows should be closed to prevent draughts.	To prevent any unnecessary airborne exposure from possible powder or droplet aerosols released.
2 While reconstitution is in progress no other activities should be carried out within the area. Movement in and out of the area should be restricted.	As above.
3 The area should contain a sink and running water.	To clean surfaces and/or skin if spillage or contamination occurs.
4 The work surface should be smooth and impermeable.	To enable cleaning of surfaces to be undertaken easily and quickly.

5 Reconstitution should take place in plastic tray or equivalent.

To enable containment of spillage and ease of cleaning.

6 Nursing staff should receive instruction in the techniques of reconstitution and the reasons for these recommendations.

To ensure staff are safe to practise and are aware of the risks involved.

7 Direct contact with the drug solution can be entirely avoided by good technique and the use of thick latex/PVC gloves.

Latex is impermeable to most cytotoxic drugs and is therefore most suitable for this purpose. PVC offers most protection to mustard-type drugs (mustine, dacarbazine) and should be used when handling these agents.

8 All cuts and scratches should be covered.

To prevent infiltration of the skin if damage to gloves occurs.

9 Use protective goggles or glasses.

To prevent contact between drugs and the eyes. If the nurse wears glasses these should provide approximately 90% protection.

10 Wash after use.

To prevent cross-contamination and/or cross-infection.

11 Use a good-quality surgical face mask when reconstituting dry powder, especially if presented in an ampoule, e.g. bleomycin.

To prevent inhalation of any powder released during reconstitution.

12 Put on a disposable plastic apron or tabard.

To provide a barrier between the drug and the handler.

13 Ampoules should be held away from the face and covered with a sterile topical swab when breaking them.

To prevent contamination of the gloves and skin. To prevent formation of aerosols or liberation of powder.

14 Luer-locking syringes should be used.

To reduce the incidence of accidental disconnection and spillage of drug.

15 The use of a second needle as an air inlet is recommended. (Filter or air-venting needles may be provided.)
The alternative 'no airway' technique involves a 'push-pull' use of the syringe to add cyclically small quantities of diluent to, and remove air from, the closed vial. This technique is not recommended (see the section on preparation of injections, pp. 134–9).

To prevent the development of pressure differentials between syringe and vial.

In inexperienced hands, the 'no airway' technique results in the danger of contamination. In extreme circumstances the vial and closure may separate, the syringe/needle junction may leak (especially if Luer slip syringes are used), or the vial may explode.

16 The diluent should be slowly introduced down the wall of the vial or ampoule.

To ensure that the powder is thoroughly wet before agitation, and is not released into the atmosphere.

17 Needles should be capped before the explusion of air or the tip should be covered with a sterile swab or the air should be expelled into the vial or ampoule.

To prevent aerosol formation.

18 Gloves, eye protection and apron/tabard should continue to be worn during administration as the nurse is still handling the drugs and may become contaminated. Gloves and aprons should be washed.

To prevent contamination at a later stage in the procedure.

Action	Rationale
19 Contamination of the skin, mucous membranes and eyes should be treated promptly. All areas should be washed with copious amounts of tap water or normal saline. Eye wash may be available.	To prevent any local damage to tissue.
20 Accidental infiltration of the skin with a vesicant drug should be treated as an extravasation and the appropriate procedure followed (see pp. 104–6).	To prevent any local damage to tissue.
21 If erythema and/or other local reaction occurs in any circumstances, contact the occupational health unit or a member of the medical staff so that appropriate treatment may be advised.	To prevent further damage and/or complications.
22 It is *essential* after any accident involving direct contact with a cytotoxic drug, or if any local or systemic symptoms occur after handling such a drug, that the occupational health unit is informed immediately.	To assist with recording and monitoring of staff exposure.
23 If pregnancy is suspected or intended, the occupational health unit should be contacted.	To discuss future work patterns and any anxiety that may be felt.

GUIDELINES: INTRAVENOUS ADMINISTRATION OF CYTOTOXIC DRUGS

The most frequently used route for administration of cytotoxic drugs is intravenously. This ensures rapid, reliable delivery of agents to the patient and the tumour site. In addition, many drugs have to be administered into a vein where rapid dilution by the blood can occur, as they are irritant to soft tissue and capable of causing necrosis. These drugs are called 'vesicant agents'. The aim of the procedure for administration of chemotherapy intravenously is to protect both nurse and patient from contamination and also to prevent extravasion of drugs which could result in local tissue damage.

The large majority of cytotoxic agents will be delivered to the ward/unit individually packaged for delivery to a named patient, by injection or infusion. If this is not so, the Guidelines for protection of nursing staff should be followed (pp. 100–2).

Action	Rationale
1 Put on gloves, eye protection and an apron or tabard before commencing the procedure.	To protect the nurse from local contamination of skin, eyes, or clothing. *Note:* With careful handling technique, this risk is minimal but sprays or splashes can occur when changing syringes/infusion containers.
2 Prepare necessary equipment for an aseptic administration procedure, and ensure that this is followed carefully. (For further information on intravenous management, see p. 179.)	To prevent local and/or systemic infection. Patients are frequently immunosuppressed and at greater risk.

3 Check that all details on the syringe or infusion container are correct when compared with the patient's prescription, prior to opening the sterile packaging.

To ensure the patient is given the correct drug which has been dispensed for him/her. To prevent wastage.

4 Explain the procedure to the patient.

To obtain the patient's consent and co-operation.

5 Inspect the infusion or injection site, and consult the patient about sensation around the device instertion site.

To detect any phenomena, e.g. phlebitis, which would render the vein unusable.

6 Establish the patency of the vein using normal saline.

To determine whether the vein will accommodate the extra fluid flow and irritant drugs and remain patent.

7 Ensure the correct administration rate.

To prevent speed shock. To prevent extra pressure and irritation within the veil.

8 Be aware of the immediate effects of the drug.

To know what to observe during administration. To be prepared to manage any side-effects which occur.

9 Administer drugs in the correct order, i.e. vesicants first.

To ensure that those agents likely to cause tissue damage are given when venous integrity is greatest, i.e. at the beginning. *Note:* Because of their irritant nature (approx. pH3–3.5) anti-emetics should be given half an hour prior to chemotherapy administration or at the end of the sequence.

10 Observe the vein throughout.

To detect any problems at the earliest moment.

11 Observe for signs of extravasation, e.g. swelling or leakage at the site of injection. Note the patient's comments about sensation at the site, e.g. pain.

To prevent any unnecessary damage to soft tissue, and to enable the remainder of the drug(s) to be given correctly at another site. To enable prompt treatment to be given, thus minimizing local damage, and possibly preserving venous access for future treatment. (For further information see the management of extravasation of vesicant drugs, pp. 104–6).

12 Flush the line between drugs and after administration.

To prevent drug interaction. To prevent leakage along the path of the cannula or from the puncture site.

13 Be aware of the patient's comfort throughout the procedure.

To minimize trauma to the patient. To involve the patient in treatment and detect any side-effects and/or problems that may then be avoided at the next treatment.

14 Record details of the administration in the appropriate documents.

To prevent any duplication of treatment to provide a point of reference in the event of queries.

15 Protect the patient from contact with the drugs by:
  (a) Placing a plastic sheet or small incontinece pad or equivalent under the sterile towel.

  To provide a waterproof barrier and protect the skin.

  (b) Inserting the needle carefully into the injection site of the giving set, extension set or cannula stopper.

  To prevent exiting on the other side and contaminating or inoculating the patient.

  (c) Careful removal of the blind hub and changing of needles/syringes plus care when insterting the administration set into the infusion container or changing bags.

  To avoid leakage or splashes and contamination of the nurse or patient.

Action	Rationale
(d) Securing a good bond between needle and syringe.	To prevent leakage or separation, which may occur due to pressure during administration, resulting in spray and contamination. To ensure that there is no leakage.
(e) Checking the injection site or stopper at the end of the procedure. (f) Acting promptly if any contamination is noted and washing the area with cold water or saline.	To prevent any local reaction on skin, mucous membranes, etc.

MANAGEMENT OF EXTRAVASATION OF VESICANT DRUGS

REFERENCE MATERIAL

The treatment of extravasations of chemotherapeutic agents is controversial. The procedure detailed here represents the policy of The Royal Marsden Hospital for the management by nursing staff of extravasion injury, drawn up with the assistance of pharmacy and medical colleagues.

Prior to administration of cytotoxic drugs the nurse should know which agents are capable of producing tissue necrosis. The following is a list of those in common use:

carmustine (concentrated solution)	mitomycin C
dacarbazine (concentrated solution)	mustine
dactinomycin	rubidazone
daunorubicin	vinblastine
doxorubicin	vincristine
epirubicin	vindesine.
mithramycin	

If in any doubt, the drug data sheet should be consulted or reference made to a trial protocol. Drugs should not be reconstituted to give solutions that are higher than the manufacturers' recommended concentration, and the method of administration checked, e.g. infusion, injection.

A variety of non-cytotoxic agents in frequent use are also capable of causing severe tissue damage if extravasated. They include:
vasoconstrictors e.g. adrenaline
antibiotics e.g. erythromycin
antivirals e.g. acyclovir
electrolytes e.g. sodium bicarbonate 8.4% injection.

This potential hazard should always be remembered. The actions listed in this procedure may not be appropriate in all these instances. Drug data sheets should always be checked and if the information is insufficient, the pharmacy departments should be consulted.

Extravasation should be suspected if:
1   the patient complains of burning, stinging pain or any other acute change at the injection site. This should be distinguished from a feeling of cold which may occur with some drugs;
2   induration, swelling or leakage at the injection site is observed. There may be redness or 'blistering' with doxorubicin and other red drugs – the 'nettle rash' effect. this is normal;
3   no blood return is obtained. (If found in isolation this should not be regarded as an indication of a non-patent vein.);
4   a resistance is felt on the plunger of the syringe if drugs are given by bolus;
5   there is absence of free flow when administration is by infusion.

Note: One or more of the above may be present. If extravasion is suspected or confirmed, action must be taken immediately.

References and further reading

Oncology Nursing Society (1984) *Cancer chemotherapy guidelines and recommendations for nursing education and practice,* Oncology Nursing Society, Pittsburgh, USA

Smith, R. (1985a) Extravasation of intravenous fluids, *British Journal of Parenteral Therapy*, Vol. 6, no. 2, pp. 30–5/42.

Smith, R. (1985b) Prevention and treatment of extravasation, *British Journal of Parenteral Therapy*, Vol. 6, no. 5, pp. 114–20.

GUIDELINES: MANAGEMENT OF EXTRAVASATION

Equipment

To assist the nurse, an extravasion kit should be assembled and should be readily available in each ward/unit. It contains:

1. Instant cold pack × 1
2. Dexamethasone injection 8 mg in 2 ml × 1
3. Hydrocortisone cream 1% 15-g tube × 1
4. 2-ml syringes × 2
5. 19G needles × 2 (for drawing up)
6. 25G needles × 4 (for injection)
7. Alcohol swabs
8. Documentation slips × 2
9. Copy of extravasation management procedure.

Procedure

Action	Rationale
1 Explain the procedure to the patient.	To obtain the patient's consent and co-operation.
2 Stop injection *immediately*, leaving the cannula or winged infusion device in place.	To minimize local injury. To allow aspiration of the drug to be attempted.
3 Aspirate any residual drug and blood from the device and suspected infiltration site.	To minimize local injury by removing as much drug as possible. Subsequent damage is related to the volume of the extravasation, in addition to other factors.
4 Remove the cannula or winged infusion device.	To prevent the site from being used as an intravenous route.
5 Apply cold pack or ice instantly.	To localize the area of extravasation, slow cell metabolism and decrease the area of tissue destruction. To reduce local pain.
6 Inform a member of the medical staff.	To enable actions differing from agreed policy to be taken if considered in the best interests of the patient. To notify the doctor of the need to prescribe drugs.
7 Draw up a dexamethasone injection 8 mg in 2 ml and inject 0.1–0.2 ml subcutaneously at the points of the compass around the circumference of the area of extravasation. Ensure the whole area is infiltrated.	To reduce local inflammation and improve the survival of tissues, especially those marginally injured.
8 Reapply a long-lasting cold pack or ice for 24 hours.	To localize the steroid effect in the area of extravasation. To reduce local pain and promote patient comfort.
9 Elevate the extremity and/or encourage movement.	To minimize swelling and to prevent adhesion of damaged area to underlying tissue, which could result in restriction of movement.
10 Apply hydrocortisone cream 1% twice daily, and instruct the patient how to do this. Continue as long as erythema persists.	To reduce local inflammation and promote patient comfort.

Action	**Rationale**
11 Provide analgesia as required.	To promote patient comfort. To encourage movement of the limb as advised.
12 Document the following details, in duplicate, on the form provided: (a) patient's name/number (b) ward/unit (c) date, time (d) needle size and type (e) venepuncture site (on diagram) (f) drug sequence (g) drug administration technique, i.e. 'bolus', infusion (h) approximate amount of the drug extravasated (i) diameter of erythematous area (j) appearance of the area (k) nursing management/action taken/medical officer notified (l) patient's complaints, comments, statements (m) signature of the nurse.	To provide an immediate full record of all details of the incident, which may be referred to if necessary. To provide a baseline for future observation and monitoring of its condition.
13 Explain to the patient that the site may remain sore for several days.	To reduce anxiety and ensure continued co-operation.
14 Observe the area regularly for erythema, induration, blistering or necrosis. Inpatients: monitor daily.	To detect any changes at the earliest possible moment.
15 Request outpatients to observe the area daily and to report immediately any increased discomfort, peeling or blistering of the skin.	To detect any changes as early as possible, and allow for a review of future management. This may include referral to a plastic surgeon.
16 If blistering or tissue breakdown occurs, begin sterile dressing techniques.	To prevent a superimposed infection.
17 If a shallow, clean ulcer develops, consider attempting to heal it using a starch-hydrogel type dressing.	To promote healing and avoid unnecessary surgery. This type of dressing has been observed to have a beneficial effect in some instances.
18 Consider referral for plastic surgery if no healing occurs and the patient's condition permits.	To prevent further pain or other complications as chemically induced ulcers rarely heal spontaneously.

ADMINISTRATION OF CYTOTOXIC DRUGS BY OTHER ROUTES

ORAL ADMINISTRATION

Nurses dispensing tablets or capsules should do this using a non-touch technique. If tablets have to be counted, this should be done using a triangle, which should be washed after use.

Many tablets are coated and this protects the drug in its inner core. There is no handling risk if these coatings are not broken.

A small number of tablets are compressed powders, but where there is no free powder visible there is no risk. It is important that these tablets are not crushed.

Capsules are free from risk if they have not been opened or have not been either broken or leaked. They should not be crushed or opened.

Any visible spillage should be dealt with as previously directed (see p. 99).

INTRAMUSCULAR AND SUBCUTANEOUS INJECTION

The local tissue toxicity of many cytotoxic drugs limits the use of this route. Drugs frequently administered in this way are:

methotrexate
bleomycin
cytosine arabinoside
L-asparaginase.

Intramuscular and subcutaneous injections are often used for patient convenience, if regular administration is required and journeys to the hospital are impractical. Community nurses are responsible for administration and must be supplied with adequate information when the patient is discharged.

Although the volume of drug and diluent handled is less than for the intravenous route, preparation and reconstitution of the agents should be in line with the preceding guidelines (see pp. 100–2). The nurse should continue to wear gloves during administration. Spillage and disposal of equipment should be dealt with as previously directed (see p. 99) and systems of work modified to ensure this is possible.

Recommendations about administration should be carefully followed, e.g. deep intramuscular injection using a Z-track technique to prevent leakage onto the skin; rotation of sites to prevent local irritation developing.

INTRAPLEURAL INSTILLATION
Definition

Introduction of cytotoxic drugs, or other substances, into the pleural cavity following drainage of an effusion to prevent or delay a recurrence.

REFERENCE MATERIAL

Pleural effusion is a common complication of malignant disease and may pose a considerable management problem.

The most common neoplasms associated with the development of malignant pleural effusions are those of the:

breast
lung
gastrointestinal tract
prostate
ovary

The incidence varies, but may be as high as 50% in patients with primary lung or breast carcinoma. Such effusions can be very distressing to the patient, causing progressive discomfort, inanition, dyspnoea and death from respiratory insufficiency.

The alteration in normal lung anatomy due to the pressure of an effusion is illustrated in Figure 9.1. In health less than 5 ml of transudate fluid are present between the visceral and parietal pleurae. This fluid acts as a lubricant and hydraulic seal. Infections and malignancies disrupt this mechanism, often repeatedly. Patients may survive for months or years; therefore, effective palliation is important in maintaining or improving their quality of life.

Several methods have been used to treat pleural effusions including surgical techniques, such as ablation of the pleural space, radiotherapy and systemic chemotherapy. In addition, instillation of sclerosing agents into the pleural space has been used for three decades. These agents have included talc, radioactive phosphorus, tetracycline and, more recently, cytotoxic drugs. Those must frequently instilled are thiotepa, nitrogen mustard and bleomycin.

Recently, methylprednisolone has been used and its effectiveness is comparable with that of cytotoxic agents, that is approximately 60% response, but no local or systemic side-effects were experienced. Patients remained free of recurrent fluid for between 4 and 7 months.

Cytology may show the presence of tumour cells in effusion fluid but even when these are absent, instillation of drugs may be effective in preventing recurrence due to the inflammatory reaction which obliterates the pleural space.

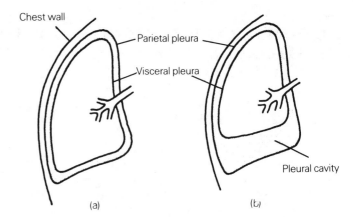

Figure 9.1 Lung anatomy. *a*, Normal lung anatomy showing pleura. *b*, Lung demonstrating presence of pleural effusion.

Improvements in equipment used, for example flexible cannulae or catheters, and lengthening of both the initial drainage period and that following instillation of the drug, have contributed to increased patient comfort plus greater effectiveness.

All studies recommend that the patient should be turned regularly following instillation of the drug to ensure its complete distribution over the pleural surfaces. The recommended timing varies and only one paper (Wood, 1981) provides a detailed procedure. The rationale for such turning is based on clinical observation and there is a lack of work comparing patients who were turned with those who were not.

Adequate analgesia and nursing measures must be provided to ensure patient comfort. The procedure and turning techniques may cause considerable distress to patients experiencing other signs and symptoms of metastatic disease.

References and further reading

Anderson, C. *et al.* (1972) The treatment of malignant pleural effusions, *Cancer*, Vol. 33, pp. 916–22.

Bartal, A.H. *et al.* (1987) Corticosteroids administration into pleural effusions in cancer patients: a novel and effective therapy. *Proceedings of the American Society of Clinical Oncology*, Vol. 6, Abstract no. 672.

Groesteck, H. *et al.* (1962) Intracavitary thio-tepa for malignant effusions, *Surgery*, Vol. 28, pp. 90–5.

Paladine, W. *et al.* (1976) Intracavity bleomycin in the management of malignant effusions, *Cancer*, Vol. 38, pp. 1903–8.

Taylor, L. (1962) A catheter technique for intrapleural administration of alkylating agents: a report of ten cases, *American Journal of the Medical Sciences*, Vol. 244, no. 6, pp. 706–16.

Wallach, H. (1975) Intrapleural tetracycline for malignant pleural effusions, *Chest*, Vol. 68, pp. 510–12.

Wood, H. (1981) Developments in the support of patients with malignant pleural effusions, in R. Tiffany (ed.) *Cancer Nursing Update*, Baillière Tindall, London.

GUIDELINES: ADMINISTRATION OF INTRAPLEURAL DRUGS

The procedure and nursing care plans related to intrapleural drainage (see Chapter 16) should be consulted for all aspects of thoracic drainage. The following information covers specific points regarding drug instillation.

Procedure

INSTILLATION OF DRUG

Action

1   Explain the procedure to the patient.

Rationale

To obtain the patient's consent and co-operation.

2 Administer, premedication to the patient, if prescribed.	To relieve anxiety and pain.
3 Prepare the required equipment (see p. 134) and cytotoxic drug with protective wear as necessary.	To ensure the procedure goes smoothly without interruption.
4 Assist the doctor with the installation and provide support for the patient.	To increase the efficiency of the procedure and reduce discomfort for the patient.
5 At the end of the procedure clamp the drainage tube and leave for the desired period.	To prevent backflow of the drug.

ROTATION OF THE PATIENT

Action	**Rationale**

1 Assess the clinical status of the patient and his/her ability to tolerate the desired rotation.	To prevent undue discomfort the patient may feel and to ensure that the doctor is informed of the patient's inability to comply.
2 Turn the patient in the following rotation: (a) left side (b) supine (c) right side (d) prone.	To ensure that the drug coats and washes the pleural cavity completely
3 Carry out the rotations as instructed. Examples are as follows: (a) Five minutes in each position, repeated once, equals 40 minutes. (b) Thirty minutes in each position, repeated once, equals 4 hours. (c) One hour in each position equals 4 hours.	As above.
4 Check if the patient is comfortable every 2–4 hours. Administer analgesia as required.	To keep the patient comfortable and free from pain.
5 Record the patient's vital signs every 15 minutes for 1 hour, then every hour until stable, then 4-hourly.	To observe for pyrexia, a common side-effect that may indicate a developing infection or a reaction to chemotherapy.

DRAINAGE OF THORACOTOMY TUBE

Rationale

Action

1 Ensure the patient is in a comfortable position, and is aware of any limitations about movement.	To prevent discomfort or dislodgement of the drainage tube.
2 Unclamp the chest tube.	To allow drainage of the drug instilled.
3 Maintain the underwater seal until a volume of less than 50 ml is drained during 24 hours for 2 consecutive days or for a maximum of 7 days.	To allow complete drainage of the drug instilled, and any additional fluid.

Action	Rationale
4 Record the colour and amount of fluid drained on the appropriate documents.	To monitor the immediate effectiveness of therapy.

NURSING CARE PLAN

Problem	Cause	Suggested action
Local or systemic effects associated with specific cytotoxic drugs, e.g. rigors due to bleomycin.	Absorption of the drug into circulation in sufficient quantities to cause toxicity.	Be aware that this can occur. Initiate preventive action, e.g. corticosteroid cover to prevent rigors, or observe for a reaction and treat symptomatically.

INTRAVESICAL INSTILLATION
Definition
The instillation of chemotherapeutic agents directly into the bladder, via a urinary catheter.

Indications
This therapy has been shown to be effective in the treatment of superficial papillary carcinoma of the bladder.

REFERENCE MATERIAL
Systemic chemotherapy has repeatedly produced disappointing results in bladder carcinoma although some recent combined modality studies have produced improved response rates. However, instillation of cytotoxic agents into the bladder via a urinary catheter has been used for many years in selected cases with some success.

A high concentration of drug bathes the endothelium. Local toxicity is not a major problem, being mainly confined to burning on urination, and there are minimal general side-effects.

The use of this method of therapy is limited to two clinical situations:
1 small, multiple, superficial, well-differentiated, non-invasive papillomatous carcinomas;
2 prophylaxis, to minimize recurrence in patients with a history of multiple tumours known readily to seed locally.

In the latter instance, the rationale is to treat subcys-
toscopic tumours.

Treatment protocols vary. Contact time with the bladder endothelium may be 1 or 2 hours and therapy may be repeated every 2–4 weeks.

In measurable disease, however, response rates are similar with an average of 60% effectiveness. Approximately 30% of patients experience a complete response.

Cytotoxic drugs most frequently used are:
thiotepa
mitomycin C
doxorubicin.
A recent paper (Garnick *et al.*, 1987) has questioned the criteria on which efficacy of treatment is based and has suggested that the primary measure of success should be the development or not of invasive bladder carcinoma.

References and further reading
Carter, S.K. and Wasserman, T.H. (1975) The chemotherapy of urologic cancer, *Cancer*, Vol. 36, pp. 729–47.

Dorr, R.T. and Fritz, W.L. (1980) *Cancer Chemotherapy Handbook*, Kimpton, London.

Garnick, M.B. *et al.* (1987) A determination of appropriate endpoints in assessing efficacy of intravesical therapies in superficial bladder cancer, *Proceedings of the American Society of Clinical Oncology*, Abstract no. 412.

Manual of Cancer Chemotherapy (1981) UICC Technical Reports 56, pp. 223–4.

GUIDELINES: INTRAVESICAL INSTILLATION OF CYTOTOXIC DRUGS

Other relevant procedures are urinary catheterization (see Chapter 41, p. 393) and bladder lavage and irrigation (see Chapter 4, p. 44). Details of required procedure and problems which may be encountered are given in these chapters. The following guidelines and care plan deal with specific aspects of chemotherapy administration.

Equipment
1   Urotainer containing prescribed drug in clinically clean tray (delivered from pharmacy reconstitution unit)
2   Sterile, latex gloves
3   Disposable apron and eye protection
4   Gate clip or equivalent clamp for catheter
5   Catheter drainage bag, if catheter is to remain in position
6   10- or 20-ml sterile syringe
7   Small dressing pack, containing sterile field, topical swabs, wool balls.

Procedure

Action	Rationale
1 Explain the procedure to the patient.	To obtain the patient's consent and co-operation.
2 Check the patient's full blood, as instructed by the medical staff, and inform them of any deficit prior to administration	Absorption of the drug through the bladder wall may cause some myelosuppression. However, there are differing opinions as to whether regular checks are necessary.
3 Check all the details on the container of cytotoxic drug against the patient's prescription chart.	To minimize the risk of error and comply with legal requirements.
4 Assemble all necessary equipment, including the cytotoxic drug container, and proceed to the patient.	To ensure that the instillation proceeds smoothly and without interruption.
5 Screen the patient's bed/couch.	To ensure privacy during the procedure.
6 Catheterize the patient, as necessary.	To enable the instillation of the drug.
7 Ensure the bladder is empty of urine.	To prevent dilution of the drug.
8 Put on an apron/eye protection.	To protect the nurse from contact with the cytotoxic drugs. With correct technique the risk of contamination is minimal, but splashes can occur.
9 If the catheter is already in place, using aseptic technique and sterile latex gloves, proceed to place sterile towel under the end of the catheter, clamp the catheter and disconnect the drainage bag.	To protect the patient from infection. To protect the nurse from drug spillage. To gain access to the catheter. To prevent urine from soiling the bed.
10 Remove the cover from the urotainer, connect to the catheter and release the clamp.	To facilitate drug instillation.
11 Gently squeeze the urotainer to administer the cytotoxic agent. Do not use force.	Rapid instillation would be uncomfortable for the patient, especially if the bladder is small or scarred from previous treatment or disease.

Action	Rationale
12 When the correct volume has been instilled, clamp the catheter.	To prevent drainage of drug from the bladder.
13 (a) If the catheter is to stay in position, connect the catheter to a new drainage bag but do not unclamp it. (b) If the catheter is to be removed, withdraw the water from the catheter balloon using the sterile syringe and remove the catheter using gentle traction.	To create a closed system, reducing the risk of bacterial contamination, and to retain the drug in the bladder. The catheter may not be required for continued urinary drainage, and may have been inserted to facilitate drug administration, particularly in the outpatient department. The risk of infection is greater if the catheter remains *in situ*.
14 Make the patient comfortable and instruct him/her about changes of position required during the time the drug is *in situ*.	Frequent changes in position ensure the drug bathes all of the bladder mucosa.
15 If the patient is unable to turn himself/herself, nursing assistance must be provided.	As above. To prevent the development of pressure sores.
16 Provide outpatients with information about the amount of movement required.	Following outpatient instillation, the journey home is usually sufficient to coat the bladder mucosa.
17 When the drug has been in the bladder for 1 hour, request the patient to micturate *or* release the clamp on the catheter to allow the drug and urine to drain into the bag.	One hour is the usual time specified for intravesical drugs to ensure the maximum therapeutic effect with minimum toxicity.
18 Advise the patient on fluid intake, suggesting ways in which he or she may increase it in the following 24-hour period. Patients should be aware that their urine may be cloudy.	To provide a good fluid output, washing out the bladder and reducing the likelihood of local irritation or difficulty in urination due to débris from the tumour.
19 Instruct the patient to report any discomfort or inability to pass urine immediately to ward staff or GP/district nurse, or to phone the hospital if anxious.	To detect any problems at the earliest moment. To reduce anxiety experienced by the patient.

NURSING CARE PLAN

Problem	Cause	Suggested action
No drainage of urine when the catheter is inserted.	Bladder is empty or the catheter is in the wrong place, e.g. in the urethra or in a false track. False tracks may develop after repeated cystoscopy or bladder surgery.	Do not inflate the balloon but tape the catheter to the skin to keep it in position. Check when the patient last micturated. Encourage the patient to drink a few glasses of fluid. Do not give the drug until urine flow is seen or correct positioning of the catheter is established. Inform a doctor if no urine has drained during the next 30 minutes.

Haematuria.	Trauma of catheterization or loosening of blood clots following cystoscopy by fluid injected into the bladder.	Inform a doctor. Observe the patient for signs of clot retention, shock, haemorrhage or fluid retention. Encourage the patient to drink fluids.
Leakage from around the catheter following administration of the drug.	Catheter slipping out of the bladder or bladder spasm caused by the drug.	Check the position of the catheter. Inform a doctor if leakage persists. Protect the patient's skin by wrapping sterile topical swabs around the catheter. Estimate the volume lost by leakage.
Patient unable to retain the requisite drug volume in the bladder for the time required	Low bladder capacity; weak sphincter muscles; unstable detrusor muscle causing uncontrolled bladder contractions.	Note actual duration of the drug in the bladder and inform a doctor.
Patient has pain during instillation of the drug or while the drug is in the bladder.	Drug injected too quickly; volume of drug and diluent too great for comfort; drug painful to raw areas in the bladder; drug causes painful spasm of the bladder.	Allow the drug to drain out and/or stop instillation if the pain is severe. Inform a doctor. Administer Entonox if appropriate (see pp. 147–8) and have analgesics prescribed for subsequent administration.
Patient unable to pass urine after the drug has been *in situ* for the required length of time.	Anxiety; poor bladder tone; prostatism.	Reassure the patient. Encourage the patient to drink fluids.
Urine does not drain from the catheter when the clamp is released.	Catheter wrongly placed. Catheter blocked with clots and/or débris.	Check the position of the catheter. Perform bladder lavage.

INTRA-ARTERIAL CHEMOTHERAPY

Definition

Delivery of high doses of cytotoxic drugs to the tumour site by catheterization of the artery providing the blood supply to the affected organ.

Drugs may be administered by slow push injection or infusion, the latter being most common. Frequency of administration is determined by the doctor in charge.

REFERENCE MATERIAL
Indications

Intra-arterial chemotherapy has been used to treat a variety of malignancies at a number of different sites during the past two decades. These include:

head and neck lesions;
liver metastases from colorectal cancer;
sarcomas/melanomas of upper and lower limb (including isolated limb perfusion);
carcinoma of the stomach;
carcinoma of the breast;
carcinoma of the cervix.

Intra-arterial chemotherapy is possible when the regional artery can be easily isolated and catheterized. Confirmation that the artery supplies the desired area can be achieved by installation of methylene blue dye if the tumour site is visible, or contrast medium if an internal organ such as the liver is the target area.

Once the catheter is in place and secured, cytotoxic drugs may be administered by:

1 injection, using a syringe;
2 small volume infusion using a syringe pump/

microvolume pump/infusor (Travenol);

3   large volume infusion using a volumetric or drop-counting peristaltic pump.

Other variations on the delivery system include the Port-a-Cath implantable infusion system and the Infusaid implantable infusion pump.

All delivery systems must be under pressure to combat arterial pressure, i.e. 300 mm Hg. The majority of infusion pumps meet this requirement.

The cytotoxic drugs used vary with the histology and site of the tumour. The following have all been used for intra-arterial administration:

actinomycin D	5-FUDR (floxuridine)
BCNU (carmustine)	methotrexate
bleomycin	melphalan
cisplatin	mitomycin C
5-FU (5-Fluorouracil)	vincristine

A high concentration of drug can be delivered to the primary or secondary tumour mass. A reduction in systemic circulating levels of drugs has been shown to occur in many circumstances resulting in a corresponding reduction in side-effects to the patient, although this is difficult to predict.

Principles of nursing care

Insertion is an operative procedure and consent must be obtained. Adequate explanation to the patient is essential, especially what to expect on return to the ward.

The area should be shaved or otherwise prepared and the period of fasting should be checked with the doctor.

The catheter is inserted in theatre or in the X-ray department and its position checked at that time. The catheter will be secured and an occlusive dressing applied. This should *not* be touched as it is essential that the catheter is *not* displaced.

A three- or one-way tap is connected to the catheter and it is at this point that all manipulations take place. An extension set should be connected to this at the time of insertion or on return to the ward to prevent unnecessary handling near the skin exit site.

The system will consist of: catheter/tap/extension set/administration set or infusion device (e.g. Infusor).

Certain general rules apply:

1   the dressing must not be touched but should be observed regularly for signs of bleeding. This should be reported immediately to the medical staff, including the radiologist;

2   all procedures or manipulations associated with the pathway must use aseptic technique;

3   all connections must be Luer locking to prevent exsanguination/air embolism or disconnection under pressure;

4   the line must be clamped securely or switched off using the tap *in situ* before any equipment changes;

5   positive pressure, greater than arterial pressure, must be maintained at all times;

6   when chemotherapy is not being infused, heparinized saline must be used to maintain patency. This should be via a syringe/syringe pump during transfer between wards or departments, or via a syringe pump/infusion pump in the ward. A nurse escort may be necessary for transfers.

The concentration of heparin should be 1 unit/ml, i.e.
   1000 i.u./1 litre of fluid
    500 i.u./500 ml of fluid
     50 i.u./50 ml of fluid.

It should be delivered at the minimum rate sufficient to combat arterial pressure and maintain patency, approximately 5 ml per hour or 10 drops per minute, dependent on the device used. If a special delivery system is used, e.g. Infusor, manufacturers' instructions should be followed.

7   the patient must be instructed on the amount of mobility allowed. This may vary depending on the site of the catheter. Assistance may be needed to maintain personal hygiene and relieve pressure. Aids may be required to prevent the development of pressure sores on all points of contact;

8   the position of the catheter may be checked daily by X-ray, which will be performed on the ward. Fluoroscopy and installation of dye are other methods of confirming position;

9   at the end of treatment, patency of the arterial line should be maintained using heparinized saline until a decision has been made about removal. Instructions for this and the amount of heparin to be used should be prescribed in advance to enable the nurse to initiate the procedure when appropriate;

10 prior to removal, the tap may be switched off and the catheter allowed to clot. The catheter should be removed by a doctor and firm pressure applied for at least 5 minutes or until all bleeding has ceased. A dressing should be applied to the site. Pressure dressings are not indicated if bleeding has ceased and can obscure the formation of a haematoma.

Any problems should be referred to the medical staff and the radiologist.

Conclusion

The administration of intra-arterial chemotherapy is an infrequent occurrence but it has been used to achieve significant reductions in tumour size and improved survival. A decrease in systemic circulating levels of drugs and a lessening of side-effects to patients has been shown although this is variable.

Do not hesitate to contact a radiologist if a problem is suspected as he/she is the expert in catheter placement and management of complications.

References and further reading

Bedford, R.F. (1978) Percutaneous radial artery cannulation, *Surgical News*, no. 4.

Dorr, R.T. and Fritz, W.L. (1980) *Cancer Chemotherapy Handbook*, Kimpton, London.

Gilbertson, A.A. (1984) *Intravenous Technique and Therapy*, Heinemann, London.

Plumer, A.L. (1982) *Principles and Practice of Intravenous Therapy*, Little, Brown & Co, Boston, USA.

Taylor, I. (1985) Hepatic arterial infusion of anti-cancer drugs, *Cancer Topics*, Vol. 5, no. 5, pp. 50–1.

NURSING CARE PLAN

Problem	Action	Rationale
Haemorrhage	Observe the dressing at regular intervals. Monitor pulse and blood pressure at least 4-hourly.	To prevent blood loss or detect haemorrhage at the earliest possible moment.
	Instruct the patient on the amount of movement permitted and to report any feeling of faintness, or oozing noted on dressing.	
	After removal of the catheter, vital signs and the dressing should be observed every 15 minutes for 2 hours. The patient should remain on bedrest for 24 hours but may be allowed up for toilet purposes, with assistance.	
	If bleeding does occur, this is an emergency; pressure should be applied immediately and a member of the medical staff contacted.	
Displacement of the catheter	Do not disturb the dressing placed in the X-ray department.	To prevent displacement or detect it as early as possible, so reducing the likelihood of extravasion of drugs (see pp. 105–6).
	Instruct the patient on amount of movement permitted.	
	Check position daily, if requested by the doctor.	
Arterial occlusion	Check vessel patency daily, if instructed to do so by medical staff. This may be done using a Doppler flowmeter or by manual location of distal pulses.	To prevent this occurring and ensure continued delivery of therapy to the patient.
	Report any abnormality to the doctor or radiologist.	
Infection	Strict asepsis must be maintained for all procedures and manipulations of the arterial line. The administration set must be changed every 24 hours, as for venous lines. Temperature must be taken every 4 hours and any pyrexia investigated.	To provent both localized infection and septicaemia.

Problem	Action	Rationale
Exsanguination/ air embolism	Luer-lock connections must be used throughout the pathway. These should be checked at regular intervals, and continuous flow maintained. Care must be taken when changing equipment to prevent blood loss occurring or air entering the line, e.g. shut off tap, firm clamping, if necessary. Care must be taken when injecting medications, as above. The seriousness of an air embolus depends on the siting of the arterial line and whether it is a direct route to the carotid artery and so to the brain.	To prevent a major blood loss progressing to shock. To prevent an air embolus, although this is less likely.
Thrombosis/ emboli	The literature indicates that thrombosis occurs in over 40% of arteries catheterized for over 48 hours. However, this is dependent on the vessel used. Most used for chemotherapy delivery pose no problem and will remain patent for the treatment period. However, a resulting thrombus may embolize causing vascular insufficiency, distal or central embolism. When occlusion occurs due to thrombus formation or spasm, blood flow is usually maintained by collaterals until the vessel recovers. Presence of a pulse and the colour of the area should be checked daily or a Doppler flowmeter may be used. Any abnormality should be reported to the medical staff and radiologist. The catheter should be removed by the doctor using firm, steady traction, in an attempt to prevent dislodging any thrombus present. The condition of the patient and the limb/area should be observed carefully at the time that vital signs are measured.	To detect this problem at the earliest possible moment, so preventing reduced blood flow to the limb or organ.
Damage to the artery, arteriovenous fistula, aneurysm formation	The incidence of these is low and the likelihood of them occurring can be minimized by gentle handling of the catheter and immobilization of the limb/area as soon as appropriate.	To reduce the incidence of these complications, however rare, and to ensure that the medical staff are notified immediately.
Extravasation of drugs/failure of drug to reach target area	Both of these are very rare but can lead to significant morbidity. The incidence can be reduced by careful placement of the catheter and verification by X-ray or installation of dye.	As above.

Problem	Action	Rationale
	If there is any doubt concerning the placement of the catheter the doctor and radiologist should be notified, as extravasation of the drug may lead to ulceration and necrosis.	
Chemical hepatitis/bilary sclerosis	The occurrence of these will be evident from elevated liver enzymes. Therefore, monitoring of liver function tests is important. Any elevation is usually transient.	To be aware that this may occur and of the significance.

10

Discharge Planning

Historical perspective
The discharge of patients into the community continues
to remain an area of concern. Research first conducted
in the late 1960s (Noble, 1967; Hockey, 1968) found that
little communication between hospital and community
nurses actually took place. Skeet (1971) found that
patients interviewed at home after their return from
hospital had at least half their health care needs unplan-
ned for and unmet.

The situation has not improved significantly in the
past 20 years. There is considerable evidence (Altschul,
1984; Jones, 1984; Armitage, 1985; Saddington, 1985)
that a patient's discharge from hospital is often unplan-
ned and little attention is paid to attempting to arrange
appropriate community nursing assistance. Inadequate
communication networks, or lack of interpersonal co-
operation, has been identified as contributing to these
problems, resulting in the needs of patient and family
being ignored and inappropriate assistance being en-
gaged.

Lack of discharge planning and its consequences may
result in physiological and psychosocial problems for
both cancer patients and their families (Edstrom and
Miller, 1981). Sque (1985) has identified that the chro-
nicity of the disease process, coupled with episodes of
acute life-threatening illness, often necessitates frequent
admission to hospital, complex treatment procedures
and the involvement of domiciliary services. This may
have a profound effect on the quality of life for patients
and their families (Giacquinta, 1977). Disruptions can
be reduced, however, if care is planned and is continuous between hospital and home (Jupp and Sims,
1987). The decision to discharge a patient from hospital
often depends on many factors other than medical considerations; individualized care planning is, therefore,
essential. Continuity of care 'only occurs when all health
providers make a concerted effort to link their plan of
care to the whole plan of care for the patient' (Marquez,
1980).

Definition
Discharge planning is the plan evolved prior to a patient
being transferred from one environment to another.
This process involves the patient, his/her family and
the health care team. An individual assessment of the
patient in the presence of the nurse to determine actual
or potential problems begins on admission. This enables
formulation of a plan which promotes continuity and
co-ordination of health care on discharge from hospital.
Discharge planning is an integral part of the continuity
of nursing care for patients throughout their hospital
stay.

Aims and objectives
1 To prepare the patient and his/her family physically
   and psychologically for transfer home.
2 To promote the highest possible level of independence for the patient and his/her family by encouraging self-care activities.
3 To provide continuity of care between the hospital
   and the community by facilitating effective communication.
4 To encourage a safe, ordered transfer home by ensuring that all necessary health care facilities are
   prepared to receive the patient.

REFERENCE MATERIAL
Assessment of patients' needs prior to discharge
Research has shown (Ferguson, 1961; Skeet, 1971;
Barnes, 1984) that many patients are readmitted to
hospital because their health care needs are not being
met in the community. Despite the considerable pub-
licity given to the need for effective discharge planning,
the trend towards lack of planning remains disturbingly
apparent (Saddington, 1985). Assessment of the
patient's needs at home is a continuous process that
begins on admission to hospital. Planning care to meet
those needs is initiated at the same time.

Table 10.1   Assessment of a Patient's Needs on Discharge Home Using Orem's (1980) Self-Care Model

Six universal self-care needs for all healthy individuals
1 Sufficient intake of air, water, nutrition.
2 Satisfactory eliminative functions.
3 Activity balanced with rest.
4 Time spent alone balanced with time spent with others.
5 Prevention of danger to the self.
6 Being 'normal'.

Table 10.1 summarizes the assessment factors to be considered prior to discharge planning. Assessment can be conducted within any relevant model of nursing care. The following assessment outline is based on Orem's Self-Care Model (1980), which attempts to encourage the patient and his/her family to make the best use of their most immediate resource in health care – themselves.

Healthy individuals have sufficient self-care ability to be able to meet the fundamental needs listed. In Table 10.1 individuals who experience illness or injury are subject to additional demands for self-care. They may be able to meet those needs with nursing assistance or require a nurse to meet those needs for them until they are capable of resuming their own self-care.

FIRST STAGE OF THE ASSESSMENT
Is there a deficit between the individual's self-care abilities and the demands for self-care.
Yes?   No?
             Nursing intervention not required.
(If patients cannot carry out their self-care activities *safely* then nursing will be required.)

SECOND STAGE OF THE ASSESSMENT
If patients cannot carry out their self-care activities, then why is there a self-care deficit?
1 Lack of knowledge?
   (a) Physical and psychological needs that are unfamiliar to the patient and his/her family.
   (b) Knowledge of specialist health care activities, e.g. dressing techniques, catheter management, etc.
   (c) Patient's and family's understanding of illness and tretment.
   (d) Specific aids and equipment that will facilitate health care.
   (e) Community resources available.
2 Lack of skill?
   (a) Techniques of physical and psychological care.
   (b) Ability to learn to manage health care problems.

   (c) Lack of contact with similar health care problems prior to discharge.
   (d) Inappropriate teaching or experience regarding health care activities prior to this admission.
3 Lack of motivation?
   (a) Willingness of patient and family to undertake self-care activities.
   (b) Willingness of patient and family to accept help and their ability to assist in care-giving.
   (c) Are the self-care activities culturally and socially acceptable e.g. self-administration of suppositories, stoma care, etc.?
4 Limited range of behaviour?
   (a) Physical limitations, e.g. effects of disease process and treatment:
        respiration
        eating and drinking
        elimination
        posture
        rest and sleep
        dressing and undressing
        temperature control
        personal hygiene
        protection from danger
        communication
        religion
        work
        recreation
        education (Henderson, 1977).
   (b) Psychological limitations.
   (c) Social limitations, e.g. resources within the family/friends, occupational and financial resources.
   (d) Is the patient safe to engage in self-care activities?
5 Potential for re-establishing self-care in the future.
   (a) Activities which will lead to the patient and family being able to take over self-care activities again.

Conclusion

From the patient's perspective, discharge remains one of the most important events of the hospital stay. The way in which the patient is transferred into the community directly influences the patient's and his/her family's ability to cope at home. It is, therefore, essential that discharge planning is considered an integral part of the nursing process. Assessment, planning, implementation and evaluation of care from the time of hospital admission, up to and including discharge, are essential if care is to be individualized and continuity of care achieved.

References and further reading

Altschul, A. (1984) Safe journey home, *Nursing Times*, Vol. 80, no. 42, pp. 18–19.

Armitage, S. (1985) Hospital to home: discharge referrals, who's responsible? *Nursing Times*, Vol. 81, no. 7, pp. 26–38.

Ashley, J.S.A. (1977) Community care; continuing or alternative care? *Royal Society of Health Journal*, Vol. 97, no. 3, pp. 127–9.

Barnes, A. (1984) Narrowing the gap, *Journal of District Nursing*, Vol. 2, no. 8, pp. 6–8.

Bend, J. (1983) Teaching for all, *Community Forum*, Vol. 7, pp. v–viii.

Bowling, A. and Betts, G. (1984a) From hospital to home 2: Communication on discharge, *Nursing Times*, Vol. 80, no. 29, pp. 31–3.

Bowling A. and Betts, G. (1984b) From hospital to home 5: Communication on discharge, *Nursing Times*, Vol. 80, no.30, pp. 44–6.

Edstrom, S. and Miller, M. (1981) Preparing the family to care for the cancer patient at home: a home care course, *Cancer Nursing*, Vol. 5, no. 2, pp. 49–52.

Ferguson T. (1961) Aftercare of the hospitalised patient, *British Medical Journal*, Vol. 1, no. 5234, pp. 1242–4.

Giacquinta, B. (1977) Helping families to face the crisis of cancer, *American Journal of Nursing*, Vol. 77, no. 10, pp. 1585–8.

Henderson, V. (1977) *Basic Principles of Nursing Care*, International Council of Nurses/Kruger.

Hockey, L. (1968) *Care in the Balance*, Queen's Institute of District Nursing, London.

Ilett, J. (1984) Community nursing 1: Liaison health visitor, *Nursing Times*, Vol. 80, no. 17, pp. 46–9.

Jones, I.H. (1984) Cause for complaint 2: Lack of communication, *Nursing Times*, Vol. 80, no. 32, pp. 51–2.

Jupp, M. and Sims, S. (1987) Going home, *Nursing Times*, Vol. 82, no. 33, pp. 40–2.

Marquez, S. (1980) A community homecare coordination programme, in S.R. Beatty S R (ed.), *Continuity of Care Between the Hospital and the Community*, Grune & Stratton, New York, Chap. 11, pp. 147–63.

Noble, M. (1967) Communication in the National Health Service – a survey of some published findings, *International Journal of Nursing Studies*, Vol. 4, pp. 15–28.

O'Leary, J. and Thacker, P. (1985) Blueprint for liaison, *Community Outlook*, Vol. 40, p. 43.

Orem, D. (1980) *Nursing: Concepts of Practice*, McGraw-Hill, New York.

Parnell, J. (1982) Continuity and communication, *Nursing Times*, Vol. 78, no. 12, pp. 37–40, no. 13, pp. 37–40.

Potterton, D. (1984) From hospital to home 3; The yawning gap, *Nursing Times*, Vol. 80, no. 29, pp. 34–5.

Roper, M. (1984) Cooperation to the end, *Journal of District Nursing*, Vol. 2, no. 8, pp. 9–10.

Saddington, N. (1985) A communication breakdown, *Nursing Times*, Vol. 81, no. 8, p. 31.

Skeet, M. (1971) *Home from Hospital*, Dan Mason Nursing Research Committee/Macmillan Press, London.

Sque, M. (1985) What's in a name? *Nursing Mirror*, Vol. 160, pp. 28–30.

Webster, S. (1984) Transfer not discharge, *Journal of District Nursing*, Vol. 3, no. 4, pp. 12–14.

GUIDELINES: DISCHARGE PLANNING

Guidelines for the planning of a patient's discharge from hospital are outlined in this care plan. The first section refers to steps that are relevant for all patients being discharged from hospital and the second section includes additional steps for patients who require referral to the primary health care team (district nurse, health visitor, community psychiatric nurse, etc.).

Procedure (after Jupp and Sims, 1987)

ALL PATIENTS

Action	Rationale
1 Assess and formulate a plan of care to meet the individual physiological and psychosocial needs of the patient and family. This is an ongoing process from the time of his/her admission.	In order to determine any nursing or social problems well in advance of discharge home.

2 Involve other members of the health care team, e.g. physiotherapist, occupational therapist, speech therapist, social worker, chaplain, if appropriate.

In order to promote the highest level of independence and offer support and guidance.

3 Discuss the patient's discharge plans with others involved in his/her care; this includes the patient, family or significant other.

To ascertain whether the patient is ready for discharge and how the patient, family or significant other views discharge planning.

4 If possible set a discharge date, taking into account the availability of family or significant other.

This will enable consultation with the family, etc. well before the event and ensures support will be available in the immediate post-discharge period.

5 Book transport if required.

Patients may not have private transport facilities, or may feel too weak to use public transport.

6 Teach the patient, his/her family or significant other any necessary skills; allow sufficient time for practising these skills prior to discharge.

To enable the patient, family or significant other to be as independent as possible and to promote understanding of self-care techniques.

7 Inform the patient, his/her family or significant other of any side-effects of treatment.

To alleviate anxiety and promote patient comfort and knowledge.

8 Give medications to be taken at home and explain dosage, route, frequency and side-effects.

To promote compliance and understanding of treatment.

9 If the patient presents with depression or confusion it is necessary to ascertain whether these symptoms existed prior to admission.

To promote comfort. To alleviate depression or confusion.

10 Arrange for nursing aids, such as catheter bags, syringes, surgical dressings or oxygen, etc. to be available on the day of discharge.

These items are not readily available in the community. The equipment and oxygen can be arranged through the patient's general practitioner.

11 Arrange rehabilitation equipment, such as commodes, urinals, walking frames, to be available in the community. (Liaise with occupational therapist.)

If family or significant other are unable to collect such items, time is required to order and arrange home delivery.

12 Reinforce any special instruction by completing a patient information sheet or by giving an approved education booklet.

To promote a knowledgeable understanding of disease and treatment.

13 Anticipate any fears about the journey home, e.g. jolting, and take steps to overcome them.

To promote patient comfort and alleviate anxiety.

14 Make an outpatient appointment and give the patient the card.

To ensure the patient is followed up.

15 Give the patient, his/her family or significant other the hospital telephone number.

In case the patient wants to contact the hospital. To alleviate anxiety.

16 Instruct the patient to inform the general practitioner of his/her discharge home.

To alert the general practitioner of patient's home-coming.

ADDITIONAL STEPS FOR PATIENTS REQUIRING REFERRAL TO THE PRIMARY HEALTH CARE TEAM

Action	Rationale
1 Determine whether the patient has had community nursing services before.	Community nurses need to be informed of the patient's admission to avoid unwanted visits. Contact with the community nurse may provide valuable information at this stage.
2 Inform the community liaison nurse of the patient's home-care needs and proposed discharge date, as soon as possible.	In order to plan for the patient's home-care needs the community liaison nurse needs to meet the patient, his/her family or significant other well in advance of discharge.
3 Assess whether a home visit by an occupational therapist is required.	To determine the extent of community support and the rehabilitation equipment needed.
4 Formulate a nursing action plan using a separate problem page in the nursing care plan.	To facilitate planning, co-ordination and communication.
5 Following discussion with the patient, his/her family or significant other and ward staff, the community liaison nurse will contact the appropriate nursing office by telephone to request a visit. In his/her absence, ward staff may obtain the appropriate telephone number from the community handbook.	In order to alert community nurses in advance of patient's discharge. To establish a link between hospital and community.
6 Referral to special support groups and organizations in the community should be considered when making the discharge plan.	To offer extra support to the patient in the community.
7 A community care referral request should be filled in by the primary nurse and the patient and placed in an envelope. This is given to the patient with instructions to give it to the community nurse.	This enables the community nurse to obtain a more in-depth knowledge of the patient's medical and nursing history and present requirements.
8 A copy of the community care referral should be kept on the ward.	In order to allow effective answers to queries from the patient or community nurse after discharge.
9 When the patient leaves the ward the primary nurse should check all necessary equipment, medications, community care sheet and outpatients appointment goes with him/her.	To avoid the patient being discharged without the appropriate equipment and medications, etc. To ensure a smooth transition home.
10 If the patient is not discharged, inform the community liaison nurse, or telephone the appropriate community nursing office so that they may be informed.	In order to avoid wasted visits and to promote community relations.

11

Drug Administration

REFERENCE MATERIAL
Legislation

The range of substances which are controlled in some way or other by law is extensive. Three broad categories may be identified:

1 opioid drugs;
2 poisons;
3 medicines.

In the United Kingdom substances intended for medicinal use must conform to certain standards as specified in the British Pharmacopoeia (BP) or the British Pharmaceutical Codex (BPC).

The law relating to the above-mentioned categories is contained in three statutes. Anyone working in the National Health Service will require a working knowledge of these three statutes, and of the body of regulations made under them, if they are to meet their legal obligations in their particular fields.

THE MISUSE OF DRUGS ACT, 1971

This Act lists the drugs to be controlled and classifies them for the purpose of the Act. It prohibits virtually all activities with controlled drugs and thereby creates a series of criminal offences for which it specifies penalties and law enforcement procedures. It authorizes certain activities with controlled drugs for professional medical (including dental and veterinary) use which would otherwise be unlawful. These authorized activities are themselves subject to control.

In addition, the Act confers on the Secretary of State at the Home Office a variety of powers made under the Act to prevent the misuse of drugs, and it creates the Advisory Council on the Misuse of Drugs.

The level of control to be exercised, which is related to the potential for abuse or misuse of the drugs concerned, is specified by dividing them into five schedules. The requirements of the Act as they apply to nurses working in a hospital with a pharmacy department are summarized in Table 11.1.

Summary

Hospital wards and departments are authorised to hold a stock of controlled drugs. These are obtained by the use of a special duplicate order form signed by the nurse in charge who is then responsible for them. They should be stored in a locked cupboard used exclusively for this purpose. They may be administered only to a patient in that ward or department when prescribed by a doctor. Appropriate records of their use must be maintained. Completed registers and copies of orders should be kept for 2 years. Unwanted drugs should normally be destroyed in the pharmacy but may, under some circumstances be disposed of on the ward under the supervision of a pharmacist. An appropriate entry should then be made in the ward register.

THE POISONS ACT, 1972

This Act deals only with non-medicinal poisons. However toxic a substance may be, it is not considered to be a poison for the purpose of this Act if it is not on the Poisons List. The Act deals with four related aspects of poison control:

1 the establishment of a Poisons Board;
2 the listing of controlled poisons;
3 the control of the sale of listed poisons;
4 the system of inspection to enforce the provisions of the Act.

Some substances on the Poisons List also have medicinal uses. When sold as medicinal products they are controlled under the Medicines Act, 1968.

THE MEDICINES ACT, 1968

This Act covers both human and animal medicines. The Act is comprehensive, covering virtually every possible activity concerned with a medicinal product and also some related areas such as retail pharmacies and the British Pharmacopoeia. In National Health Service hospitals adherence to the Act means that purchase of medicines is normally by a pharmacist or, failing this, by

Table 11.1   Summary of the Legal Requirements for the Handling of Controlled Drugs as They Apply to Nurses in Hospitals with a Pharmacy

	Schedule 1	Schedule 2	Schedule 3	Schedule 4	Schedule 5
Drugs in schedule	Cannabis + derivatives but excluding nabilone LSD	Most opioids in common use including: alfentanl amphetamines cocaine diamorphine methadone morphine papaveretum fentanyl phenoperidine pethidine codeine dihydrocodeine pentazocine	Minor stimulants. Barbiturates (but excluding: hexobarbitone thiopentone methohexitone). Diethylpropion } injec- tions only	Benzodiazepines	Some preparations containing very low strengths of: cocaine codeine morphine pholcodine and some other opiods
Ordering	Possession and supply permitted only by special licence from the Secretary of State issued (to a doctor only) for scientific or research purposes	A requisition must be signed in duplicate by the nurse in charge. The requisition must be endorsed to indicate that the drugs have been supplied. Copies should be kept for 2 years	As Schedule 2	No requirement[1]	No requirement[1]
Storage[5]	As Schedule 2	Must be kept in a suitable locked cupboard to which access is restricted	Diethylpropion: as Schedule 2. All other drugs: no requirement	No requirement[1]	No requirement[1]
Record keeping	As Schedule 2	Controlled Drugs[3] Register must be used	No requirement	No requirement[1]	No requirement[1]
Prescriptions	As Schedule 2	See below for detail of requirements[4]	As Schedule 2 except for phenobarbitone[2]	No requirement[1]	No requirement[1]
Administration to patients	As Schedule 2. Under special licence only	A doctor or dentist or anyone acting on their instructions may administer these drugs to anyone	As Schedule 2	No requirement[1]	No requirement[1]

Table 11.1   (*contd.*)

	Schedule 1	Schedule 2	Schedule 3	Schedule 4	Schedule 5
		for whom they have been prescribed			

1 'No requirement' indicates that the Misuse of Drugs Act imposes no legal requirements additional to those imposed by the Medicines Act 1968.

2 All references to phenobarbitone should be taken to include all preparations of phenobarbitone and phenobarbitone sodium. Because of its use as an anti-epileptic, phenobarbitone is exempt from the handwriting requirements only of the full prescription requirements (see 4 below).

3 *Record keeping*.

There is no legal requirement for the nurse in charge or acting in charge of a ward or department to keep a record of Schedule 1 or 2 Controlled Drugs obtained or supplied. However the Aitken Report recommended that this should be done and in practice a Controlled Drug Register is invariably kept according to the following guidelines:

(a)   Each page should be clearly headed to indicate the drug and preparation to which it refers. Records for different classes of drug should be kept on separate pages.

(b)   Entries should be made as soon as possible after the relevant transaction has occurred and always within 24 hours.

(c)   No cancellations or obliteration of an entry should be made. Corrections should be made by means of a note in the margin or at the foot of the page and this should be signed, dated and cross-referenced to the relevant entry.

(d)   All entries should be indelible.

(e)   The Register should be used for Controlled Drugs only and for no other purposes.

(f)   A completed register should be kept for 2 years from the date of the last entry.

4 *Prescription requirements*.

(a)   The prescription *must* state:

(i)   The name and address of the patient.

(ii)   The drug, the dose, the form of preparation (e.g. tablet).

(iii)   The total quantity of drug, or the total number of dosage units to be supplied. This quantity must be stated in *words* and *figures*.

All the above must be indelibly written in the prescriber's own handwriting and he/she must sign the prescription.

(iv)   The date of the prescription.

(v)   If the prescription is to be dispensed in instalments, the number of instalments and the intervals between them.

It is illegal to write or dispense a prescription which does not comply with these requirements.

(b)   The full handwriting requirements and statement of quantity to be supplied do not apply to prescriptions for hospital inpatients if the Controlled Drugs concerned are administered from ward or department stocks. They do, however, apply to prescription for drugs 'to take home' or for outpatients.

5 *Storage and safe custody*.

(a)   All Controlled Drugs should be stored in a suitably secure (usually metal) cupboard which is kept locked and to which access is restricted. This cupboard (which may be within a second outer cupboard) should be used only for the storage of Controlled Drugs.

(b)   The Aitken Report recommends that all Controlled Drug record entries be checked by two nurses. In conjunction with the pharmacy a procedure should be developed to ensure regular checking of records and reconciliation of receipts and issues.

(c)   A programme for regular stock checking should be established and adhered to.

6 *Destruction*.

Unwanted or unused Controlled Drugs in Schedule 2 must not be destroyed on the ward but should be returned to the pharmacy.

a nurse or doctor. Medicines must be stored in a suitable environment so that they reach the patient in a stable condition. Containers must be labelled according to the law and issued and administered in accordance with a written prescription signed by a doctor or dentist. The adverse use or misuse of medicines is thus prevented by having trained health care professionals involved in their control and administration. The Act may be divided into seven broad categories:

1   the administrative system;
2   the licensing system;
3   the sale and supply of medicines to the public;
4   the retail pharmacies;
5   packing and labelling;
6   the promotion of medicines;
7   the British Pharmacopoeia.

Section 2 of the licensing system of this Act permits a registered nurse or a certified midwife to assemble a medicinal product without the need for a manufacturer's licence. 'Assembly' is defined as either enclosing a medicinal product (with or without other medicinal products of the same description) in a container to be labelled before supply or, if it is already in the container, labelling it before supply.

Types of medicinal preparations of drugs

PREPARATIONS FOR ORAL ADMINISTRATION

Tablets

These come in a great variety of shapes, sizes, colours and types. The formulation may be very simple and result for instance in a plain, white, uncoated tablet, or complex and designed with specific therapeutic aims. Sugar coatings are used to improve appearances and palatability. In cases where the drug is a gastric irritant or is broken down by gastric acid, an enteric coating may be used. This is designed to allow the tablet to remain intact in the stomach and to pass unchanged into the small bowel where the coating dissolves and hence the drug is released and absorbed. Sustained-release tablets may be formulated in many ways but all with the object of producing a slow continuous rate of drug release as the tablet passes along the alimentary tract. Tablets may also be specifically formulated to dissolve readily ('soluble' or 'effervescent'), to be chewed or to be held under the tongue ('sublingual'). Unscored or coated tablets should not be crushed or broken, nor should most 'slow-release' or 'sustained action' tablets.

Capsules

These consist of a gelatin shell in which is contained the drug powder or granules. They offer a useful method of formulating drugs which are difficult to make into a tablet or are particularly unpalatable. Slow-release capsule formulations also exist. Capsules should not normally be broken or opened.

Lozenges and pastilles

These are designed to be sucked for local treatment of the mouth and throat.

Linctuses, elixirs, syrups

These are usually sweet, syrup-like solutions used to treat coughs or where, in children for instance, a tablet or capsule may be inappropriate.

Mixtures

These are flavoured solutions or suspensions of drugs. It is particularly important the suspensions are thoroughly mixed by shaking before each dose is measured. This ensures that the measured volume always contains the correct amount of drug.

RECTAL AND VAGINAL PREPARATIONS

Enemas

These are solutions which are instilled into the rectum as laxatives or to obtain other localized therapeutic effects, or for diagnostic purposes.

Suppositories

These are solid wax pellets for rectal administration. They may either melt at body temperature or dissolve or disperse in the mucous secretions of the rectum. They may be used to obtain local effect (e.g. as laxatives) or for systemic therapy. Many drugs, such as the opioids for example, are well absorbed when administered this way. Suppositories sometimes offer a useful alternative to injections for very sick patients unable to take drugs orally.

Pessaries

These are solid pellets for vaginal administration and are usually designed to have a local therapeutic action.

TOPICAL APPLICATIONS

Creams

These are semisolid emulsions containing a high proportion of water. When applied they are quickly absorbed into the skin leaving little or no greasy residue. They may be used as a 'base' in which a variety of drugs may be applied for local therapy.

Ointments

These are similar to cream but contain a higher proportion of oil. They are more slowly absorbed into the skin and leave a greasy residue. They have similar uses to creams, and are particularly suitable for dry, scaly lesions.

INJECTIONS

Injections are defined by the BPC as: 'sterile solutions, suspensions, or emulsions which contain one or more medicaments in a suitable aqueous or non-aqueous vehicle; they are intended to be administered parenterally to produce a localized or systemic, rapid or sustained response'. The parenteral route of administration is often adopted for medicaments which cannot be given orally because of patient intolerance or because of instability, therapeutic inactivity or poor absorption. In an emergency, an injection can provide a rapid and effective response.

Subcutaneous injection
This is given into the highly vascular layer beneath the epidermis and drugs are fairly rapidly absorbed by this route.

Intradermal injection
This is used mainly for diagnostic tests.

Intramuscular injection
Many drugs may be administered by this route provided they are not irritant to soft tissues and are sufficiently soluble. Absorption is usually rapid and can produce blood levels comparable to those achieved by intravenous bolus injection. Intramuscular injections should, where possible, be avoided in thrombocytopaenic patients.

Intravenous injection
This type of injection ranges from small volumes for 'bolus' or 'push' administration to large-volume infusions.

Intrathecal injection
This may be used when the drug concerned does not penetrate the blood/brain barrier.

Intra-articular injection
This term refers to the injection of a solution into a joint.

Intra-arterial injection
This special technique allows delivery of a high concentration of drug to the tissues supplied by a particular artery.

Subconjunctival injection
Some drugs may be given by this procedure in ophthalmology.

INHALATIONS

The term 'inhalation' once referred solely to the inhalation of volatile constituents of such preparations as compound tincture of benzoin. In modern therapeutics two techniques – nebulization and aerosolization – permit the inhalation of a range of drugs with the aim of a localized therapeutic effect.

Nebulization involves the passage of air (or sometimes oxygen) through a solution of the drug concerned to create a fine spray. Some antibiotics and bronchodilators may be given in this way.

Aerosolization involves the use of a solution of drug in an inert diluent. Passing a metred volume of this solution through a valve under pressure allows the delivery to the patient of a measured dose of drug in a very fine spray of controlled particle size. Bronchodilators and steroids are commonly administered in this way. Although a very small total dose of drug is administered the concentration achieved at the site of action is high. Rapid and effective control of symptoms is achieved but without the side-effects commonly associated with an equivalent systemic (oral or parenteral) dose of the drug(s).

Storage
Certain general principles apply to the storage of medicinal preparations.

Principle	Rationale
1 *Security*: locked cupboards. When not in use drug trolleys should not only be kept locked but should also be secured to a wall and thus immobilized.	To prevent unauthorized access and deter abuse and/or misuse.
2 *Separate storage*: for medicines and non-medicines.	To prevent confusion and hence danger to patients.
Separate storage: for preparations for oral use and those for topical use.	To prevent errors and therefore danger to the patient.

Principle	Rationale
3 *Stability*: no medicinal preparation should be stored where it may be subject to substantial variations in temperature, e.g. not in direct sunlight or over a radiator.	To maintain efficacy of the medicines.
Stability: some preparations require storage under well-defined conditions, e.g. 'below 10 °C' or 'store in a refrigerator'.	To maintain efficacy of the medicines.
4 *Labelling*: the wording of labels is carefully chosen to convey clearly all essential information. Printed labels should always be used.	To ensure that the user has all the necessary information.
5 *Containers*: the type of container used may have been chosen for specific reasons.	The design and material of which the container is made may significantly influence the stability of the contents.
Medicinal preparations should never be transferred (in bulk) from one container to another except in the pharmacy.	As above. Inadequate labelling of repackaged medicines is dangerous.
6 *Stock control*: a system of stock rotation must be operated (e.g. 'first in, first out') to ensure that there is no accumulation of 'old' stocks. Regular stock checks should be carried out, if possible by pharmacy staff.	All medicinal preparations, even when correctly stored, retain activity only for a limited period of time.

The label on the pack should in most cases give guidance about storage conditions for individual preparations. The term 'a cool place' is normally interpreted as meaning between 1° and 15° C for which a refrigerator will normally suffice. 'Room temperature' allows a range of approximately 15°–25° C.

If you are in any doubt about the storage requirements for any preparation you should check with a pharmacist, but the following points are noteworthy:

1 aerosol containers should not be stored in direct sunlight or over radiators – there is a risk of explosion if they are heated;
2 creams may deteriorate rapidly if subjected to extremes of temperature;
3 eye drops and ointments may become contaminated with micro-organisms during use, and hence pose a danger to the recipient. Hence, in hospitals, eye preparations should be discarded 7 days after they are first opened. For use at home this limit is extended to 28 days;
4 mixtures may have a relatively short shelf-life. Most antibiotic mixtures require refrigerated storage and even then have a shelf-life of only 7–14 days. Always check the label for details;
5 tablets and capsules are relatively stable but are susceptible to moisture unless correctly packed. They should be stored only in the containers in which they were supplied by the pharmacy;
6 vaccines and similar preparations usually require refrigerated stored and may deteriorate rapidly if exposed to heat.

Administration

The effective and safe administration of drugs to patients demands a partnership between the various health professionals concerned, i.e. doctors, pharmacists and nurses. The nurse is responsible for the correct administration of prescribed drugs to patients in his/her care. To achieve this the nurse must have a sound knowledge of the use, action, usual dose and side-effects of the drugs being administered. Various studies have shown that this is not always the case. Markowitz *et al.* (1981) came to the conclusion that not only nurses but doctors and pharmacists in the survey hospital needed to upgrade their knowledge of the drugs they prescribed or administered. They then went on to suggest that inadequate practitioner knowledge may contribute to the incidence of preventable adverse drug reactions in hospitals. Francis (1980) examined the number of 'hidden', i.e. undeclared, medication errors committed by nurses. In the survey hospital it was found that nurses made ten times more of such errors than they reported.

Observation of the patient receiving medication is important. No drug produces a single effect. The combined effect of two or more drugs taken together may be different from the effects when taken separately. The effectiveness of any drug should be noted and any signs of resistance or dependence reported. Side-effects may vary from slight symptoms to severe reaction and any signs must be brought to the attention of the appropriate personnel.

The nurse must also be aware of the hazards involved in handling drugs, detergents and alcohols. Nurses Action Group (1981) attempts to highlight some hazards and offers advice on how nurses should protect themselves from some of the more common preparations found in hospitals.

Wherever possible, patients should be encouraged to be responsible for storing and administering their own medication. Falconer (1971), in her study, found that patients were able to cope proficiently with the administration of their medication. Even mildly confused patients, who were, initially, judged to be unsuitable for self-medication, were able to become independent after a period of instruction and supervision. Roberts (1978), in her study of self-medication in the elderly, reported that no patient took another's medication. Most patients kept their medicines in handbags or other places of safety. The common factor among those who failed to comply was that of ignoring the tablets altogether. There was no evidence of overdosage.

Injections

Injection is defined as the act of giving medication by use of a syringe and needle.

Newton and Newton (1979) identify eight routes for the use of parental injection:

1	intra-arterial	5	intralesional
2	intra-articular	6	intramuscular
3	intracardiac	7	intravenous
4	intradermal	8	subcutaneous.

Intrathecal routes are employed when the prescribed drug is unable to cross the blood/brain barrier. These authors also include a useful table of the tissues, sites and types of needle used, the amount of medication usually injected and the medications commonly administered via these routes.

SITES OF INJECTION

Site selection is predetermined for intra-arterial, intra-articular, intracardiac, intralesional and intrathecal injections. The choice of the remaining sites will normally depend on the desired therapeutic effect and the patient's safety and comfort.

Intradermal

Chosen sites are the ventral forearms and the scapulae. Observation of an inflammatory reaction is a priority, so the best sites are those that are highly pigmented, thinly keratinized and hairless.

Subcutaneous

Chosen sites are the lateral aspects of the upper arms, and thighs, the abdomen in the umbilical region, the back and the lower loins. Slow absorption is a priority so ideal sites are those poorly supplied with sensory nerves. Rotation of these sites decreases the likelihood of irritation and ensures improved absorption.

Intramuscular

Intramuscular injections are given at five sites (see Figure 11.1):

1 *Mid-deltoid*: used for the injection of such drugs as narcotics, sedatives, absorbed tetanus toxoid, vaccines, epinephrine in oil and vitamin B_{12}. It has the advantage of being easily accessible whether the patient is standing, sitting or lying down. It is also a better site than the gluteal muscles for small-volume (less than 2 ml), rapid-onset injections. Because the area is small, it limits the number and size of the injections that can be given at this point.

2 *Gluteus medius*: used for deep intramuscular and Z-track injections. The gluteus muscle has the lowest drug absorption rate. The muscle mass is also likely to have atrophied in elderly, non-ambulant and emaciated patients. This site carries with it the danger of the needle hitting the sciatic nerve and the superior gluteal arteries.

3 *Gluteus minimus*: used for antibiotics, anti-emetics, deep intramuscular and Z-track injections in oil, narcotics and sedatives. It is best used when large-volume intramuscular injections are required and for injections in the elderly, non-ambulant and emaciated patient as the site is away from major nerves and vascular structures.

4 *Rectus femoris*: used for anti-emetics, narcotics, sedatives, injections in oil, deep intramuscular and Z-track injections. It is the preferred site for infants and for self-administration of injections.

5 *Vastus lateralis*: used for deep intramuscular and Z-track injections. This site is free from major nerves and blood vessels. It is a large muscle and can accommodate repeated injections.

SKIN PREPARATION

McConnell (1982) quotes the two most common solutions for preparing the skin for injection as ethyl alcohol and the iodophors, such as povidone-iodine (Betadine). If using the iodophors, the nurse must check beforehand

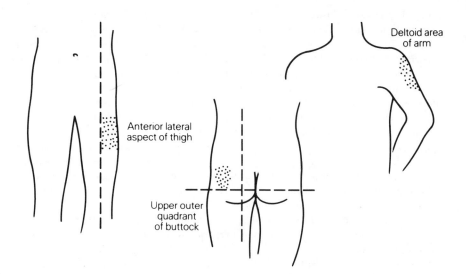

Figure 11.1 Sites for intramuscular injections.

that the patient is not allergic to iodine. An iodophor must not be used to prepare the skin for an intradermal injection as the solution discolours the skin and this makes it difficult to assess any expected reaction.

When cleaning the skin, the use of friction together with a circular motion is recommended. The nurse should begin at the centre of the chosen site and progress outwards. The antiseptic must be allowed to dry thoroughly before injection, otherwise the antiseptic may be forced into the tissue with the injection.

Research, however, has questioned the value of skin preparation prior to injection. Dann (1969) has shown that there is no experimental evidence that skin bacteria are introduced into the deeper tissues by injection, thereby causing infection. Antiseptics in current use cannot act in the time allowed in practice (5 seconds on average) and cannot possibly cause complete sterility. Over a period of 6 years, during which time more than 5,000 injections were given to unselected patients via all the injection routes, without using any form of skin preparation, no single case of local and/or systemic infection was reported. Only before injections where strict asepsis is needed, as in intrathecal or intra-articular injections, is skin preparation required. Koivistov and Felig (1978) carried out a survey into the need for skin preparation before giving an insulin injection and found that skin preparation did reduce skin bacterial count but was not necessary to prevent infection at the injection site.

NEEDLE BEVEL
Three categories of needle bevel are available:

1 *regular*: for all intramuscular and subcutaneous injections;

2 *intradermal*: for diagnostic injections and other injections into the epidermis;

3 *short*: tends to be used rarely. It is recommended only for transferring medication from container to syringe.

NEEDLE SIZE
Lenz (1983) states that when choosing the correct needle length for intramuscular injections it is important to assess the muscle mass of the injection site, the amount of subcutaneous fat and the weight of the patient. Without such an assessment, most injections intended for gluteal muscle are deposited in gluteal fat. The following are suggested by the author as ways of determining the most suitable size of needle to use:

Deltoid and vastus lateralis muscles
The muscle to be used should be grasped between thumb and forefinger to determine the depth of the muscle mass or the amount of subcutaneous fat at the injection site. One half of the distance between thumb and forefinger will be the appropriate length of the needle required to penetrate into that muscle.

Gluteal muscles
The layer of fat and skin above the muscle should be gently lifted with the thumb and forefinger for the same reasons as before. Use the patient's weight to calculate the needle length required. Lenz recommends (1983) the following guide:

31.5–40 kg	2.5-cm needle
40.5–90 kg	5–7.5-cm needle
90+ kg	10–15-cm needle.

INJECTIONS AND PAIN

McConnell (1982) and Newton and Newton (1979) set out, in point form, techniques which may reduce the discomfort experienced by the patient. Kruszewski *et al.* (1979) focus on ways in which positioning can help to minimize pain. Field (1981), in an interesting article, attempts to answer the question of what it is like to give an injection, and goes on to explore the meaning and use of language relating to injections, the feelings involved in preparing and administering injections, and the meaning of the patient's response to the nurse.

Intravenous drug administration

The administration of intravenous medications is an area in which the role of the nurse is being increasingly extended. For further information on intravenous drug administration see pp. 179–204.

Intra-arterial drug administration

Injection of drugs into an artery is a rare and hazardous procedure. The introduction of the cannula or catheter must be performed with care as the vessel may go into spasm, causing pain and occlusion. This could result in necrosis of an organ or part of a limb. Injection of irritant chemicals increases the risk of spasm and its sequentiae. In patients with some forms of cancer, however, arterial catheterization is occasionally performed when it is desirable to deliver a high concentration of a drug to a tumour mass. The most common procedures are catheterization of the hepatic artery and isolated limb perfusion.

References and further reading

Adamson, L. (1978) Control of medicines in the UK, *Nursing Times*, Vol. 74, pp. 973–5.

Bayliss, P.F.C. (1980) *Law on Poisons, Medicines and Related Substances*, 3rd edn, Ravenswood Publications, London.

Central Health Services Council (1958) *Report of Joint Sub-Committee on the Control of Dangerous Drugs and Poisons in Hospitals* (Chairman J.K. Aitken), HMSO, London.

Dale, J.R. and Appelbe, G.E. (1983) *Pharmacy, Law and Ethics*, 3rd edn, The Pharmaceutical Press, London.

Dann, T.C. (1969) Routine skin preparation before injection: an unnecessary procedure, *Lancet*, Vol. ii, pp. 96–7.

David, J.A. (1983) *Drug Round Companion*, Blackwell Scientific, Oxford.

Dorr, R. and Fritz, W. (1980) *Cancer Chemotherapy Handbook*, Kimpton, London.

Downie, G. *et al.* (1987) *Drug Management for Nurses*, Churchill Livingstone, Edinburgh.

Drugs and Therapeutics Bulletin (1977) Storage and shelf life of drugs: when is it important? *Drugs and Therapeutics Bulletin*, Vol. 15, no. 21, pp. 81–3.

Falconer, M. (1971) Self administered medication, *Hospital Administration in Canada*, Vol. 13, no. 5, pp. 28–30.

Field, P.A. (1981) A phenomenological look at giving an injection, *Journal of Advanced Nursing*, Vol. 6, no. 4, pp. 291–6.

Fink, J.L. (1983) Preventing lawsuits, *Nursing Life*, Vol. 3, no. 2, pp. 27–9.

Francis, G. (1980) Nurses' medication 'errors': a new perspective, *Supervisor Nurse*, Vol. 11, no. 8, pp. 11–13.

Hopkins, S.J. (1987) *Drugs and Pharmacology for Nurses*, 9th edn, Churchill Livingstone, Edinburgh.

Koivistov, V.A. and Felig, P. (1978) Is skin preparation necessary before insulin injection? *Lancet*, Vol. i, pp. 1072–3.

Kruszewski, A.Z. *et al.* (1979) Effect of positioning on discomfort from intramuscular injections in the dorsogluteal site, *Nursing Research*, Vol. 28, no. 2, pp. 103–5.

Lenz, C.L. (1983) Make your needle selection right to the point, *Nursing (US)*, Vol. 13, no. 2, pp. 50–1.

Loebl, S. *et al.* (1980) *The Nurse's Drug Handbook*, 2nd edn, John Wiley, Chichester, pp. 10–22.

Lydiate, P.W.H. (1977) *The Law Relating to the Misuse of Drugs*, Butterworth, London.

McConnell, E.A. (1982) The subtle art of really good injections, *Research Nurse*, Vol. 45, no. 2, pp. 25–34.

Markowitz, J.S. *et al.* (1981) Nurses, physicians, and pharmacists: their knowledge of hazards of medication, *Nursing Research*, Vol. 30, no.6, pp. 366–70.

Marks, M. (no date) *Neoplatin Cisplatin: A Nurse's Guide*, Mead Johnson.

Newton, D.W. and Newton, M. (1979) Route, site and technique: three key decisions in giving parenteral injections, *Nursing (US)*, Vol. 9, no. 7, pp. 18–25.

Nurses Action Group (1981) Health and safety 3. Beware the drug, *Nursing Mirror*, Vol. 152, pp. 22–5.

Pearson, R.M. and Nestor, P. (1977) Drug interactions, *Nursing Mirror*, Vol. 145, Suppl. XI.

Roberts, R. (1978) Self medication trial for the elderly, *Nursing Times*, Vol. 74, no. 23, pp. 976–7.

Thomas, S. (1979) Practical nursing – medicines: care and administration, *Nursing Mirror*, Vol. 148, pp. 28–30.

Wade, A. (1980) *Pharmaceutical Handbook*, 19th edn, The Pharmaceutical Press, London.

Whincup, M.H. (1982) *Legal Rights and Duties in Medical and Nursing Service*, 3rd edn, Ravenswood Publications, London.

Wieck, L. *et al.* (1986) *Illustrated Manual of Nursing Techniques*, 3rd edn, J.B. Lippincott, Philadelphia.

GUIDELINES: ORAL DRUG ADMINISTRATION

Equipment
1   Medicine trolley
2   Jug of water
3   Tumblers
4   Graduated medicine containers
5   Bowl with warm soapy water
6   Roll of paper towel
7   Disposable waste bag
8   Two spoons.

Procedure

Action	**Rationale**
1 Wash hands.	To prevent cross-infection.
2 Ensure that the medicine trolley is prepared before beginning the procedure.	To prevent interruption of the procedure once it has begun.
3 It is usual to carry out the procedure in the company of another nurse. One nurse should be a qualified nurse. The other nurse, preferably, should be a student.	To minimize error. To create a learning situation.
4 Before administering any prescribed drug, check that it is due and has not been given already. Check that the information contained in the prescription chart is complete, correct and legible.	To protect the patient from harm.
5 Select the required medication and check the expiry date.	Treatment with medication that is outside the expirty date is dangerous. Drugs deteriorate with storage. The expiry date indicates when a particular drug is no longer pharmacologically efficacious.
6 Empty the required dose into a medicine container. Avoid touching the preparation.	To prevent cross-infection. To prevent harm to the nurse.
7 Take the medication and the prescription chart to the patient. Check the patient's identity and the dose to be given.	To prevent error.
8 Evaluate the patient's knowledge of the medication being offered. If this knowledge appears to be faulty or incorrect, offer an explanation of the use, action, dose and potential side-effects of the drug or drugs involved.	A patient has a right to information about treatment.
9 Administer the drug as prescribed.	
10 Offer a glass of water, if allowed, to facilitate swallowing the medication.	

11 Record the dose given in the prescription chart and in any other place made necessary by legal requirement or hospital policy.	To meet legal requirements and hospital policy.
12 Place the used medicine container and tumbler in the bowl of warm, soapy water.	
13 Administer irritating drugs with meals or snacks.	To minimize their effect on the gastric mucosa.
14 Administer drugs that interfere with foods, or drugs destroyed in significant proportions by digestive enzymes, between meals or on an empty stomach.	To prevent interference with the absorption of the drug.
15 Do not break a tablet unless it is scored. Break scored tablets with a file.	Breaking may cause incorrect dosage, gastrointestinal irritation or destruction of a drug in an incompatible pH.
16 Do not interfere with time-release capsules and enteric coated tablets. Instruct patients to swallow these whole and not to chew them.	The absorption rate of the drug will be altered.
17 Sublingual tablets must be placed under the tongue and buccal tablets between gum and cheek.	To allow for correct absorption.
18 When administering liquids to babies and young children, or when an accurately measured dose in multiples of 1 ml is needed for an adult, an oral syringe should be used in preference to a medicine spoon or measure.	A syringe is much more accurate than a measure or a 5-ml spoon.
	Use of a syringe makes administration of the correct dose much easier in an unco-operative child.
	Special syringes are available for this purpose:
	(a) They are washable and re-usable; the graduations do not readily rub off.
	(b) They have a non-Leur fitting to which it is impossible to attach a needle in error.
19 In babies and children especially, correct use of the syringe is very important. The tip should be gently pushed into and towards the side of the mouth. The contents are then *slowly* discharged towards the inside of the cheek, pausing if necessary to allow the liquid to be swallowed. In difficult children it may help to place the end of the barrel between the teeth!	To prevent injury to the mouth and eliminate the danger of choking the patient.
	To get the dose in and to prevent the patient spitting it out.

CONTROLLED DRUGS

Action	**Rationale**
1 Two nurses should be involved in the administration of a controlled drug, one of whom must be a registered general nurse.	To comply with the legal obligations and hospital policy.
2 Select the correct drug from the controlled drug cupboard.	

Action	**Rationale**
3 Check the stock against the last entry in the ward record book.	To comply with the legal obligations and hospital policy.
4 Check the appropriate dose against the prescription sheet.	
5 Return the remaining stock to the cupboard and lock the cupboard.	
6 Enter the date and the patient's name in the ward record book.	
7 Take the prepared dose to the patient, whose identity is checked.	
8 Administer the drug after checking the prescription chart again. Once the drug has been administered, the prescription chart is signed by the nurse responsible for administering the medication.	
9 The dose, time of administration and the signatures of the two nurses are entered against the patient's name in the ward record book.	

GUIDELINES: ADMINISTRATION OF INJECTIONS

Equipment
1   Clean tray or receiver in which to place drug and equipment
2   19G needle(s) to ease reconstitution and drawing up
3   21, 23 or 25G needle, size dependent on route of administration
4   Syringe(s) of appropriate size for amount of drug to be given
5   Swabs saturated with isopropyl alcohol 70%
6   Sterile topical swab, if drug is presented in ampoule form
7   Drug(s) to be administered
8   Patient's prescription chart, to check dose, route, etc.
9   Recording sheet or book as required by law or hospital policy
10   Any protective clothing required by hospital policy for specified drugs, such as antibiotics or cytotoxic drugs.

Procedure

Action	**Rationale**
1 Collect and check all equipment.	To prevent delays and enable full concentration on the procedure.
2 Check that the packaging of all equipment is intact.	To ensure sterility. If the seal is damaged, discard.
3 Wash hands.	To prevent contamination of medication and equipment.

4   Prepare needle(s), syringe(s), etc. on a tray or receiver.

5   Inspect all equipment.

To check that none is damaged; if so, discard.

6   Consult the patient's prescription sheet, and ascertain the following:
  (a)   drug
  (b)   dose
  (c)   date and time of administration
  (d)   route and method of administration
  (e)   diluent as appropriate
  (f)   validity of prescription
  (g)   signature of doctor.

To ensure that the patient is given the correct drug in the prescribed dose using the appropriate diluent and by the correct route.

7   Check all details with another nurse if required by hospital policy.

To minimize any risk of error.

8   Select the drug in the appropriate size of container, and check the expirty date.

To reduce wastage.
To prevent an ineffective or toxic compound being administered to the patient.

9   Proceed with the preparation of the drug, using protective clothing if advisable.

SINGLE DOSE AMPOULE: SOLUTION

Action

Rationale

1   Inspect the solution for cloudiness or particulate matter. If this is present, discard and follow hospital guidelines on what action to take, e.g. return drug to pharmacy.

To prevent the patient from receiving an unstable or contaminated drug.

2   Tap the neck of the ampoule gently.

To ensure that all the solution is in the bottom of the ampoule.

3   Cover the neck of the ampoule with a sterile topical swab and snap it open. If there is any difficulty a file may be required.

To aid asepsis. To prevent aerosol formation or contact with the drug which could lead to a sensitivity reaction. To prevent injury to the nurse.

4   Inspect the solution for glass fragments; if present, discard.

To prevent injection of foreign matter into the patient.

5   Withdraw the required amount of solution, tilting the ampoule if necessary.

To avoid drawing in any air.

6   Replace the guard on the needle and tap the syringe to dislodge any air bubbles. Expel air.

To prevent aerosol formation, etc.
To ensure that the correct amount of drug is in the syringe.

7   Alternatives to expelling the air with the needle guard in place include the following:
  (a)   Covering the needle tip with sterile cotton wool or topical swab.
  (b)   Using the ampoule or vial to receive any air and/or drug.

Action	Rationale
8 Change the needle.	To reduce the risk of infection. To avoid tracking medications through superficial tissues. To ensure that the correct size of needle is used for the injection.

SINGLE DOSE AMPOULE: POWDER

Action	Rationale
1 Tap the neck of the ampoule gently.	To ensure that any powder lodged here falls to the bottom of the ampoule.
2 Cover the neck of the ampoule with a sterile topical swab and snap it open. If there is any difficulty a file may be required.	To aid asepsis. To prevent contact with the drug which could cause a sensitivity reaction. To prevent injury to the nurse.
3 Add the correct diluent carefully down the wall of the ampoule.	To ensure that the powder is thoroughly wet before agitation and is not released into the atmosphere.
4 Agitate the ampoule and inspect the contents.	To dissolve the drug. To detect any glass fragments or particulate matter. If present, continue agitation or discard as appropriate.
5 When the solution is clear withdraw the prescribed amount, tilting the ampoule if necessary.	To avoid drawing in air.
6 Replace the guard on the needle and tap the syringe to dislodge any air bubbles. Expel air.	To prevent aerosol formation, etc. To ensure that the correct amount of drug is in the syringe.
7 Change the needle.	To reduce the risk of infection. To avoid tracking medications though superficial tissues. To ensure that the correct size of needle is used for the injection.

MULTIDOSE VIAL: SOLUTION

Action	Rationale
1 Inspect the solution for cloudiness or particulate matter. If this is present, discard. Follow hospital guidelines on what action to take, e.g. return drug to pharmacy.	To prevent patient from receiving an unstable or contaminated drug.
2 Clean the rubber cap with the chosen antiseptic and let it dry.	To prevent bacterial contamination of the drug.
3 Insert a 19G needle into the cap to vent the bottle (Figure 11.2a).	To prevent pressure differentials which can cause separation of needle and syringe.
4 Withdraw the prescribed amount of solution, and inspect for pieces of rubber which may have 'cored out' of the cap (Figure 11.2b).	To prevent the injection of foreign matter into the patient.

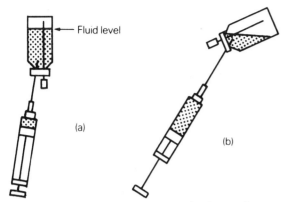

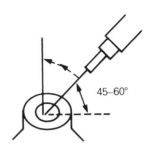

Figure 11.2   *a*, To remove reconstituted solution, insert syringe needle then invert vial. Ensuring that tip of second needle is above fluid, withdraw solution. *b*, Remove air from syringe without spraying into the atmosphere by injecting air back into vial.

Figure 11.3   Method to minimize coring.

Note: Coring can be minimized by inserting the needle into the cap, bevel up, at an angle of 45–60°. Before complete insertion of the needle tip, lift the needle to 90° and proceed (Figure 11.3).

5 Replace the guard on the needle and tap the syringe to dislodge any air bubbles. Expel air.

To prevent aerosol formation. To ensure that the correct amount of drug is in the syringe.

6 Change the needle.

To reduce the risk of infection. To avoid possible trauma to the patient if the needle has barbed. To avoid tracking medications through superficial tissues. To ensure that the correct size of needle is used for the injection.

MULTIDOSE VIAL: POWDER

Action

Rationale

1 Clean the rubber cap with the chosen antiseptic and let it dry.

To prevent bacterial contamination of the drug.

2 Insert a 19G needle into the cap to vent the bottle (Figure 11.4*a*).

To prevent pressure differentials, which can cause separation of needle and syringe.

3 Add the correct diluent carefully down the wall of the vial.

To ensure that the powder is thoroughly wet before it is shaken and is not released into the atmosphere.

4 Remove the needle and the syringe.

5 Place a sterile wool ball over the venting needle (Figure 11.4*b*).

To prevent contamination of the drug or the atmosphere.

6 Proceed to the patient.

Note: The nurse may encounter other presentations of drugs for injection, e.g. vials with a transfer needle, and should follow the manufacturer's instructions in these instances.

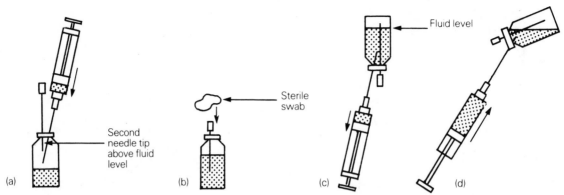

Figure 11.4   Suggested method of vial reconstitution to avoid environmental exposure, *a*, When reconstituting vial, insert a second needle to allow air to escape when adding diluent for injection, *b*, When shaking the vial to dissolve the powder, push in second needle up to Luer connection and cover with a sterile swab. *c*, To remove reconstituted solution, insert syringe needle then invert vial. Ensuring that tip of second needle is above the fluid, withdraw the solution. *d*, Remove air from syringe without spraying into the atmosphere by injecting air back into vial.

SUBCUTANEOUS INJECTIONS

Action	**Rationale**
1 Explain the procedure to the patient.	To obtain the patient's consent and co-operation.
2 Assist the patient into the required position.	
3 Expose the chosen site.	
4 Choose the correct needle size.	To minimize the risk of missing the subcutaneous tissue and any ensuing pain.
5 Clean the chosen site with a swab saturated with isopropyl alcohol 70%.	To reduce the number of pathogens introduced into the skin by the needle at the time of insertion. (For further information on this action see Reference Material, pp. 129–30.)
6 Grasp the skin firmly.	To elevate the subcutaneous tissue.
7 Insert the needle into the skin at an angle of 45° and release the grasped skin.	Injecting medication into compressed tissue irritates nerve fibres and causes the patient discomfort.
8 Pull back the plunger. If no blood is aspirated, depress the plunger and inject the drug slowly. If blood appears, withdraw the needle, replace it and begin again. Explain to the patient what has occurred.	To confirm that the needle is in the correct position. To prevent pain and ensure even distribution of the drug.
9 Withdraw the needle rapidly. Apply pressure to any bleeding point.	To prevent haematoma formation.
10 Record in the appropriate documents that the injection has been given.	
11 Dispose of the equipment in the required fashion.	To ensure safe disposal and to avoid laceration or other injury to staff.

INTRAMUSCULAR INJECTIONS

Action	Rationale
1 Explain the procedure to the patient.	To obtain the patient's consent and co-operation.
2 Assist the patient into the required position.	
3 Expose the chosen site.	
4 Clean the chosen site with a swab saturated with isopropyl alcohol 70%.	To reduce the number of pathogens introduced into the skin by the needle at the time of insertion. (For further information on this action see Reference Material, pp. 129–30.
5 Stretch the skin around the chosen site.	To facilitate the insertion of the needle and to displace the subcutaneous tissue.
6 Holding the needle at an angle of 90°, quickly plunge it into the skin. Leave a third of the shaft of the needle exposed.	To ensure that the needle penetrates the muscle. To facilitate removal of the needle should it break.
7 Pull back the plunger. If no blood is aspirated, depress the plunger and inject the drug slowly. If blood appears, withdraw the needle, replace it and begin again. Explain to the patient what has occurred.	To confirm that the needle is in the correct position. To prevent pain and ensure even distribution of the drug.
8 Withdraw the needle rapidly. Apply pressure to any bleeding point.	To prevent haematoma formation.
9 Record in the appropriate documents that the injection has been given.	
10 Dispose of the equipment in the required fashion.	To ensure safe disposal and to avoid laceration or other injury to staff.

GUIDELINES: ADMINISTRATION OF RECTAL AND VAGINAL PREPARATIONS

Equipment
1   Disposable glove
2   Topical swabs
3   Lubricating jelly
4   Prescription chart.

Procedure
RECTAL PREPARATIONS
For further information about the administration of rectal medication see the relevant sections in the Procedure, Bowel Care (pp. 56–70).

VAGINAL PESSARIES

Action	Rationale
1 Explain the procedure to the patient.	To obtain the patient's consent and co-operation.

Action	Rationale
2 Select the appropriate pessary and check it with the prescription chart and another nurse.	To ensure that the correct medication is given to the correct patient at the appropriate time.
3 Assist the patient into the appropriate position, either left lateral with buttocks to the edge of the bed or supine the knees drawn up and legs parted.	To facilitate the correct insertion of the pessary.
4 Wash hands and put on gloves.	To prevent cross-infection.
5 Apply lubricating jelly to a topical swab and from the swab on to the pessary.	To facilitate insertion of the pessary and ensure the patient's comfort.
6 Insert the pessary along the posterior vaginal wall and into the top of the vagina. *Note*: This procedure is best performed late in the evening when the patient is unlikely to get out of bed.	To ensure that the pessary is retained and that the medication can reach its maximum efficiency.
7 Wipe away any excess lubricating jelly from the patient's vulval and/or perineal area with a topical swab.	To promote patient comfort.
8 Make the patient comfortable and apply a fresh sanitary pad.	To absorb any excess discharge.
9 Record in the appropriate documents that the pessary has been given.	

GUIDELINES: TOPICAL APPLICATIONS OF DRUGS

Equipment
1 Flat wooden spatulae.
2 Sterile topical swabs.
3 Applicators.

Procedure

Action	Rationale
1 Explain the procedure to the patient.	To obtain the patient's consent and co-operation.
2 Use aseptic technique if the skin is broken.	To prevent local or systemic infection.
3 Remove semisolid or stiff preparations from their containers with a flat wooden spatula. Use a different spatula each time if more of the preparation is required.	To prevent cross-infection.
4 If the medication is to be rubbed into the skin, the preparation should be placed on a sterile topical swab. The wearing of gloves may be necessary.	To prevent cross-infection. To protect the nurse.
5 If the preparation causes staining, advise the patient of this.	To ensure that adequate precautions are taken beforehand and to prevent unwanted stains.

GUIDELINES: ADMINISTRATION OF DRUGS IN OTHER FORMS

Procedure

INHALATIONS

Action	Rationale
1 Seat the patient in an upright position if possible.	To permit full expansion of the diaphragm.
2 Administer only one drug at a time unless specifically instructed to the contrary.	Several drugs used together may cause undesirable reactions or they may inactivate each other.
3 Measure any liquid medication with a syringe.	To ensure the correct dose.
4 Clean any equipment used after use.	To prevent infection.
5 Correct use of aerosol inhalers is essential and will only be achieved if this is carefully explained and demonstrated to the patient.	Incorrect use may result in most of the dose remaining in the mouth and/or being expelled almost immediately. This renders treatment ineffective.

GARGLES

Action	Rationale
1 Throat irrigations should not be warmer than 49 °C.	Any liquid warmer than 49 °C will destroy or damage tissue.

NASAL DROPS

Action	Rationale
1 Have paper tissues available.	To wipe away secretions and/or medication.
2 Clean the patient's nasal passages.	To ensure maximum penetration for the medication.
3 Hyperextend the patient's neck.	To obtain the best position for insertion of the medication.
4 Avoid touching the external nares with the dropper.	To prevent the patient from sneezing.
5 Request the patient to maintain his/her position for 1–2 minutes.	To ensure full absorption of the medication.
6 Each patient should have his/her own medication and dropper.	To prevent cross-infection.

EYE MEDICATIONS
For information on Eye Care see pp. 156–64.

EAR DROPS

Action	Rationale
1 Ask the patient to lie on his/her side with the ear to be treated uppermost.	To ensure the best position for insertion of the drops.

Action	Rationale
2 Warm the drops to body temperature if allowed.	To prevent trauma to the patient.
3 Pull the cartilagenous part of the pinna backwards and upwards.	To prepare the auditory meatus for instillation of the drops.
4 Allow the drops to fall in the direction of the external canal.	To ensure that the medication reaches the target.
5 Request the patient to remain in this position for 1–2 minutes.	To allow the medication to reach the eardrum and be absorbed.

SINGLE-NURSE ADMINISTRATION OF DRUGS

Certain nurses may administer drugs by themselves provided it is the policy of the health authority by whom they are employed and they have received specific training, both in theory and practice, and are in possession of a certificate stating their proficiency in the technique.

It is felt that this will result in greater care being given since that one nurse will be aware that she/he is solely responsible and accountable.

Those nurses who wish or need to have their administration supervised will retain the right to do so until such time as all parties agree that the requested level of proficiency has been achieved.

SELF-ADMINISTRATION OF DRUGS

Definition
Patients are responsible for taking their own prescribed drugs. The self-administration of prescribed drugs should not be confused with self-medication using over-the-counter drugs.

Indications
Ideally self-administration is practised when:
1 there is a safe locked place in which to store drugs;

2 pharmacy staff are able to dispense the drug individually;
3 the drug regimen is not subject to frequent adjustments.

For patients who have psychological or physical problems with taking drugs, the development of an education and training programme for self-administration needs to be undertaken prior to discharge. This will improve compliance.

REFERENCE MATERIAL
Research has concentrated on the advantages of self-administration for the elderly, mainly because this group have greater educational needs and frequently take two or more different drugs. Errors in compliance have been shown to increase with the number of drugs having to be taken (Garland, 1979). An increase in compliance has been demonstrated when training and memory aids are given to patients prior to discharge from hospital (Wandless, 1977). Such benefits are of equal advantage to other patient groups and are in line with self-care models of nursing. For patients who take drugs long term (for example endocrine replacement drugs) the removal of their drug-taking responsibility on hospital admission is humiliating, making them immediately dependent on nursing staff. They are also controlled by the timing of drug administration in hospital which may well produce physiological changes in the drug response.

Aids to self-administration are available for those with physical problems such as opening containers, measuring liquids as well as problems with remembering when drugs have to be taken (Williams, 1984).

References and further reading
Brock, A.M. (1979) Self administration of drugs in the elderly, *Nursing Forum*, Vol. 18, no. 4, pp. 340–57.
Central Health Services Council (1958) *Report of the Joint Sub-Committee on the Control of Dangerous*

Drugs and Posions in Hospitals (Chairman J.K. Aitken), HMSO, London.

David, J.A. (1983) *Drug Round Companion*, Blackwell Scientific, Oxford, Chs 3, 7 and 8.

Falconer, M. (1971) Self-administered medication, *Hospital Administration in Canada*, Vol. 13, no. 5, pp. 28–30.

Garland, M.H. (1979) Drugs and the elderly *Nursing Times*, Vol. 75, pp. 3–6.

Powys Health Authority (1984) *All Wales working party of Review of the Administration of Drugs by Nurses*, Powys Health Authority, Bronllys.

Roberts, R. (1978) Self-medication trial for the elderly, *Nursing Times*, Vol. 74, no. 23, pp. 976–7.

Royal College of Nursing (1983) *Drug Administration: A Nursing Responsibility*, 2nd edn, Royal College of Nursing of the United Kingdom, London.

Shannon, M. (1983) Self-medication in the elderly, *Nursing Mirror* Vol. 157; 12th October. *Clinical Forum*, Vol. 9, pp. i–iii, vi–viii.

Wandless I. and Davie, J.W. (1977) Can drug compliance in the elderly be improved? *British Medical Journal*, Vol. i, pp. 359–61.

Williams, A. (1984) Medicine management, *Nursing Mirror*, Vol. 159, no. 12, Suppl. 1 pp. i–viii.

GUIDELINES: SELF-ADMINISTRATION OF DRUGS

Equipment

1 Individually issued prescribed drugs in suitable containers
2 Locked drawer or locker for storage
3 Drug administration record prepared for self-administration.

Procedure

Action	Rationale
1 Take a drug history from the patient on admission.	This will record any drugs (prescribed or over the counter) being taken, allergies or idiosyncrasies to drugs, problems with self-administration and the patient's current understanding of his/her drugs.
2 Discuss the selection of the patient for self-administration with the charge nurse and pharmacist.	To ensure that the patient is suitable and that the drug can be supplied for self-administration from the pharmacy.
3 Explain self-administration to the patient, making a joint plan for education, storage and recording.	The patient is contracted to self-administer, education can be undertaken and co-operation ensured.
4 Check that drugs are taken correctly.	Checking drugs daily with the patient ensures compliance, offers educational opportunities and enables the nurse to record that drugs have been taken.
5 Ensure that new supplies are ordered for the patient, particularly if discharge is anticipated.	To continue administration without problems.
6 Evaluate the patient's capability to self-administer and the effectiveness of drug education.	To allow for a new plan if required and to set long-term goals.

NURSING CARE PLAN

Problems	Cause	Suggested action
Patient unwilling to self-administer.	Anxiety about drugs or present medical condition. Does not see the value of self-administration. Unsure of capabilities.	Discuss the problem, educate the patient and answer questions. Explain how self-administration can establish a routine. Work with the patient gradually giving more responsibility.
Failing memory.	Old age, confusion, anxiety.	Plan memory aids, timing of drug-taking linked to events. Diary or pad to tick off drugs taken. Drugs packed for daily administration, e.g. in Dosette box (Cow and Gate Ltd).
Physical problems: dexterity, vision, communication.	Arthritis, old age, does not speak English.	Make use of aids (Williams, 1984), an interpreter and the adaptation of practice to meet the individual patient's needs.
Special technique required for administration.	Drug to be given via central line, rectally or vaginally. Drugs to be given by relative (children).	Introduce the technique to the patient (relative) and gradually involve in administration. Remain available once competence is achieved.

12

Entonox Administration

Definition

Entonox is a gaseous mixture of 50% oxygen and 50% nitrous oxide which acts as an analgesic agent when inhaled. The mixture remains stable at temperatures of above −6°C.

The Entonox cylinder is coloured blue and has white segments on the shoulder. The apparatus consists of the cylinder, the Bodok seal, inhalation tubing and the handpiece. Either a mask or a mouthpiece may be used (Figure 12.1).

Indications

The use of Entonox is indicated prior to or during a number of painful procedures:

1   changing packs, drains and dressings;
2   removal of sutures from sensitive areas, e.g. the vulva;
3   re-dressing burns, where an occlusive or open technique is not used;
4   invasive procedures such as catheterization and sigmoidoscopy;
5   childbirth;
6   removal of radioactive intracavity gynaecological applicators;
7   following myocardial infarction (Entonox provides safe analgesia as well as supplementary oxygen);
8   altering the position of a patient who is in pain;
9   manual evacuation of the bowel to relieve constipation;
10 traumatic injuries;
11 applying orthopaedic traction;
12 physiotherapy procedures, particularly postoperatively.

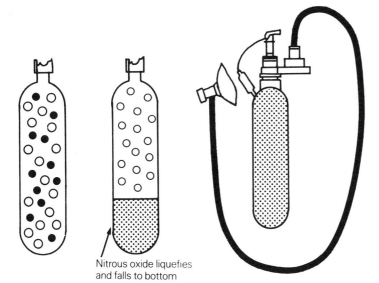

Nitrous oxide liquefies and falls to bottom

Figure 12.1   Entonox cylinder. The apparatus consists of the cylinder, the Bodok seal, inhalation tubing and the handpiece. Either a mask or a mouthpiece may be used.

Contraindictions

Its use is contraindicated in the following cases and situations:

1. maxillofacial injuries, as the patient may not be able to hold the mask tightly to the face or to use the mouthpiece adequately;
2. head injuries with impairment of consciousness;
3. heavily sedated patients;
4. intoxicated patients;
5. pneumothorax, as it will increase the problem;
6. the 'bends', as nitrous oxide escapes into the bloodstream and increases the size of the nitrogen bubbles in the tissues;
7. laryngectomy patients, as they will be unable to use the apparatus;
8. administration over continuous periods of longer than 48–72 hours as leucopenia may occur;
9. temperatures below −6 °C as separation of the gases occurs.

REFERENCE MATERIAL

The relief of pain for patients undergoing painful procedures is often not adequately met. The reasons for this are varied and range from the inability of professional personnel to measure adequately how much pain a patient is suffering to the difficulty of judging at the outset how painful a procedure will prove to be for a patient. Nurses are able to administer analgesics only if the doctor has specifically prescribed their use. Many procedures can only be assessed as painful once their performance has begun. At this stage it is difficult either to wait for a doctor to prescribe analgesics or to wait for a prescribed analgesic to take effect. In these situations an analgesic that could be prescribed and administered by nurses, would take rapid effect, would be equally rapidly excreted from the body and would have few side-effects is the ideal. Entonox meets all these criteria. See Table 12.1 for a comparison between opiates and Entonox.

Principle of administration

Entonox is designed for self-administration by the patient. The apparatus works as a demand unit, i.e. gas can only be obtained by the patient inhaling and producing a negative pressure. When the patient exhales, the gas flow stops. The patient must hold the mask firmly over his/her face to produce an airtight fit before the gas will flow. Expired gases escape by the expiratory valve on the handpiece. Alternatively, a mouthpiece can be used. It is essential to adhere to this method of self-administration as it is impossible for the patient to overdose him/herself because if he/she becomes drowsy he/she will relax his/her grip on the hand set and the gas flow will cease when no negative pressure is applied.

A smaller dose than normal of an opiate may be given to augment the effects of Entonox. This should be given in sufficient time to take effect before the procedure begins.

Table 12.1 Comparison of Opiates and Entonox

Opiates	Entonox
1 Usually have to be given by injection – an added discomfort for the patient. There is also the risk of local or systemic infection.	Inhaled, i.e. a painless procedure.
2 May take up to 1 hour to become effective.	Rapid onset, i.e. 1½–2 minutes.
3 Effects that last for approximately 1 hour or more.	Effects wear off rapidly, i.e. in approximately 2–5 minutes.
4 Need to be prescribed by a doctor.	Can be prescribed by an appropriately qualified trained nurse or physiotherapist.
5 Side-effects include respiratory and cardiovascular depression, emesis, drowsiness and thus an inability to co-operate.	Side-effects are few and self-limiting as the gas is self-administered. Recovery from side-effects such as drowsiness and amnesia is rapid.
6 Tend to decrease peripheral circulation in patients suffering from shock due to their effect on the cardiovascular system.	The extra oxygen in Entonox increases peripheral circulation oxygenation in patients suffering from shock.

Entonox has an oxygen content two and a half times that of air and is, therefore, a good way of giving extra oxygen as well as providing analgesia.

Personnel qualified to teach and supervise the use of Entonox

Only those staff who have been trained and supervised in the use of Entonox should be allowed to train and supervise patients. Usually these will be:
1   registered general nurses or certified midwifes;
2   physiotherapists.

References and further reading

Diggory, G. (1979) Entonox and its role in nursing care, *Nursing*, April, pp. 28–31.

Entonox (1975) Abstracted proceedings of the symposium on Entonox organized by the Department of Anaesthesia, St Bartholomew's Hospital, London.
Msi, J. (1981) The use of Entonox for the relief of pain experienced by cancer patients, in R. Tiffany (ed.) *Cancer Nursing Update*, Baillière Tindall, London.

Audiovisual aids

Entonox in Hospitals, BOC's Audio Visual Services, 42 Upper Richmond Road, West London SW14 8DD.

GUIDELINES: ENTONOX ADMINISTRATION

Equipment

1   Entonox cylinder and head
2   Face mask or mouthpiece.

Procedure

Action	**Rationale**
1 Check to see if there is gas in the Entonox cylinder by turning the tap in an anticlockwise (⌒) direction.	
2 Examine the gauge to determine how much gas is in the cylinder.	To ensure an adequate supply of gas throughout the procedure.
3 Ensure that the patient is in as comfortable a position as possible.	
4 Demonstrate how to use the apparatus by holding the mask tightly to your face and breathing in and out regularly and deeply. A hissing sound will indicate that the patient is inhaling the gas.	To ensure that the patient understands what to do before any painful procedure commences. To reassure the patient of the non-toxic effects of the gas. To provide a correct role model.
5 Allow the patient to practise using the apparatus.	To enable the patient to adopt the correct technique and observe the analgesic effect of the gas before the procedure commences.
6 Encourage the patient to breathe gas in and out for at least 2 minutes prior to commencing any painful procedure.	To allow sufficient time for an adequate circulatory level of nitrous oxide to provide analgesia. (When the patient inhales, gas enters first the lungs then the pulmonary and systemic circulations. It takes 1–2 minutes to build up reasonable concentrations of nitrous oxide in the brain.)

7 During the procedure keep encouraging the patient to breathe in and out regularly and deeply.

To maintain adequate circulatory levels, thus providing adequate analgesia.

8 At the end of the procedure observe the patient until the effects of the gas have worn off.

Some patients may feel a transient drowsiness or giddiness and should be discouraged from getting out of bed until these effects have worn off. It is rare for the patient to experience transient amnesia.

9 Turn off the Entonox supply from the cylinder by turning the tap in a clockwise ( ) direction. The gauge should then read 'Empty'.

To avoid potential seepage of gas from the apparatus.

10 Depress the diaphragm under the valve to express residual gas.

11 Wash the face mask, expiratory valve and handpiece in a neutral detergent.

To minimize the risk of cross-infection.

NURSING CARE PLAN

Problem	Cause	Suggested action
Patient not experiencing adequate analgesic effect.	Entonox cylinder empty. Apparatus not properly connected. Patient not inhaling deeply enough.	Check before procedure commences. Encourage the patient to breathe in until a hissing noise can be heard from the cylinder.
	Patient inhaling pure oxygen, i.e. cylinder has been stored below −6°C and nitrous oxide has liquified and settled at the bottom of the cylinder. (All cylinders should be stored horizontally at a temperature of 10°C or above for 24 hours before use.)	Initially safe, but later the patient may inhale pure nitrous oxide and be asphyxiated. Discontinue the procedure. Ensure adequate warming of the cylinder and inversion of the cylinder to remix the gases adequately.
	Not enough time has been allowed for nitrous oxide to exert its analgesic effect.	Allow at least 2 minutes of Entonox use before commencing the procedure.
Patient experiences generalized muscle rigidity.	Hyperventilation during inhalation.	Discontinue Entonox and allow the patient to recover. Explain the procedure again, stressing deep and regular inspiration. Try a mouthpiece instead of a mask.
Patient unable to tolerate a mask.	Smell of rubber, feeling of claustrophobia.	Try a mouthpiece.
Patient feels nauseated, drowsy or giddy.	Effect of nitrous oxide accumulation.	Discontinue Entonox administration – the effect will then rapidly disappear.

| Patient afraid to use Entonox. | Associates gases with previous hospital procedures, e.g. anaesthesia before surgery. | Demonstrate use and thus its non-toxic effects. |

13

Epidural Analgesia

Definition

Epidural analgesia provides blockage of nerve roots outside the dura. This technique provides analgesia, reflex muscle flaccidity, a degree of hypotension and consequent ischaemia secondary to sympathetic blockage, while allowing spontaneous respiration to continue relatively unimpaired.

Indications

Epidural (extradural) analgesia is indicated for the following purposes:

1 to provide analgesia during labour;
2 for patients undergoing surgery who are considered to be an anaesthetic risk, i.e. patients with respiratory disease or severe cardiovascular disease;
3 as a supplement to general anaesthesia;
4 to provide postoperative pain control;
5 to provide pain relief for patients suffering from rib fractures enabling them to maintain adequate respiratory function;
6 to provide relief from intractable pain, i.e. severe pain from bone metastases;
7 to enable individuals whose airway is difficult to intubate when surgery is required.

Contraindications

The procedure is contraindicated in the following cases:

Absolute

In individuals with coagulation problems due to risk of spinal haematoma.

1 iatrogenic, i.e. low platelet count, anticoagulated patients;
2 congenital, i.e. haemophiliacs;
3 local sepsis due to risk of meningitis, or epidural abscess;
4 allergy to local anaesthetic agents or opiates;
5 unstable spinal fractures;
6 patient does not consent.

Relative

1 cardiovascular disease;
2 spinal deformity;
3 patients with neurological problems.

REFERENCE MATERIAL
Anatomy and physiology

The epidural space lies between the spinal dura and the vertebral canal. Its average diameter is 0.5 cm and it is widest in the midline posteriorly in the lumbar region. The contents of the epidural (extradural) space include the dural sac and the spinal nerve roots, the extradural plexus of veins and the spinal arteries, lymphatics and fat. The usual distance between skin and epidural (extradural) space is 4–5 cm (see Figure 13.1).

Principle

A catheter is passed via a Tuohy needle to lie outside the dura in the space usually between L3 and L4 through which drugs may be given producing an effect on nerves coming off the cord plus some penetration. The following fibres are blocked: (1) anterior nerve roots; (2) posterior nerve roots and their ganglia; (3) mixed spinal nerves; (4) white and grey rami communicantes; (5) visceral afferents accompanying sympathetic fibres (6) certain descending pathways in the spinal cord.

A number of factors influence the spread of solution. These include the volume of solution injected, the age of the patient (elderly patients requiring less than young ones), the force of injection, drug used and level injected. Gravity (a head-down tilt) aids upward diffusion and vice versa. A high concentration solution spreads further than a similar volume of a low concentration solution.

Common solutions used

Lignocaine 0.5–2% has a rapid onset of about 10 minutes and provides good relaxation. The duration of effect is 1½–2 hours depending on the strength of solution employed.

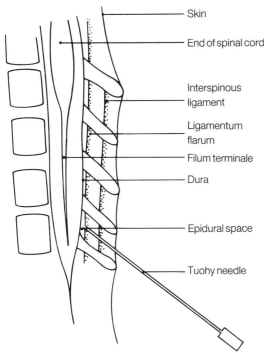

Skin

End of spinal cord

Interspinous ligament

Ligamentum flarum

Filum terminale

Dura

Epidural space

Tuohy needle

Figure 13.1   Diagrammatic section of lower vertebrae and spinal cord showing Tuohy needle *in situ*.

Bupivacaine (Marcaine) 0.25–0.75% is a long-acting drug giving analgesia for up to 8 hours.

Morphine sulphate 2–4 mg given in 5–10 ml of saline into the epidural (extradural) space can provide analgesia for up to 10 hours.

Other drugs used include amethocaine hydrochloride, prilocaine, adrenaline, and other opiates such as fentanyl. The duration of action is dependent on the drug used.

Complications of epidural analgesia

1   *Paraplegia* is a rare occurrence. It may be caused by cord infarction, stenosis of the vertebral canal or extradural spinal cord tumour.

2   *Intraocular haemorrhage* has been reported after rapid injection of 30 ml of fluid. This is thought to raise cerebrospinal fluid pressure with resultant intraocular bleeding.

3   *Backache* has occasionally been produced from local irritation of the needle or catheter.

4   *Extradural abscess* may take up to 16 days to develop. Extradural abscess or haematoma should be drained immediately after diagnosis otherwise paraplegia may result.

References and further reading

Atkinson, R.S. *et al.* (1982) *A Synopsis of Anaesthesia*, 9th edn, John Wright, Bristol.

Bibbings, J. (1984) Epidural analgesia, *Nursing Times*, Vol. 80, no. 35, pp. 53–5.

Sheargold, L. (1986) Epidural and spinal anaesthetics, *Nursing Times*, Vol. 82, no. 27, pp. 44–5.

Ward, M.E. (1978) Epidural analgesia, *Nursing*, no. 2, pp. 78–81.

GUIDELINES: EPIDURAL ANALGESIA

Note: Patients undergoing epidural analgesia should always have venous access/intravenous infusion prior to the procedure.

Equipment

1   Antiseptic skin-cleansing agent
2   Local anaesthetic
3   Selection of needles and syringes
4   Sterile dressing pack
5   Sterile gloves
6   Face mask
7   Tuohy needle or assorted gauge lumbar puncture needle
8   Epidural catheter
9   Bacterial filter such as Millipore
10   Waterproof plastic dressing, plastic dressing spray such as Sleek.

Procedure

Action	Rationale
1 Explain the procedure to the patient.	To obtain the patient's consent and co-operation.

2 Assist the patient into the required position:
(a) Lying:
        One pillow under his/her head.
        Firm surface.
        On side with knee drawn up to the abdomen and clasped by the hands.
        Support the patient in his/her position.
	To ensure maximum widening of the intervertebral spaces providing easier access to the epidural space.
	
	To prevent sudden movement.

(b) Sitting: Patient sits on firm surface with arms resting on a table resting head on arms.	Allows accurate identification of the spinal processes and therefore intervertebral spaces.
3 Support, encourage and observe the patient throughout procedure.	
4 Assist the doctor as required. The doctor will proceed as follows: (a) Clean the skin with antiseptic agent. (b) Identify the area to be punctured and inflitrate the skin and subcutaneous layers with local anaesthetic. (c) Introduce Tuohy or spinal needle usually between 3rd and 4th lumbar vertebrae. (d) Ensure epidural space has been entered. (e) Inject test dose of drug (may be performed). (f) Thread epidural catheter through barrel of Tuohy needle. (g) Attach the bacterial filter. (h) Apply dressing and sleek to catheter insertion site. (i) Inject solution into epidural space via catheter.	To maintain sterility. To prevent anaesthesia being given directly into spinal cord or intravenously via dural veins. To ensure the position of the needle. To facilitate intermittent topping up of anaesthesia and to allow greater control. To prevent injection of contaminants into epidural space. To prevent the catheter being dislodged. To provide anaesthesia.
5 Position the patient according to the doctor's instructions, tilting if appropriate.	To ensure spread of solution to provide optimum effect.
6 Take vital signs observations: blood pressure and respirations every 5 minutes for 30 minutes and then every 15 minutes for next 1½ hours. Pulse every 15 minutes for 2 hours.	To monitor for signs of hypotension and respiratory depression.
7 Make the patient comfortable. Usually the patient is nursed flat for the first 3–6 hours, then slowly elevated into a sitting position. Bedclothes should not constrict the feet.	To prevent the development of footdrop.

GUIDELINES: TOPPING UP EPIDURAL ANALGESIA

Usually performed by the doctor but may be performed by nursing staff as part of an extended role according to local policy.

Equipment
1 Antiseptic cleansing agent
2 Syringes and needles
3 Drug as prescribed
4 Water or saline for injection as necessary
5 Patient's prescription chart
6 Sterile hub/bung.

Procedure

Action	Rationale
1 Wash hands.	To prevent cross-infection.
2 Check the drug to be administered and dilutants according to policy.	To ensure the correct drug, amount and concentration is administered to the patient.
3 Draw up the drug.	
4 Clean access portal of the bacterial filter.	To prevent introduction of contaminants/micro-organisms into the epidural space.
5 Dispose of the equipment.	
6 Make the patient comfortable.	
7 Monitor vital signs: blood pressure and respirations every 5 minutes for 30 minutes then every 15 minutes for 1½ hours. Pulse every 15 minutes for 2 hours.	To monitor for signs of hypotension and respiratory depression.

GUIDELINES: REMOVAL OF AN EPIDURAL CATHETER

Equipment
1 Dressing pack
2 Skin-cleansing agent, i.e. normal saline
3 Povidone-iodine spray
4 Collodion
5 Occlusive dressing.

Procedure

Action	Rationale
1 Wash hands.	To minimize cross-infection.
2 Open the dressing pack.	
3 Remove the tape and dressing from catheter insertion site.	

Action	Rationale
4 Clean the area around the insertion site.	
5 Gently, in one swift movement, remove catheter. Check that it is removed intact by observing marks along the barrel.	To ensure the catheter is removed intact.
6 Spray insertion site with povidone-iodine spray.	As prophylaxis against infection along the catheter tract.
7 Apply collodion to the puncture site.	To provide closure/occlusion of the puncture site.
8 Apply an occlusive dressing and leave *in situ* for 24 hours.	To prevent inadvertent access for micro-organisms along the tract.

NURSING CARE PLAN

Problem	Cause	Suggested action
Rapid fall in blood pressure.	Sympathetic blockade producing hypotension.	If systolic blood pressure falls below 85mmHg; Summon medial aid. Tilt the patient's head down unless contraindicated. Give oxygen 4 litres/minute. To prevent hypoxia caused by pulmonary hypotension. Fully open intravenous infusion. To increase circulatory volume and blood pressure. Prepare 15–30 mg of ephedrine for intravenous injection which may be required by the doctor. Ephedrine increases heart rate/cardiac output and produces vasoconstriction by direct and indirect action on sympathetic nervous system.
Respiratory depression.	Medullary depression due to morphine/local anaesthetic drug.	Call for medical assistance. Prepare naloxone (Narcan) 0.4 mg intravenous. If prescribed give dose according to criteria i.e. respiratory rate < 8/min. Dosage counteracts respiratory depression but not the analgesic effect. If no improvement administer second dose. A further 0.4 mg naloxone intravenously can be given 5–10 minutes after first.

Prepare emergency equipment to
support respiration.

Total spinal anaesthesia.

Call for medical assistance.
Turn the patient into the supine position.
Ventilate the lungs.
Elevate the legs.
Prepare emergency drugs.
Open intravenous infusion.
Prepare equipment for intubation.

Total central neurological blockade:

(a)   Marked hypotension
(b)   Apnoea
(c)   Dilated pupils
(d)   Loss of consciousness.

Toxicity due to injected drug:

(a)   Disorientation
(b)   Twitching
(c)   Convulsions
(d)   Apnoea.

Call medical assistance.
Institute emergency measures.

14

Eye Care

Indications

Eye care may be necessary under the following circumstances:

1   to relieve pain and discomfort;
2   to prevent infection.

REFERENCE MATERIAL

The patient can be instructed to carry out many of the procedures involved in eye care him/herself. However, the nurse is often involved in caring for the postoperative, very ill or unconscious patient. Infection can easily be transmitted, by careless technique, from one eye to the other. In some cases this can lead to loss of sight.

Anatomy and physiology

The eyeball is protected from injury by the bony cavity of the orbit, the conjuctiva, the lacrimal apparatus, the eyebrows, the eyelids and eyelashes.

The eyeball itself has three layers (see Figure. 14.1):

1   the outermost, composed of the cornea and sclera;
2   the middle, composed of the choroid, ciliary body and iris (uveal tract);
3   the innermost, composed of the retina, macula lutea (yellow spot) and fovea centralis.

The function of the outer coat is protective. The middle layer is vascular and pigmented, while the innermost contains the light-sensitive nerve endings which are concerned with vision, i.e. the rods and cones.

The blood vessels of the retina are readily seen with an ophthalmoscope. Abnormal changes in these vessels can be indicative of both generalized diseases, such as diabetes and hypertension, and diseases of the eye itself.

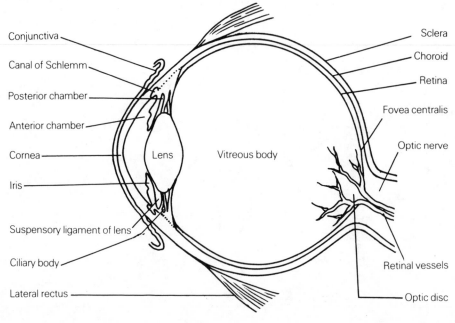

Figure 14.1 Anatomy and physiology of the eye.

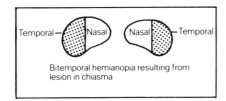

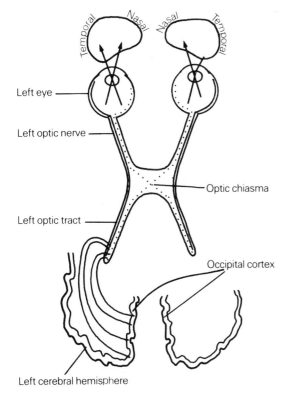

Figure 14.2 Visual pathways and visual fields.

The optic nerve (cranial nerve II) has two tracts which cross over at the optic chiasma. Each tract supplies the opposite side of the body. These tracts enter the eyeball to the side of the macula lutea. This area is known as the optic disc and is an area of no vision (blindspot) (see Figure 14.2).

The inside of the eyeball is divided by the lens into an anterior and posterior chamber. The anterior chamber is filled with a clear, watery fluid called the aqueous humour and the posterior chamber by a jelly-like substance called the vitreous humour which gives the eyeball its shape.

The tears are produced in the lacrimal gland (Figure 14.3). Their function is to wash over the eyeball, removing any foreign substances and providing antisepsis by the action of the enzyme lysozyme. Lysozyme ruptures the cell walls of bacteria and causes their lysis or death. The tears drain through the lacrimal puncti into the nasolacrimal duct. In health, the surface of the eye should always be slightly moist.

The cornea has no blood vessels and is dependent on the tears and aqueous humour for its nourishment.

General principles of eye care

Aseptic technique is not always essential when performing eye care, but the positions of the patient and the nurse in relation to the light source are vital in order for the procedure to be carried out safely and efficiently.

POSITION OF THE PATIENT

Where possible the patient should be lying down with his/her head tilted backwards and his/her chin pointing upwards. This enables ease of access to the eyes. It is also easier for the patient to maintain the head in this position when lying down.

POSITION OF THE NURSE

If possible the nurse should work from behind the patient's head. This gives him/her ease of access to both eyes and any equipment used can be kept out of the

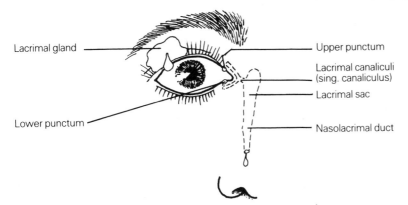

Figure 14.3 Lacrimal apparatus.

patient's line of vision. With the nurse behind him/her the patient is also more able to co-operate and less likely to try to follow the nurse's movements with his/her eyes.

POSITION OF THE LIGHT SOURCE

A good light source before commencing eye procedures is necessary in order to be able to assess carefully the state of the eyes and to avoid damaging their delicate structures during the procedure. The light should be above and behind the nurse or to his/her side. Light should never be allowed to shine directly into the patient's eyes as this will be painful and harmful to the patient.

Instillation of drops

Most types of drops are instilled into the outer side of the lower fornix as the conjuctiva is less sensitive than the cornea and the outer side avoids loss of the drops into the nasolacrimal passage. Exceptions to this are as follows:

1 *Drops used to lubricate the cornea*: these should be directed onto the cornea. Oil-based drops produce less corneal reaction than aqueous ones as they do not feel as cold to the cornea when administered.
2 *Anaesthetic drops*: the first drops should be instilled into the conjunctiva and then directly on to the cornea until the patient is no longer able to feel the drops.
3 *Drops used to treat the nasal passages*: these should be instilled at the punctal end of the eye.

The number of drops to be instilled depends on the type of solution used and its purpose. Usually one drop only is ordered and will be sufficient if it is instilled in the correct manner. The exceptions to the 'one drop' rule are:

1 *Oil-based solutions, e.g. paroleine*: this is used for lubricating the eyeball and several drops are usually ordered.
2 *Anaesthetic drops*: it is usual to instil two or three drops at a time at intervals, until the drop cannot be felt on the eye.

The dropper should be held as close to the eye as possible without touching either the lids or the cornea, i.e. approximately 2.5 cm. This will avoid corneal damage and the risk of infection. If the drop falls from too great a distance it is difficult to control and will also be uncomfortable for the patient.

There are a variety of droppers and bottles, including pipettes, pipettes incorporated into the eye drop bottle, plastic bottles and single dose packs. Pipettes are easy to use but need drying and sterilizing between doses. The disposable varieties are also expensive. The bottles that incorporate a pipette have an advantage in that the flow drops are easily controlled. Plastic bottles can be squeezed and so avoid the need for a pipette but again, they are

expensive. Ideally, single-dose containers should be used if they do not prove too expensive for routine use.

Eye irrigation

The most common use of eye irrigation is for the removal of a caustic substance from the eye. This should be done as soon as possible to minimize damage. The procedure is also used as a preoperative preparation or to remove infected material. The lotion most commonly ordered is normal saline. Boracic lotion in a solution of 4% may also be used. In an emergency, water may be used.

Care of an insensitive eye

Any interference with the sensory nerve supply to the eye, such as unconsciousness, will cause the eye surface to become insensitive. The blink reflex is often lost, the eye surface becomes dry and the cornea may be damaged. Corneal ulcers, scarring and loss of vision may be the end result.

When a patient has lost these protective reflexes it is the duty of the nurse to institute measures to replace them. The treatment aims at keeping the eye surface clean by swabbing, lubricating the surface, the instillation of oil-based drops, such as paroleine, and protecting the cornea by closing the eyelids. In certain cases the lids may be kept closed by the use of a non-allergenic tape. Eye pads should be avoided as the eye may open beneath them, rubbing or scratching the cornea. Frequency of care is determined by the needs of the individual patient.

Eye medications

Drugs may be given either systemically or topically to exert an effect on the eye. However, if given systemically the prescribing doctor needs to take account of the physiological barrier and the blood/aqueous barrier which exists within the eye and which is selective in allowing drugs to pass into the intraocular fluids. Permeability of this barrier may be altered in inflammatory conditions and following paracentesis.

Drugs applied locally meet some resistance at the tear film. The cornea allows the passage of water but not of drugs. This resistance may alter where there are corneal epithelial changes. Wetting agents may be employed to alter corneal permeability.

Many drugs will produce similar effects on a diseased or a healthy eye. Drugs for use in the eye are usually classified according to their action:

MYDRIATICS AND CYCLOPLEGICS

These drugs produce their effects by paralysing the sphincter, by stimulating the dilator muscle of the pupil or by a combination of both (see Figure 14.4). Atropine 1% is the most commonly used mydriatic. It is usually administered as drops but can be used as an ointment. It

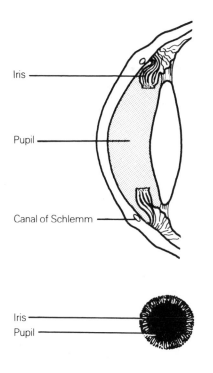

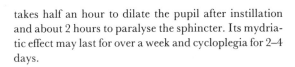

Figure 14.4 Effect of mydriatics.

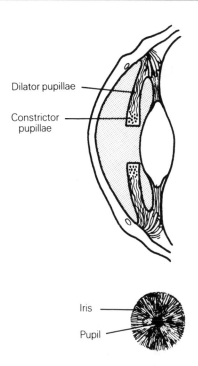

Figure 14.5 Effect of miotics.

takes half an hour to dilate the pupil after instillation and about 2 hours to paralyse the sphincter. Its mydriatic effect may last for over a week and cycloplegia for 2–4 days.

MIOTICS
These drugs produce their effects by constricting the pupil and contracting the ciliary muscle (Figure 14.5). Miotics are used primarily in the treatment of glaucoma.

LOCAL ANAESTHETICS
These render the eye and the inner surfaces of the lids insensitive. They are used prior to minor surgery, removal of foreign bodies and tonometry. Cocaine is less used now as some patients develop an idiosyncrasy to it and may suddenly collapse after its use. Its effects do not wear off for at least half an hour after administration.

ANTI-INFLAMMATORIES
These may be steroids, antihistamines or pyrazole derivatives, such as oxyphenabutazone 10%.

ANTIBIOTICS
Antibiotics can be used in the active treatment of infection and as prophylactics both pre- and postoperatively, following removal of a foreign body or following an injury. Antibiotic preparations in common use are framycetin 0.5%, sulphacetamide 10, 20 and 30%, neomycin 0.5% and chloramphenicol 0.5%.

ARTIFICIAL TEARS
Where tear deficiency exists due to disease processes, treatment with radiation or reduction of the blink reflex, artificial lubricants such as methyl cellulose or hypromellose may be used.

Toxic effects of common systemic drugs on the eye
As the eye may be the first place to show signs of systemic disease, so some systemic drugs may now show their toxic effects in the eye. These effects range from pruritis, irritation, redness, excess tear formation with overflow (epiphora), photophobia and blapharoconjunctivitis to disturbance of vision.

1 *Methotrexate and related antimetabolites*: these drugs affect the Meibornian glands, aggrevate seborrhoeic blepharitis, and produce photophobia, epiphora, periorbital oedema and conjunctival hyperaemia.

2 *5-Fluorouracil (5-FU)*: 5-FU causes canalicular fibrosis and oculomotor disturbances (probably secondary to a local neurotoxicity affecting the brainstem).

3 *Antihistamines*: these drugs decrease tear production

and may lead to 'dry eye', especially in patients with Sjogren's syndrome or ocular pemphigus, in patients who wear contact lenses and in the elderly.

4   *Tamoxifen*: this drug can cause subepithelial, whirl-like, corneal deposits and retinal lesions.

5   *Indomethacin*: this can cause corneal deposits and retinal pigmentary toxicity.

6   *Oral contraceptives*: these can stimulate corneal steeping and intolerance to contact lenses.

7   *Atropine, scopalamine and belladonna-like substances*: such drugs cause mydriasis and cycloplegia.

8   *Corticosteroids*: prolonged use of corticosteroids produces posterior subcapsular cataracts.

9   *Chloramphenicol*: chloramphenicol treatment can lead to optic neuritis.

10 *Ethambutol*: this drug can cause damage to the optic nerve.

References and further reading

Bryant, W.M. (1981) Common toxic effects of systemic drugs on the eye, *Occupational Health Nursing*, Vol. 29, pp. 15–17.

Chilman, A.M. and Thomas, M. (1987) *Understanding Nursing Care*, 3rd edn, Churchill Livingstone, Edinburgh.

Darling, V.H. and Thorpe, M.R. (1981) *Ophthalmic Nursing*, 2nd edn, Baillière Tindall, London.

Garland, P. (1975) *Ophthalmic Nursing*, 6th edn, Faber and Faber, London.

Percy, E. and Smith W.A.M. (1973) *Ophthalmology (Ophthalmic Techniques)*, William Heinemann Medical Books, London.

Phillips, M. (1982) Ophthalmic preparations, Nursing Mirror, Vol. 155, pp. 69–71.

Rooke, F.C.E., Rothwell, P.J. and Woodhouse, D.F. (1980) *Ophthalmic Nursing – Its Practice and Management*, Churchill Livingstone, Edinburgh.

Smith, J. and Nachazel, D.P. (1980) *Ophthalmologic Nursing*, Little, Brown, Boston.

Wilson, P. (1976) *Modern Ophthalmic Nursing*, Edward Arnold, London.

GUIDELINES: EYE SWABBING

Equipment

1   Sterile dressing pack
2   Normal saline solution
3   Sodium bicarbonate solution.

Procedure

Action	Rationale
1 Explain the procedure to the patient.	To obtain the patient's consent and co-operation.
2 Assist the patient into the correct position: (a) Head well supported and tilted back (b) Preferably the patient should be in bed or lying on a couch.	The patient needs to be discouraged from flinching or making unexpected movements and so should be in the most comfortable position possible at the start of the procedure.
3 Ensure an adequate light source, taking care not to dazzle the patient.	To enable maximum observation of the eyes without causing the patient harm or discomfort.
4 Wash and dry hands thoroughly.	Asepsis is essential, particularly where the patient has a damaged eye or has just had an operation on the eye. Infection can lead to loss of an eye.
5 Always treat the uninfected or uninflamed eye first.	To avoid cross-infection.

6 Using a slightly moistened lint square or wool swab, ask the patient to look up and swab the lower lid from the nasal corner outwards.	If the swab is too wet the solution will run down the patient's cheek. This increases the risk of cross-infection and causes the patient discomfort. Swabbing from the nasal corner outwards avoids the risk of swabbing discharge into the lacrymal punctum, or even across the bridge of the nose into other eye.
7 Ensure that the edge of the swab is not above the lid margin.	To avoid touching the sensitive cornea.
8 Using a new swab each time, repeat the procedure until all the discharge has been removed.	To avoid infection.
9 Swab with a dry swab.	Moist areas encourage bacterial growth.
10 Swab the upper lid by slightly everting the lid margin and asking the patient to look down. Swab from the nasal corner outwards and use a new swab each time until all discharge has been removed.	
11 Swab with a dry swab.	
12 Once both eyelids have been cleansed and dried, make the patient comfortable.	
13 Remove and dispose of equipment.	To avoid cross-infection.
14 Wash hands.	
15 Record the procedure in the appropriate documents.	To monitor trends and fluctuations.

Note: For information about obtaining an eye swab for pathological investigations, see the appropriate section in Specimen Collection (p. 337).

GUIDELINES: INSTILLATION OF EYE DROPS

Equipment
1 Sterile dressing pack
2 Normal saline solution
3 Sodium bicarbonate solution
4 Appropriate eye drops. (Any preparation must be checked against the doctor's prescription.)

Procedure

Action	Rationale
1 Explain the procedure to the patient.	To obtain the patient's consent and co-operation.
2 If there is any discharge, proceed as for eye swabbing.	To remove any infected material and thus ensure adequate absorption of the drops.

Action	**Rationale**

3 Check the following:
   (a) Prescription against bottle label.
   (b) For which eye the drops are prescribed.
 	
   (c) Expiry date on bottle.
	To ensure that appropriate drops are instilled.
	To avoid cross-infection and instillation of the drug into the wrong eye.
	To ensure that medication is potent.

4 Assist the patient into the correct position, i.e. head well supported and tilted back.	To ensure that drops are instilled beneath the lower lid into the fornix and to avoid excess solution running down the patient's cheek.
5 Wash and dry hands thoroughly.	Asepsis is essential, particularly when the patient has a damaged eye or has just had an operation on the eye. Infection can lead to loss of an eye.
6 Place a cotton wool swab on the lower lid against the lid margin.	To absorb any excess solution which may be irritating to the surrounding skin.
7 Ask the patient to look up immediately prior to instilling the drop.	This opens the eye and allows the drop to be instilled into the outer side of the lower fornix. If done too soon the patient may blink as the drop is instilled.
8 Ask the patient to close his/her eye. Keep the wool swab on the lower lid.	To ensure absorption of the fluid and to avoid excess running down the cheek.
9 Make the patient comfortable.	
10 Remove and dispose of equipment.	To avoid cross-infection.
11 Wash hands.	
12 Record the procedure in the appropriate documents.	To monitor trends and fluctuations.

GUIDELINES: INSTILLATION OF EYE OINTMENT

Equipment
1 Sterile dressing pack
2 Normal saline solution
3 Sodium bicarbonate solution may be used to soften a crusted discharge
4 Appropriate eye ointment. (Any preparation must be checked against the doctor's prescription.)

Procedure

Action	**Rationale**
1 Explain the procedure to the patient.	To obtain the patient's consent and co-operation.

2 If there is any discharge, and to remove any previous application of ointment, proceed as for eye swabbing.	To remove any infected material and previous ointment to allow for absorption of ointment.
3 Check the following: (a) Prescription against tube of ointment (b) For which eye the ointment is prescribed (c) Expiry date on tube.	To ensure that appropriate ointment is applied. To avoid cross-infection and administration of an inappropriate treatment. To ensure that medication is patent
4 Wash and dry hands thoroughly.	To avoid infection.
5 Place a wool swab on the lower lid against the lid margin.	To absorb excess ointment which may be irritating to the surrounding skin.
6 Slightly evert the lower lid by pulling on the wool swab. Ask the patient to look up immediately prior to applying the cream.	To allow the application to be made inside the lower lid into the lower fornix.
7 Apply the ointment by gently squeezing the tube and, with the nozzle 2.5 cm above the lower lid, drawing a line along the inner edge of the lower lid from the nasal corner outward.	
8 Ask the patient to close his/her eye and remove excess ointment with a new wool swab.	To avoid excess ointment irritating the surrounding skin.
9 Warn the patient that, when he/she opens his/her eye, vision will be a little blurred for a few minutes.	
10 Make the patient comfortable.	
11 Remove and dispose of equipment.	To avoid infection.
12 Wash hands.	
13 Record the procedure in the appropriate documents.	To monitor trends and fluctuations.

GUIDELINES: EYE IRRIGATION

Equipment
1 Sterile dressing pack
2 Irrigation fluid (usually sterile normal saline but, in an emergency, tap water may be used)
3 Receiver
4 Towel
5 Plastic cape
6 Irrigating flask
7 Hot water in a bowl to warm irrigating fluid to tepid temperature.

Procedure

Action	Rationale
1 Explain the procedure to the patient.	To gain the patient's consent and co-operation.
2 Prepare the irrigation fluid to the appropriate temperature.	Tepid fluid will be more comfortable for the patient. The solution should be poured across the inner aspect of the nures's wrist to test the temperature.
3 Assist the patient into the appropriate position: (a) Head comfortably supported with chin almost horizontal (b) Head inclined to the side of the eye to be treated.	To avoid the solution running either over the cheek into the eye or out of the eye and down the side of the nose.
4 Wash and dry hands.	To avoid infection.
5 Remove any discharge from the eye by swabbing.	To prevent washing the discharge down the lacrimal duct or across the cheek.
6 Ask the patient to hold the receiver against his/her cheek below the eye being teated.	To collect irrigation fluid as it runs away from the eye.
7 Position the towel and plastic cape.	To protect the patient's clothing.
8 Hold the patient's eyelids apart, using your first and second fingers, against the orbital ridge.	The patient will be unable to hold his/her eye open once irrigation commences.
9 Do not press on the eyeball.	To avoid causing the patient discomfort or pain.
10 Warn the patient that the flow of solution is going to start and pour a little on to his/her cheek first.	
11 Direct the flow of the fluid from the nasal corner outwards.	To wash away from the lacrimal punctum.
12 Ask the patient to look up, down and to either side while irrigating.	To ensure that the whole area is washed.
13 Keep the flow of irrigation fluid constant.	
14 When the eye has been thoroughly irrigated, ask the patient to close his/her eyes and use a new swab to dry the lids.	
15 Take the receiver from the patient and dry his/her cheek.	If the receiver is removed first, solution may run down the patient's neck.
16 Make the patient comfortable.	
17 Remove and dispose of equipment.	To avoid infection.
18 Wash hands.	
19 Record the procedure in the appropriate documents.	To monitor trends and fluctuations.

15

Gastric Lavage

Definition
Gastric lavage is the irrigation or washing out of the stomach with repeated flushing of an appropriate fluid. It is used to obtain a specimen of gastric contents and to remove poisons or other harmful substances, that were swallowed deliberately or accidentally, thus preventing further absorption.

Indications
Gastric lavage may be used under the following circumstances:
1 if the patient is seen within 4 hours of ingesting poisons or harmful substances;
2 if the patient is unconscious and the time of ingestion is not known;
3 in all cases of salicylate poisioning with 12 hours of ingestion;
4 for gastrointestinal haemorrhage (Evans, 1981).

REFERENCE MATERIAL
The reliability of gastric lavage is debatable, advice on its use conflicting, and its value questionable (Burstom, 1970; Matthew, 1971; Stoddart, 1975; Goth and Vesell, 1984). Blake *et al.* (1978) attempted to identify those factors that influenced the decision to perform gastric lavage in 236 cases of deliberate self-poisoning seen over a period of 6 months in one hospital. Of patients seen within 4 hours of ingesting the poison, 87% had a lavage performed irrespective of the number of tablets and the nature of the drug taken. Overall, 77% had a gastric lavage. Most of the late lavages were carried out for salicylate ingestion. The authors concluded that given the changing pattern of drugs used for attempted self-poisoning, at least 50% of patients were subjected to gastric lavage unnecessarily.

Gastric lavage is generally carried out by medical staff assisted by nurses. Registered general nurses in specialized units, mainly accident and emergency departments, may carry out the procedure without medical

involvement after initial assessment.

Gastric lavage versus induced emesis
Research has shown (Beckett and Rowland, 1965; Bell, 1969; Chazan and Cohen, 1969) that of the two methods for removing gastric contents in drug overdose, induced emesis is more effective than gastric lavage.

The issue is more complicated than this, however, for one method cannot be applied to the exclusion of the other in all cases. For drug-induced emesis, two agents are commonly used – ipecacuanha and apomorphine. Ipecacuanha is a centrally acting drug, its site of action being in the chemoreceptor zone in the medulla oblongata. As a result it takes 20–25 minutes to produce an effect. If this fact is not appreciated, repeated doses may be given before the first dose has had time to work and this may result in protracted vomiting. A sufficient quantity of water (up to 10 glasses is quoted in the literature) must be given to produce emesis. Apomorphine produces vomiting within about 5 minutes and again water must be given to produce the required effect. The drug is administered subcutaneously or intramuscularly. It possesses narcotic properties and is contraindicated in patients who have ingested sedatives or hypnotics or who have respiratory problems. Induced emesis should only be used when the patient is alert and the development of lethargy and coma is unlikely. Unless the patient is awake the cough reflex may be depressed and this may result in the patient inhaling the vomitus. When a drug with strong antiemetic properties has been ingested, e.g. chlorpromazine, induced emesis will have little or no effect and gastric lavage may become the method of choice.

Gastric lavage is contraindicated when a caustic or corrosive has been ingested because of the possibility of perforating the oesophagus when passing the tube. It is also contraindicated when strychine has been ingested since stimulation while passing the tube into the stomach may precipitate convulsions. In patients brought to a hospital's emergency department several hours (4 hours is quoted in the literature) after the ingestion of drugs, gastric lavage is held to be of little value in that after such a period of time very little if any of the drug will remain in the stomach. Any drug that does remain may then be washed into the small intestines by the procedure. Gastric lavage within 6 hours is quoted by Evans (1981) as valuable in methanol poisoning. Drugs such as aspirin and glutethimide remain in the small intestines for long periods and act as a reservoir for continued absorption. Gastric lavage is useful at any time within 12 hours of ingestion in these cases.

Gastric lavage tubes

Cosgriff (1978) gives a brief illustrated summary of some of the tubes used for gastric lavage in the United States of America. The tube of choice in the United Kingdom appears to be 30 gauge Jacques stomach tube (Matthew, 1971; Evans, 1981). This wide-bore tube enables tablets, food with tablet particles adherent, and virtually all the contents of the stomach to be evacuated through it.

References and further reading

Arena, J. (1974) *Poisoning: Toxicology, Symptoms, Treatment*, 3rd edn, Charles C. Thomas.

Beckett, A. and Rowland, M. (1965) Urinary excretion kinetics of amphetamine in man, *Journal of Pharmacy and Pharmacology*, Vol. 17, p. 628.

Bell, D.S. (1969) Dangers of treatment of status epilepticus with diazepam, *British Medical Journal*, Vol. i, p. 159.

Blake, D.R. *et al.* (1978) Is there excessive use of gastric lavage in the treatment of self-poisoning? *Lancet*, Vol. ii, pp. 1362–4.

Budassi, S.A. and Barber, J.M. (1985) *Emergency Nursing: Principles and Practice*, C.V. Mosby, St Louis.

Burstom, G.R. (1970) *Self-poisoning*, Lloyd-Luke, London.

Chazan, J. and Cohen, J. (1969) Clinical spectrum of glutethimide intoxication, *Journal of the American Medical Association*, Vol. 208, p. 837.

Cosgriff, J.H. (1978) *An Atlas of Diagnostic and Therapeutic Procedures for Emergency Personnel*, J.B. Lippincott, Philadelphia.

Cosgriff, J.H. *et al.* (1984) *The Practice of Emergency Nursing*, 2nd edn, J.B. Lippincott, Philadelphia.

Evans, R. (1981) *Emergency Medicine*, Butterworth, London.

Goth, A. (1984) *Medical Pharmacology: Principles and Concepts*, 11th edn, C.V. Mosby, St Louis.

Matthew, H. (1971) Acute poisoning: some myths and misconceptions, *British Medical Journal*, Vol. i, p. 521.

Stoddart, J.C. (1975) *Intensive Therapy*, Blackwell Scientific Publications, Oxford.

GUIDELINES: GASTRIC LAVAGE

Equipment

1   Sterile gastric tube with connector
2   Connecting tubing
3   Lubricating jelly
4   Tape
5   Syringe (50 ml)
6   Receiver
7   Litmus paper
8   Mouth gag
9   Funnel
10 Jug
11 Tepid water or prescribed irrigation fluid
12 Plastic sheet
13 Disposable paper sheets
14 Disposable plastic aprons
15 Disposable plastic gloves
16 Bucket
17 Suction equipment
18 Emergency resuscitation equipment.

Procedure

Action	**Rationale**
1 Explain the procedure to the patient when possible.	To obtain the patient's consent and co-operation. (The efficacy of explanations is questionable, however, on the basis that an adult who has ingested a toxic substance deliberately is unlikely to want to co-operate with agents whose aim is to prevent suicidal gestures. Tact must be employed in these circumstances.
2 Unconscious patients must be intubated.	To maintain a clear airway.
3 Place the patient on a firm surface, lying in the left lateral position with his/her head down (Figure 15.1). (A standard emergency department trolley should be available ideally.)	To maintain a clear airway.
4 Remove any prostheses from the buccal cavity. Remove débris and/or vomitus from the buccal cavity with suction.	To maintain a clear airway.
5 Have emergency resuscitation equipment available.	Strong vagal stimulation can induce cardiac dysrhythmias and cardiopulmonary arrest.
6 Place a disposable sheet under the patient's head and a plastic sheet over the floor.	To protect nurse and patient should vomiting occur.
7 Lubricate the tube with jelly.	To facilitate passage of the tube.
8 If the patient is able to co-operate, ask him/her to sit up and swallow sips of water.	Swallowing will cause the epiglottis to close and prevent accidental passage of the tube into the trachea.
9 Secure the tube with tape once inserted.	To prevent dislodgement of the tube.

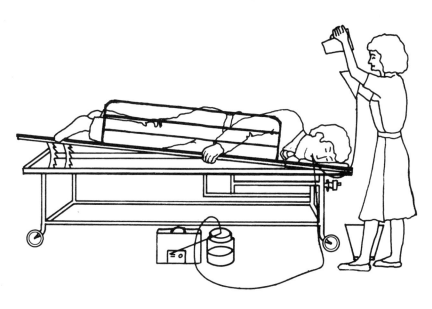

Figure 15.1   Gastric lavage.

Action	**Rationale**
10 *Either* aspirate the tube before lavage begins and test the aspirate with litmus paper, *or* listen with a stethoscope over the stomach as air is introduced into the tube via a syringe.	To ensure that the tube is in the stomach.
11 Retain a specimen of aspirate in a labelled specimen bottle.	For analysis.
12 Instil, via a funnel, water, or the prescribed irrigation fluid, in volumes of 100–500 ml.	Approximately 500 ml of fluid are necessary to flatten out the rugae of the stomach so that the fluid may reach all parts of the mucous membrane.
13 Any fluid instilled must be tepid.	To prevent a sudden lowering of body temperature and possible shock.
14 Hold the funnel below the level of the patient. Once the required amount of fluid has been poured into the funnel, raise it gradually until the fluid empties into the stomach. Do not allow the contents of the funnel to empty.	To control the rate at which the fluid is instilled. A siphoning action is needed to recall the contents of the stomach.
15 Lower the funnel and observe all the contents as they return from the stomach. Empty the contents into a bucket. If blood returns, stop the procedure and inform the medical staff. Lavage until the returning fluid is clear.	
16 Pinch the tube off and remove the tube quickly. Have suction at hand.	Gagging and possible vomiting may occur when the tube is removed. As the tube reaches the pharynx, any fluid left may escape and infiltrate into the lungs.
17 Provide oral hygiene facilities as required.	To maintani a clean, moist mouth. To prevent the accumulation of oral secretions. To prevent the development of mouth infection.

16

Intrapleural Drainage

Definition
Intrapleural drainage is an underwater-seal system of drainage that prevents the entry of air into the pleural space, thus avoiding pneumothorax.

Indications
Intrapleural drainage is indicated under two circumstances:
1. to remove matter from the pleural space or thoracic cavity:
   a. solids, e.g. fibrin or clotted blood;
   b. liquids, e.g. serous fluids, blood, pus, chyle or gastric juice;
   c. gas, e.g. air from the lungs, trachea or oesophagus;
2. to allow the lung to re-expand following surgery.

REFERENCE MATERIAL
Anatomy and physiology
The pleura is a thin sheet of tissue covering the undersurface of the ribs, diaphragm and the structures of the mediastinum. It continues over the surface of both lungs, thus forming a space known as the pleural space. The layer in contact with the surface of the lungs is known as the visceral pleura; that in contact with the thoracic wall, the parietal pleura. These two membranes are continuous with each other but are separated by a thin serous fluid that allows the pleurae to slide smoothly over each other during respiration. In health the pleural space is a potential space only. This space has a negative pressure normally. The elastic tissues of the lungs and the chest wall continually pull in opposite directions, the lungs tending to recoil inwards and the chest wall outwards. As these opposing forces attempt to pull the visceral and parietal pleurae apart, they create a negative pressure in the pleural space. Pressures in the pleural space are approximately 8 mm H_2O during inspiration and 2 mm H_2O on expiration. A negative pressure of 54 mm H_2O can be measured during forced

inspiration; during forced expiration, e.g. coughing, a positive pressure of approximately 68 mm H_2O develops.

Any opening of the thoracic cavity results in a loss of negative pressure and the lungs collapse. Collections of fluids or materials can also cause the lung to collapse as these substances take up space, restricting expansion of the lungs and inhibiting cardiopulmonary function.

When a tube is inserted to remove air it is normally inserted fairly high in the intrapleural space as air is light and will usually rise. If a tube is inserted to remove liquids or debris, it is usually inserted fairly low in the intrapleural space on the premise that the substances are relatively heavy and will therefore fall due to gravity. If more than one tube is inserted, e.g. following intrathoracic surgery, to remove both air and fluid or debris, the higher, known as the apical drain, is used to remove air, and the lower, known as the basal drain, is used to remove liquid and debris.

Types of chest drain (see Figure 16.1)
Any system must be capable of removing whatever collects in the pleural space more rapidly than it accumulates.

SINGLE BOTTLE WATER-SEAL SYSTEM
In this system the end of the drainage tube from the patient's chest is covered by a layer of water that permits drainage and prevents lung collapse by sealing out the atmosphere. Drainage depends on gravity, the mechanics of respiration and, if necessary, suction by the addition of a controlled vacuum. The tube from the patient should extend approximately 2.5 cm below the level of the water in the container.

TWO-BOTTLE WATER-SEAL SYSTEM
This system consists of the same water-seal chamber with the addition of a manometer bottle. Drainage is similar again to the single-bottle system. Suction,

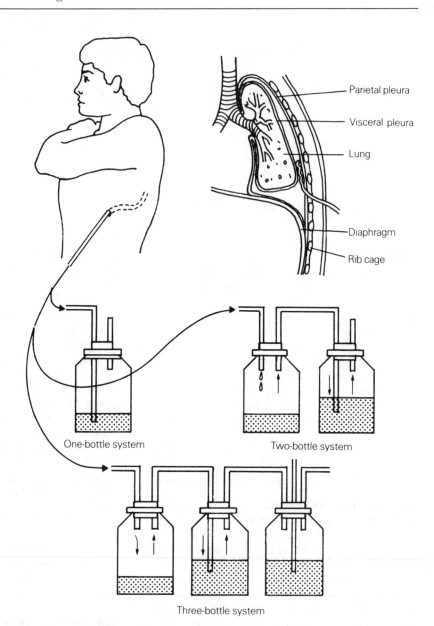

Figure 16.1 One-, two- and three-
bottle chest drainage systems.

however, is controlled by containing sufficient fluids to establish the degree of vacuum required. Effective drainage depends on gravity and the amount of suction added as controlled by the manometer bottle.

THREE-BOTTLE WATER-SEAL SYSTEM
The initial chamber in this system collects the drainage, so that the fluid in the water-seal chamber stays constant as drainage accumulates. This has an advantage over the aforementioned systems in that as the chest drainage collects in the water-seal chamber the resistance of flow from the pleural space is increased. When the fluid in the water-seal chamber equals the amount of fluid in

the manometer bottle, any effective suction is cancelled. In this system drainage depends on gravity and the amount of suction added as controlled by the manometer. The suction system maintains a negative pressure throughout the closed drainage system. The manometer bottle regulates the amount of vacuum in the system.

THE ARGYLE 'DOUBLE-SEAL' SYSTEM
This system consists of four chambers and is portable (see Figure 16.2). The second chamber is the collection chamber and is divided into three subchambers. The next chamber is the water-seal chamber. It is essentially

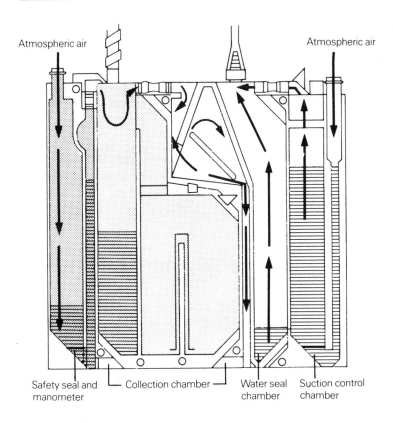

Atmospheric air   Atmospheric air

Safety seal and   └── Collection chamber ──┘   Water seal   Suction control
manometer   chamber   chamber

Figure 16.2   Argyle double-seal system.

U-shaped. The last chamber is the suction control chamber. Again this is U-shaped. The extra chamber in an Argyle unit is also a water-seal chamber. The patient's air passes through the third chamber into the suction source. If, however, the passage into the suction source is accidentally obstructed, the patient's air will pass instead through the first chamber into the atmosphere. The first chamber provides as safety vent of the patient's air.

References and further reading

Brunner, L.S. and Suddarth, D.S. (1982), *The Lippincott Manual of Medical-Surgical Nursing*, Harper and Row, London.

Brunner, L.S. and Suddarth, D.S. (1986) *The Lippincott Manual of Nursing Practice*, 4th edn, J.B. Lippincott, Philadelphia.

Cohen, S. and Stack, M. (1980) Programmed instruction: how to work with chest tubes, *American Journal of Nursing*, Vol. 80, pp. 685–712.

Erickson, R. (1981) Chest tubes: they're really not that complicated, *Nursing* (US), Vol. 11, no. 5, pp. 34–43.

Erickson, R. (1981) Solving chest tube problems, *Nursing* (US), Vol. 11, no. 6, pp. 62–8.

GUIDELINES: MANAGEMENT OF UNDERWATER-SEAL DRAINAGE

Equipment

1   Sterile chest drainage bottle
2   Sterile disposable tubing
3   Drainage bottle holder – if available
4   Suction pump – if required
5   Two pairs of artery forceps – tips to be covered with rubber.

Procedure

Action	**Rationale**

1 Attach the intrapleural drain to the drainage tube. *Note:* This should lead to the long tube whose end is under water seal.

Water-seal drainage provides for the escape of air, fluid and débris into a drainage bottle. The water acts as a seal and keeps the air from being drawn back into the pleural space.

2 Ensure that drainage tubing is 2.5 cm below the water level (Figure 16.3).

If the tube is not deep enough under the water level, there is a danger of it emerging above the water line if the bottle is moved. If the tube is too deep, a higher intrapleural pressure is required to expel air.

3 The other, shorter tube, is:
(a) Left open to the atmosphere
(b) Attached to a controlled suction apparatus.

To allow gas to escape.
Although drainage of liquids and/or débris relies on gravity and the mechanics of respiration, additional controlled suction may be necessary to accelerate the process.

4 Establish the original level of fluid by:
(a) Marking with a piece of tape
(b) Filling to a preset amount.
    Note: All bottles used should, preferably, be calibrated.

This provides a baseline for measurement of fluid drainage.

5 When recording fluid drainage:
(a) Note the date and time
(b) Mark hourly or daily increments by taping the level on the drainage bottles. *Note:* When using tape specify whether the upper, mid or lower border of the tape is the level to be measured at (Figure 16.4).

This marking will show the amount of fluid loss and how fast fluid is collecting in the drainage bottle. If the fluid is blood, it serves as a basis for retransfusion or reoperation, if following surgery. Inaccuracies of 100–200 ml can occur if the incorrect border is used.

6 Secure tubing to the bed clothes by the use of tape and safety pins.

This will prevent kinking, looping or pressure on the tubing which may cause reflux of fluid into the pleural space or impede drainage, causing blocking of the intrapleural drain by debris.

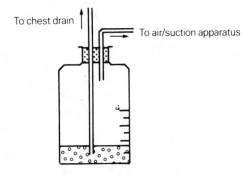

Figure 16.3   Underwater-seal drainage.

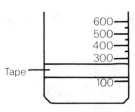

Figure 16.4   Specify whether the upper, mid- or lower level of the tape is to be measured.

7   Ensure that artery clamps are in close proximity to patient, i.e. taped to the wall, clamped to the bed clothes or on the bedside locker.

In the event of accidental disconnection of the drainage tubing from the intrapleural drain, the artery clamps should immediately be applied to the intrapleural drain to prevent entry of air (on inspiration) into the pleural space – leading to pneumothorax. When moving the patient, the drainage tubing is more likely to become disconnected, therefore the artery clamps should be readily available. There may be medical orders to apply the clamps, at set intervals, to delay drainage; e.g. following instillation of drugs or radioactive substances it is normal to clamp the tubing for 24 hours.

8   Ensure that the patient is sitting in a comfortable position which allows optimum drainage. Encourage the patient to change his/her position frequently. This may be enhanced by adequate pain control, using drugs which do not depress respiration.

Correct poisitioning aids drainage by gravity and by ensuring that the patient breathes freely, to promote gaseous exchange. Changing position also promotes better drainage as well as avoiding discomfort and pressure sores.

9   Ask the physiotherapist to help encourage the patient with mobility, chest and arm exercises.

To promote drainage and avoid the complications of pressure sores and stiffness of the arm on the side of drain insertion.

10 Ensure patency of tubing by 'milking' tubing towards the drainage bottle, if necessary. Take care not to disconnect tubing while executing this manoeuvre.
    Note: This is only necessary if draining fluid.

'Milking' the tubing prevents it from becoming clogged with clots or fibrin. Constant attention to maintaining the patency of the tube will facilitate prompt expansion of the lung and minimize complications.

11 Ensure that there is fluctuation (swinging) of the fluid level in the drainage tube under water seal.

Fluctuation of the water level in the tube shows that there is effective communication between the pleural cavity and the drainage bottle, provides a valuable indication of the patency of the drainage system, and is a gauge of intrapleural pressure.

12 Ensure that the drainage bottle remains at floor level, except when the patient is being helped to move. The drainage bottle should never be raised above the level of the intrapleural drain.

To prevent backflow of fluid into the pleural space.

13 Caution visitors and ancillary staff against handling any part of the system or displacing the drainage bottle.

To prevent backflow and to guard against accidental disconnection of the tubing which would allow air entry.

GUIDELINES: CHANGING DRAINAGE TUBING AND BOTTLES

Equipment
1   Sterile drainage bottle
2   Sterile water
3   Two pairs of artery clamps – tips covered with rubber
4   Suitable antiseptic solution, e.g. Hibisol
5   Sterile tubing.

Procedure

Action	**Rationale**
1 Explain the procedure to the patient.	To gain the patient's consent and co-operation.
2 Wash hands.	To minimize the risk of infection.
3 Prepare the drainage bottle by putting in a set amount (enough to cover the end of the long arm of the drainage tubing) of sterile water and taking note of that level. Mark this level with tape. If tubing is to be changed, attach clean tubing to the drainage bottle prepared.	To provide an underwater seal. Enough water should be in the bottle to ensure maintenance of the seal. Too much water creates pressure and reduces the capacity of the bottle for drainage. It is essential to note the amount of water added to the bottle for accurate measurement of drainage.
4 Take the equipment to the bedside.	
5 Clamp the intrapleural drain using both artery clamps, before changing the bottle or tubing.	To avoid tension pneumothorax occurring when the water seal is broken.
6 Clean hands with a suitable antiseptic solution, e.g. Hibisol.	To minimize the risk of infection.
7 Remove the bung with the drainage tubing from the underwater-seal bottle and replace it in the clean bottle. Ensure that there is an airtight connection between the bung and bottle. If tubing is being changed, the bung will already be in place in the sterile bottle.	To prevent air entry and reduce the risk of infection.
8 Take the clamps off the intrapleural drainage tube.	To re-establish drainage.
9 Make the patient comfortable.	
10 Remove equipment.	
11 Record in appropriate documentation the amount of drainage, deducting the water originally in the bottle.	For accurate recording of the amount of drainage.
12 Empty and clean the bottle and return it to the central sterile supplies department.	

Note: If an underwater-seal drain is established to drain air from the pleural space, there is probably no need to change either connection tubing or bottle. However, if fluid and debris are drained the bottle may need changing frequently (at least daily), depending on the amount drained. The tubing need only be changed if there is a copious amount of debris and there is a danger of it becoming blocked. Changing the tubing or the bottle breaks the closed system and provides a potential portal of entry for bacteria.

GUIDELINES: REMOVAL OF AN INTRAPLEURAL DRAIN

Equipment
1   Sterile dressing pack
2   Cleansing lotion
3   Surgical gloves
4   Stitch cutter
5   Collodion lotion
6   Adhesive tape
7   Plaster remover.

Procedure
This is a procedure usually carried out by a member of the medical staff, preferably the doctor who inserted the drain. However, it may be performed by a qualified nurse if he/she has been instructed and supervised in the removal of intrapleural drains.

Action		Rationale
Doctor/First Nurse	*Assisting Nurse*	
1 Explain the procedure to patient and allow the patient to practise the procedure beforehand.	Wash hands.	To obtain the patient's consent and co-operation. Speed and accuracy are essential in this procedure so all equipment must be at hand.
2 Wash hands.		To minimize the risk of infection.
3 Prepare equipment using strict aseptic technique.	Assist in preparation of equipment without causing contamination.	
4 Remove the old dressing, using forceps.		
5 Cut the knot from the purse-string suture.		Allows mobility of the suture.
6 Cut the suture holding the drain in place.	Hold the drain in place.	To prevent the drain falling out.
7 Tie the purse-string suture lightly to skin level.		To enable rapid tightening of the suture when the drain is removed.
8 Instruct the patient to breathe in to the maximum and to hold his/her breath. This manoeuvre should have been practised beforehand.		To minimize the risk of tension pneumothorax occurring as the drain is removed. Prior preparation of the patient ensures full co-operation.
	Steadily pull out the drain.	If the drain is pulled out too quickly, tension pneumothorax may occur.

Action		Rationale
Doctor/First Nurse	*Assisting Nurse*	
10 As the drain leaves the skin, tighten the purse-string suture and tie a firm double-knot. Speed is essential. Cut the ends to 1.25 cm.		The purse-string suture must be tightened immediately the drain leaves the chest to avoid tension pneumothorax.
11 Place gauze with collodion over the suture.	Strap the gauze firmly in place.	To provide a tight seal.
12 Tell the patient that he/she may exhale and relax.		
	Remove any debris from the site of the wound and ensure that the patient is comfortable.	
	Clear equipment away.	
	Wash hands.	To prevent cross-infection.
	Empty and clean the drainage bottles and send them to the central sterile supplies department.	
	Record the amount of drainage in appropriate documents.	To provide an accurate record.

NURSING CARE PLAN

Problem	Cause	Suggested action
Lack of drainage.	Kinking, looping or pressure on the tubing may cause reflux of fluid into the intrapleural space or may impede drainage, causing blocking of the intrapleural drain.	Check the system and straighten tubing as required. Secure the tubing to prevent a recurrence of the problem.
No fluctuation of fluid in tubing from the underwater seal.	Re-expansion of the lung.	Ask medical staff if the drain may be removed following chest X-ray. The purpose of the drain has been fulfilled. Keeping the drain in any longer than necessary may lead to hazards from infection or air re-entry.
	Tubing is obstructed by blood clots or fibrin.	'Milk' the tubing towards the drainage bottle to try to dislodge the obstruction and re-establish patency.
	Tubing is looped or kinked.	Straighten tubing as required. Secure the tubing to prevent a recurrence.
	Failure of the suction apparatus.	Disconnect the suction appartus and leave this tube open to the air, allowing intrapleural air to escape.

Constant bubbling of fluid in the drainage bottle.

An air leak in the system.

Clamp the intrapleural drain, momentarily, close to the chest wall and establish whether there is a leak in the rest of the system. Clamping the tubing shows whether the leak is below the level of the clamp. However, if the clamp is left on for too long, and the leak is at thoracic level, i.e. air is entering the pleura, this will increase the patient's pneumothorax. Inform medical staff as leaking and trapping of air in the pleural space can result in tension pneumothorax.

Patient shows signs of rapid, shallow breathing, cyanosis, pressure in the chest, subcutaneous emphysema or haemorrhage.

Tension pneumothorax; mediastinal shift; postoperative haemorrhage; severe incisional pain; pulmonary embolus or cardiac tamponade.

Observe, record and report any of these signs to a doctor immediately.

Incisional pain.

Provide adequate analgesia, as prescribed, to reduce the patient's discomfort and to enable him/her to perform deep breathing exercises and mobilization to ensure adequate drainage and to avoid complications.

Accidental disconnection of the drainage tubing from the intrapleural drain.

Apply an artery clamp to the drain immediately in order to avoid air entering the pleural space; this is more of a danger if the patient is exhaling at the time. Re-establish the connection as soon as possible in order to re-establish drainage. If necessary, use a clean, sterile drainage tube; tubing may have been contaminated when it became disconnected. If air entry has occurred, report this to a doctor. Record the incident in the relevant records. The patient may have been upset by the incident and will need reassurance.

Patient needs to be moved to another area, e.g. X-ray department.

Place the drainage bottle below the level of the intrapleural drain, as close to the floor as possible, in order to prevent reflux of fluid into the pleural space. Do not clamp the drain unless the doctor has ordered it; this may obstruct drainage and allow clot formation if fluid is being drained. Attach clamps to the patient's gown, in case of accidental disconnection *en route*.

Problem	Cause	Suggested action
Intrapleural drain falls out.		Pull the purse-string suture immediately to close the wound. Cover the wound with an occlusive sterile dressing. Inform a doctor. The objective is to minimize the amount of air entering the pleural space. The drain will probably need reinserting.

17

Intravenous Management

DRUG ADMINISTRATION

REFERENCE MATERIAL

The involvement of nursing staff in the administration of intravenous drugs was formally recognized in the mid-1970s following the publication of the Breckenridge Report (Department of Health and Social Security, 1976). A working party had been established in 1974 under the chairmanship of Professor Breckenridge as a result of the increasing use of the intravenous route for drug administration. There was concern that hazards such as microbial contamination and drug incompatibilities were not fully appreciated and that the staff participating were not adequately trained in the procedures used.

The terms of reference of the working party were as follows:

1 to identify and investigate the problems associated with this form of intravenous therapy;
2 to consider the responsibilities of the various parties involved;
3 to consider modification of nurse training to ensure safe practice;
4 to produce guidelines for the three main professions, i.e. doctor, pharmacists and nurses;
5 to assess the value of various aids, e.g. charts for reference.

The working party received evidence from a number of sources and considered pharmaceutical data. In 1976 the findings were published by the Department of Health and Social Security. The report proposed a rational approach to intravenous drug administration, established guidelines for documentation and outlined the responsibilities of health authorities and health professionals. The responsibility of medical staff was to ensure that the drug was administered by the most

effective and safest route and that the instructions to facilitate this were clearly written.

An intravenous additive service provided by pharmacists was favoured. In situations where this was not practical, pharmacists were to act as an information source for other personnel. It was accepted that nursing staff could undertake the addition and administration of intravenous drugs. The nurse, however, should be qualified (i.e. should be a registered general nurse or an enrolled nurse) and have undergone a period of training and assessment in both the theoretical knowledge and practical procedures involved in such drug administration. He/she should be issued with a certificate of competence and fully understand the legal implications of undertaking such an extension of the role of the nurse.

In all intravenous therapy the nurse's responsibility continued to include the following:

1 checking the infusion fluid and container for any obvious faults or contamination;
2 ensuring the administration of the prescribed fluid to the correct patient;
3 observing whether the intravenous line remains patent;
4 inspecting the site of insertion and reporting abnormalities;
5 controlling the rate of flow as prescribed;
6 monitoring the condition of the patient and reporting any changes;
7 maintaining appropriate records.

Permitted methods of intravenous drug administration by nurses were identified.

1 continuously, or intermittently, by addition to an intravenous infusion in a bottle, bag or burette. This method may include the use of a variety of equipment, e.g. a small-volume syringe pump or a Y administration set;
2 intermittently by injection into the latex rubber section of an intravenous administration set;
3 intermittently by injection into a cannula or winged

infusion device. The device's patency may be maintained by use of a stylet or by heparinization;

4   intermittently by injection via a three-way tap or stopcock. This method is not advised, however, due to the increased risk of contamination associated with these devices. Streamlined adaptors are now available and are preferred.

Additional guidelines

Certain guidelines were also issued in 1976 about general intravenous management related to the areas of nursing involvement. These included the following:

1   the infusion container should not hang for more than 24 hours. This was reduced to 8 hours in the case of blood or blood products;

2   the administration set must be changed every 24 hours. More recent research indicates that a 48-hour set change is not associated with an increase in infection. It is desirable to record the time and date when this is due;

3   the site of the infusion should be inspected at least daily for complications such as infiltration or inflammation;

4   the sterile dressing covering the insertion site must be changed daily, at the time of inspection or

whenever it is touched, e.g. at the time of administration of an intravenous injection.

In the light of more recent research, it is now possible to propose further recommendations. It is desirable that a closed system of infusion is maintained wherever possible, with as few connections or stopcocks as is necessary for its purpose. This reduces the risk of extrinsic bacterial contamination, especially if three-way taps or their equivalents are excluded. The dead space in this equipment has been identified as a reservoir for microorganisms which may be released into the circulation.

The majority of sepsis is cannula related and both infective and non-infective complications have been shown to increase substantially after the device has been in position for 48 hours. Routine testing is, therefore, advised if at all possible. Although the nurse is not normally responsible for this duty, he/she may be able to remind the doctor when this time has elapsed.

In order for the insertion site to be readily available for inspection, it may be necessary for the nurse to assume responsibility for taping the cannula in place as well as dressing the insertion site. Non-sterile tape should not cover the site, the equivalent of an open wound, and a method must be devised so that the site remains visible and the cannula is stable. The procedure

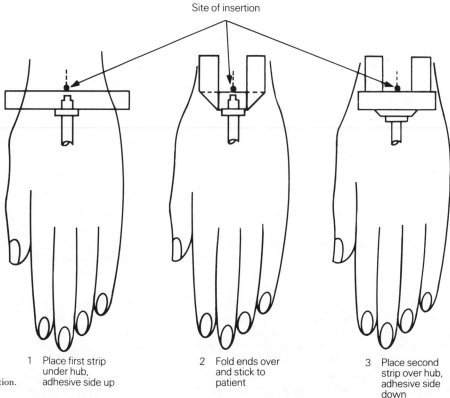

Site of insertion

1   Place first strip under hub, adhesive side up

2   Fold ends over and stick to patient

3   Place second strip over hub, adhesive side down

Figure 17.1 Site of insertion.

illustrated in Figure 17.1 is recommended.

The purpose of all recommendations is to reduce the complications associated with intravenous therapy. Competent, informed management and adherence to basic principles will ensure this.

Removal of the intravenous device or cannula should be an aseptic procedure. The cannula must be taken out gently in order to prevent damage to the vein and pressure should be applied immediately. This pressure should be firm and not involve any rubbing movement. A haematoma will occur if the needle is carelessly removed, causing discomfort and a focus for infection. Pressure should be applied until bleeding has stopped, then a light sterile dressing applied.

Drugs are used for three basic purposes:
1 diagnostic purposes, e.g. assessment of liver function or diagnosis of myasthenia gravis;
2 prophylaxis, e.g. heparin to prevent thrombosis or antibiotics to prevent infection;
3 therapeutic purposes, e.g. replacement of fluids or vitamins, supportive purposes (to enable other treatments, such as anaesthesia), palliation of pain and cure (as in the case of antibiotics).

Drugs administered intravenously also fall within the above-mentioned categories.

Advantages of using the intravenous route
1 An immediate therapeutic effect is achieved due to rapid delivery of the drug to its target site.
2 Total absorption allows precise dose calculation and more reliable treatment.
3 The rate of administration can be controlled and the therapeutic effect maintained or modified as required.
4 Pain and irritation caused by some substances when given intramuscularly or subcutaneously are avoided.
5 Intravenous administration is suitable for drugs which cannot be absorbed by any other route due to large molecular size and irritation to, or instability in, the gastrointestinal tract.

Disadvantages of using the intravenous route
1 There is an inability to recall the drug and reverse the action of it. This may lead to increased toxicity or a sensitivity reaction.
2 Insufficient control of administration may lead to speed shock. This is characterized by a flushed face, headache, congestion, tightness in the chest, etc.
3 Additional complications may occur, such as the following:

(a) microbial contamination through a point of access into the circulation for a period of time;
(b) vascular irritation, e.g. chemical phlebitis;
(c) drug incompatibilities and interactions if multiple additives are prescribed.

Principles to be applied throughout preparation and administration
ASEPSIS
Aseptic technique must be adhered to throughout all intravenous procedures to prevent extrinsic bacterial contamination. The nurse must employ good hand washing and drying techniques or use an alcohol-based skin cleanser as an alternative. Injection sites or bungs should be cleaned using an alcohol-based antiseptic, allowing time for it to dry. A non-touch technique should be employed when changing infusion bags or bottles and these procedures should be completed as quickly as possible. If asepsis is not maintained, local infection, septic phlebitis or septicaemia may result. Any indication of infection, e.g. redness at the insertion site of the device of pyrexia, requires removal of the cannula and further investigation.

Inspection of fluids, drugs, equipment and their packaging must be undertaken to detect any points where contamination may have occurred during manufacture and/or transport. This intrinsic contamination may be detected as cloudiness, discoloration or the presence of particles.

Sterility will ensure that the patient does not receive an injection or infusion of microbes.

SAFETY
All details of the prescription and all calculations must be carefully checked in accordance with hospital policy in order to ensure safe preparation and administration of the drug(s). The nurse must also check the compatibility of the drug with the diluent or infusion fluid. He/she should be aware of the types of incompatibilities, and the factors which could influence them. These include pH, concentration, time, temperature, light and the brand of the drug. If insufficient information is available, a reference book must also be checked and constant monitoring of both the mixture and the patient is important. The preferred method and rate of intravenous administration must be determined.

Drugs should never be added to the following: blood; blood products, i.e. plasma or platelet concentrate; mannitol solutions; sodium bicarbonate solution. Only specially prepared additives should be used with fat emulsions or amino acid preparations.

Accurate labelling of additives and records of administration are essential.

Any protective clothing which is advised should be worn.

COMFORT

Both the physical and psychological comfort of the patient must be considered. By maintaining high standards throughout, the patient's physical comfort should be assured. Comprehensive explanation of the practical aspects of the procedure together with balanced information about the effects of treatment will contribute to reducing anxiety.

Methods of administering intravenous drugs

Three methods are recommended: continuous infusion, intermittent infusion and intermittent injection.

CONTINUOUS INFUSION

Continuous infusion may be defined as the administration of a large volume of fluid, i.e 250–1000 ml, over a number of hours that may be repeated over a period of days. An exception of this may be a small-volume infusion (e.g. of heparin) delivered continously via a syringe pump.

A continuous infusion may be used when:

1 the drugs to be administered must be highly diluted;
2 a maintenance of steady blood levels of the drug is required.

Pre-prepared infusion fluids with additives such as those containing potassium chloride should be used whenever possible. Only one addition should be made to each bottle or bag of fluid after the compatibility has been ascertained. The additive and fluid must be mixed well to prevent a layering effect which can occur with some drugs. The danger is that a bolus injection of the drug may be delivered. To safeguard this, any additions should be made to the infusion fluid before the fluid is hung on the infusion stand. The infusion container should be clearly labelled after the addition has been made. Constant monitoring of the infusion fluid mixture and the patient should occur.

INTERMITTENT INFUSION

Intermittent infusion is the administration of a small-volume infusion, i.e. 50–250 ml, over a period of between 20 minutes and 2 hours. This may be given as a specific dose at one time or at repeated intervals during 24 hours.

An intermittent infusion may be used when,

1 a peak plasma level is therapeutically required;
2 the pharmacology of the drug dictates this specific dilution;

3 the drug is not stable for the time required to administer a large-volume infusion;
4 the patient does not require or cannot tolerate large volumes of fluid.

Delivery of the drug by intermittent infusion may utilize a system such as a Y set, if the simultaneous infusion is of a compatible fluid, or a burette set with a chamber capacity of 100 or 150 ml. A small-volume infusion may also be connected to a heparinized cannula if no fluids are required between doses.

All the points considered when preparing for a continuous infusion should be taken into account here, e.g. pre-prepared fluids, single additions, adequate mixing, labelling and monitoring.

CALCULATIONS OF ACCURATE RATE OF ADMINISTRATION (CONTINUOUS OR INTERMITTENT)

The rate of administration of a continuous or intermittent infusion may be calculated from the following equation:

$$\frac{\text{No. millilitres to be infused}}{\text{No. hours over which infusion is to be delivered}} \times \frac{\text{No. drops per millilitre}}{60}$$

$$= \frac{\text{No. drops to be delivered per minute}}{}$$

In this equation, 60 is a factor for the conversion of the number of hours to the number of minutes; the number of drops per millilitre is dependent on the administration set used and the viscosity of the infusion fluid. For example, crystalloid fluid administered via a solution set is delivered at the rate of 20 drops/ml; the rate of packed red cells given via a blood set will be calculated at 15 drops/ml.

DIRECT INTERMITTENT INJECTION

Direct intermittent injection is a procedure for the introduction of a small volume of drug(s) into the cannula or the injection site of the administration set using a needle and syringe. This may take a few seconds or a number of minutes.

A direct injection may be used when:

1 a maximum concentration of the drug is required to vital organs. This is a 'bolus' injection which is given rapidly over seconds, as in an emergency;
2 the drug cannot be diluted due to pharmacological or therapeutic reasons. This is given as a controlled 'push' injection over a few minutes. Rapid administration could result in toxic levels and an anaphylactic-type reaction. Manufacturers' re-

commendations of rates of administration (i.e. millilitres or milligrams per minute) should be adhered to. In the absence of such recommendations, administration should proceed slowly;

3   a peak blood level is required and cannot be achieved by small-volume infusion.

Delivery of the drug by direct injection may be via the cannula through a resealable latex bung, extension set or via the injection site of an administration set. Whatever method is chosen, the same procedure should be followed. This includes the following:

1   removal of any bandage or dressing present to inspect the insertion site of the cannula;
2   confirmation of the patency of the vein and its ability to accept an extra flow of fluid or irritant chemical.

Administration into the injection site of a fast-running drip may be advised if the infusion in progress is compatible. Alternatively a stop–start procedure may be employed if there is doubt about venous integrity. If the infusion fluid is incompatible with the drug, the line may be switched off and a syringe of normal saline used as a flush.

In some centres a heparin lock may be utilized. This means maintaining the patency of the cannula using a weak solution of heparin. A plug with a resealable injection cap is inserted into the end of the intravenous device. Sufficient heparin to fill the 'dead space' and of a concentration to prevent fibrin formation is injected. The cannula can then be left for a number of hours before reheparinization is required. The time is dependent on the strength of heparin used, for example Hepflush 200 i.u. every 12 hours. After every use reheparinization is obviously required.

The advantage of using a heparin lock are as follows:

1   it reduces the risk of circulatory overload;
2   it reduces the risk of vascular irritation;
3   it decreases the risk of bacterial contamination as it eliminates a continuous intravenous pathway;
4   it increases patient comfort and mobility;
5   it may reduce the cost of intravenous equipment.

An alternative method of maintaining patency is the use of a stylet which can be inserted into certain cannulae.

If a number of drugs are being administered, normal saline must be used to flush in between each to prevent interactions. This flush should also be repeated at the end of the administration.

The insertion site of the device should be observed throughout for swelling or redness. Patients must be constantly consulted about any pain or discomfort they may be experiencing. Problems that arise during administration will involve the vein. Patency throughout should not be assumed. Early detection of extravasation

of any drug, especially in concentrated form, is essential to meet the aims of therapy.

These aims can be summarized as the effective delivery of treatment without discomfort or tissue damage to the patient and without compromising venous access, especially if long-term therapy is proposed.

Summary

The nurse is responsible for administering intravenous drugs safely by the methods listed. In order to do this he/she requires a thorough knowledge of the principles and their application, and a responsible attitude which ensures that he/she does not give intravenous medications without full knowledge of immediate and late effects, toxicities and nursing implications.

Knowledge of equipment and techniques for combining multiple additives is also essential.

Only by investigating these topics can the nurse develop into a confident and safe practitioner.

References and further reading

Band, J. and Maki, D. (1979) Safety of changing intravenous delivery systems at longer than 24 hour intervals, *Annals of Internal Medicine*, Vol. 90, pp. 173–8.

British Intravenous Therapy Association (1987) *Guidelines for the Preparation of Nurses for Intravenous Drug Administration and Associated Intravenous Therapy.*

British Medical Association/Pharmaceutical Society of Great Britain (1988) *British National Formulary*, BMA, London.

Buxton, A.E. *et al.* (1979) Contamination of intravenous infusion fluid: effects of changing administration sets, *Annals of Internal Medicine*, Vol. 90, pp. 764–8.

Department of Health and Social Security (1976) Health Services Development, *Addition of Drugs to Intravenous Fluids*, HC(76)9 (Breckenridge Report), HMSO, London.

Josephson, A. *et al.* (1985) The relationship between intravenous fluid contamination and the frequency of tubing replacement, *Infection Control*, Vol. 9, pp. 367–70.

Mehtar, S. (1981) A review of bacteriological observation in the care of intravenous therapy, *British Journal of Intravenous Therapy*, Vol. 2, no. 4, pp. 16–22.

Nystrom, B. *et al.* (1983) Bacteraemia in surgical patients with intravenous devices: a European multicentre incidence study, *Journal of Hospital Infection*, Vol. 4, pp. 338–49.

Parish, P. (1982) Benefits to risks of I.V. therapies, *British Journal of Intravenous Therapy*, Vol. 3, no. 6, pp. 10–19.

Peters, J. *et al.* (1984) Peripheral venous cannulation:

reducing the risks, *British Journal of Parenteral Therapy*, Vol. 5, no. 2, pp. 56–68.

Plumer, A.L. (1987) *Principles and Practice of Intravenous Therapy*, 4th edn, Little Brown & Co, Boston, USA.

Sager, D. and Bomar, S. (1980) *Intravenous Medications*, J.B. Lippincott, Philadelphia.

Sager, D. and Bomar, S. (1983) *Quick Reference to Intravenous Drugs*, J.B. Lippincott, Philadelphia.

Smith, R. (1985a) Extravasation of intravenous fluids, *British Journal of Parenteral Therapy*, Vol. 6, no. 2, pp. 30–5.

Smith, R. (1985b) Prevention and treatment of extravasation, *British Journal of Parenteral Therapy*, Vol. 6, no. 5, pp. 114–19.

Speechley, V. (1984) The nurse's role in intravenous management, *Nursing Times* 2 May, pp. 31–2.

Speechley, V. (1986) Intravenous therapy: peripheral/central lines, *Nursing* Vol. 3, no. 3, pp. 95–100.

Speechley, V. and Toovey, J. (1987) Factsheets: problems in I.V. therapy 1, 2, 3, *The Professional Nurse*, Vol. 2, no. 8, pp. 240–2; no. 12, p. 413; Vol. 3, no. 3, pp. 90–1.

United States Department of Health and Human Services (PHS) (1982) *Guidelines for Prevention of Intravenous Therapy-Related Infections*, Centers for Disease Control, Atlanta.

Walrath, J.M. *et al.* (1979) Stopcock, bacterial contamination in invasive monitoring systems, *Heart and Lung*, Vol. 8, no. 1, pp. 100–3.

GUIDELINES: ADMINISTRATION OF DRUGS BY CONTINUOUS INFUSION

This procedure may be carried out by the infusion of drugs from a bag, bottle or burette.

Equipment

1 Clinically clean receiver or tray containing the prepared drug to be administered
2 Patient's prescription chart
3 Recording sheet or book a required by law or hospital policy
4 Protective clothing as required by hospital policy for specific drugs
5 Container of appropriate intravenous infusion fluid
6 Swab saturated with isopropyl alcohol 70%
7 Drug additive label.

Procedure

Action	Rationale
1 Explain the procedure to the patient.	To obtain the patient's consent and co-operation.
2 Inspect the infusion.	To check it is running satisfactorily and that the patient is not experiencing any discomfort at the site of insertion.
3 Wash hands and assemble the necessary equipment.	
4 Prepare the drug for injection described in the procedure.	
5 Check the name, strength and volume of intravenous fluid against the prescription chart.	To ensure that the correct type and quantity of fluid are administered.
6 Check the expiry date of the fluid.	To prevent an ineffective or toxic compound being administered to the patient.
7 Check that the packaging is intact.	To maintain asepsis.
8 Inspect the container and contents in a good light for cracks, punctures, air bubbles, discoloration, haziness and crystalline or particulate matter.	To maintain asepsis. To prevent any toxic or foreign matter being infused into the patient.

9 Check the identity and amount of drug to be added. Consider:
   (a) Compatibility of fluid and additive
   (b) Stability of mixture over the prescription time
   (c) Any special directions for dilution, e.g. pH, optimum concentration, etc.
   (d) Sensitivity to external factors such as light
   (e) Any anticipated allergic reaction.
   If any doubts exist about the listed points, consult the pharmacist or appropriate reference works.

To minimize any risk of error. To ensure safe and effective administration of the drug. To enable anticipation of toxicities and the nursing implications of these.

10 Any additions must be made immediately prior to use.

To prevent any possible microbial growth or degradation.

11 Wash hands thoroughly.

To maintain asepsis.

12 Expose the injection site on the container by removing any seal present.

13 Clean the site with the swab and allow it to dry.

To maintain asepsis.

14 Inject the drug using a new sterile needle into the bag, bottle or burette. A 23 or 25G needle should be used.

To enable resealing of the latex or rubber injection site.

15 If the addition is made into a burette at the bedside:
   (a) Avoid contamination of the needle and inlet port.
   (b) Check that the correct quantity of fluid is in the chamber.
   (c) Switch the infusion off briefly so that a bolus injection is not given.

To maintain asepsis and prevent incompatibility, etc.

16 Invert the container a number of times, especially if adding to a flexible infusion bag.

To ensure adequate mixing of the drug.

17 Check again for haziness, discoloration, etc. This can occur even if the mixture is theoretically compatible, thus making vigilance essential.

To detect any incompatibility or degradation.

18 Complete the drug additive label and fix it on the bag, bottle or burette. Complete the patient's recording chart and other hospital and/or legally required documents.

To maintain accurate records. To provide a point of reference in the event of any queries. To prevent any duplication of treatment.

19 Place the container in a clinically clean receptacle. Wash hands and proceed to the patient.

To maintain aspesis.

20 Check again that the infusion is running well and that the contents of the previous container have been delivered.

To confirm that the vein and/or cannula remain patent. To ensure that the preceding prescription has been administered.

21 Switch off the infusion and hang the new container quickly using a non-touch technique.

To achieve a safe and aseptic change-over.

22 Restart the infusion and adjust the rate of flow as prescribed.

To deliver the mixture accurately.

Action	Rationale
23 If the addition is made into a burette, the infusion can be restarted immediately following mixing and recording and the infusion rate adjusted accordingly.	
24 Ask the patient if he/she is experiencing any abnormal sensations, etc.	To ascertain whether there are any problems. If so, investigate.
25 Discard waste, making sure that it is placed in the correct containers, e.g. 'sharps' into a designated receptacle.	To ensure safe disposal and avoid injury to staff. To prevent re-use of equipment.

GUIDELINES: ADMINISTRATION OF DRUGS BY INTERMITTENT INFUSION

This procedure is carried out via a heparinized cannula or when patency is maintained by a stylet.

Equipment

Equipment for this procedure is as described for the previous procedure (i.e. items 1–7, p. 184) together with the following:

 8 Intravenous administration set
 9 Intravenous infusion stand
10 Clean dressing trolley
11 Clinically clean receiver or tray
12 Sterile needles and syringes
13 Normal saline 0.9%, 20 ml for injection
14 Heparin, in accordance with hospital policy, plus sterile bung or sterile stylet
15 Alcohol-based lotion for cleaning injection site
16 Alcohol-based hand wash solution
17 Sterile dressing pack
18 Hypo-allergenic tape.

Procedure

Action	Rationale
1 Explain the procedure to the patient.	To obtain the patient's consent and co-operation.
2 Prepare the intravenous infusion and additive as described previously (see items 2–11, pp. 184–5).	
3 Prime the intravenous administration set with infusion fluid mixture and hang it on the infusion stand.	
4 Draw up 10 ml of normal saline 0.9% for injection in two separate syringes, using an aseptic technique.	
5 Draw up heparin, as required by hospital policy, and check.	
6 Place the syringes in a clinically clean receiver or tray on the bottom shelf of the dressing trolley.	

7	Collect the other equipment and place it on the bottom shelf of the dressing trolley.	
8	Place a sterile dressing pack on the top of the trolley.	
9	Check that all necessary equipment is present.	To prevent delays and interruption of the procedure.
10	Wash hands thoroughly before leaving the clinical room.	To maintain asepsis.
11	Proceed to the patient.	
12	Open the sterile dressing pack.	To maintain asepsis.
13	Add lotion for cleaning the skin to the gallipot in order to wet the cotton wool balls.	
14	Wash hands with soap and water or with an alcohol-based hand wash solution.	To maintain asepsis.
15	Remove the patient's bandage and dressing.	To observe the insertion site.
16	Inspect the insertion site of the cannula.	To detect any signs of inflammation, infiltration, etc. If present, take appropriate action.
17	Wash hands or clean them with an alcohol-based hand wash solution.	To maintain asepsis.
18	Place a sterile towel under the patient's arm.	To create a sterile field.
19	Remove the injection bung or stylet from the cannula while applying digital pressure at the point when the vein where the cannula tip rests. This may be achieved easier using a sterile cotton wool ball.	To prevent blood spillage.
20	Inject gently 10 ml of normal saline 0.9% for injection.	To confirm the patency of the cannula.
21	If no resistance is met, no pain or discomfort is felt by the patient, no swelling is evident, no leakage occurs around the cannula and there is a good backflow of blood on aspiration, it can be assumed that the cannula is patent.	
22	Connect to the infusion.	To commence treatment.
23	Open the control valve.	To check free flow.
24	Check the insertion site and ask the patient if he/she is comfortable.	To confirm that the vein can accommodate the extra fluid flow and that the patient experiences no pain, etc.
25	Adjust the flow rate as prescribed.	To ensure that the correct speed of administration is established.
26	Tape the administration set in a way that places no strain on the cannula.	To reduce the risk of mechanical phlebitis or infiltration.

Action	**Rationale**
27 Cover the cannula with a sterile topical swab and tape it in place.	To maintain asepsis.
28 If the infusion is to be completed within 40 minutes, bandaging is unnecessary and the patient may be instructed to keep the arm resting on the sterile field.	
29 Cover the dressing trolley and equipment with a sterile towel and leave by the bedside.	To maintain asepsis.
30 Return at frequent intervals.	To check the flow rate, the patient's comfort and for signs of infiltration.
31 If the infusion is to be in progress for longer than 40 minutes, a bandage should be applied. The equipment may be cleared away and reassembled at the end of the infusion.	To provide support and to promote patient comfort.
32 When the infusion is complete, wash hands and recheck that all the equipment required is present.	To maintain asepsis and ensure that the procedure runs smoothly.
33 Stop the infusion when all the fluid has been delivered.	To ensure that all of the prescribed mixture has been delivered.
34 Wash hands or clean them with an alcohol-based hand wash solution.	To maintain asepsis.
35 Disconnect the infusion set and flush the cannula with 10 ml of normal saline 0.9% for injection. (A 'minibag' may be used to flush the drug through the tubing but the cost implications of this should be considered before this is routinely adopted.)	To flush any remaining irritating solution away from the cannula.
36 Insert a new sterile bung or stylet.	
	To maintain the patency of the cannula for future use.
37 If a new sterile bung is inserted, heparinization must follow.	
38 Clean the injection site of the bung with a swab saturated with isopropyl alcohol 70%.	To maintain asepsis.
39 Administer heparin, as prescribed, using a 23 or 25G needle.	To maintain the patency of the cannula and enable resealing of the latex injection site.
40 Cover the insertion site and cannula with a new sterile topical swab. Tape it in place.	To maintain asepsis.
41 Apply a bandage.	To provide support and increase the patient's comfort.
42 Ensure that the patient is comfortable.	
43 Discard waste, placing it in the correct containers, e.g. 'sharps' into a designated container.	To ensure safe disposal and avoid injury to staff. To prevent re-use of equipment.

GUIDELINES: ADMINISTRATION OF DRUGS BY DIRECT INJECTION, BOLUS OR PUSH

This procedure may be carried out via any one of the following:

1   the injection site of an intravenous administration set;
2   an adaptor or injectable plug into a cannula or winged infusion device (patency may be maintained by stylet or by heparinization);
3   an extension set, multiple adaptor or stopcock (one-, two- or three-way).

Equipment

1   Clinically clean receiver or tray containing the prepared drug(s) to be administerd
2   Patient's prescription chart
3   Recording sheet or book as required by law or hospital policy
4   Protective clothing as required by hospital policy or specific drugs
5   Clean dressing trolley
6   Clinically clean receiver or tray
7   Sterile needles and syringes
8   Normal saline 0.9%, 20 ml for injection
9   Heparin, in accordance with hospital policy, or a sterile intravenous stylet
10 Alcohol-based lotion for cleaning injection site
11 Sterile dressing pack
12 Hypo-allergenic tape

Procedure

Action	**Rationale**
1 Explain the procedure to the patient.	To obtain the patient's consent and co-operation.
2 Check any infusion in progress.	To see if it is running satisfactorily, and that the patient is not experiencing any discomfort at the site of insertion.
3 Wash hands and assemble necessary equipment.	
4 Prepare the drug for injection as per procedure.	
5 Prepare a 20-ml syringe of normal saline 0.9% for injection, as described, using aseptic technique.	
6 Draw up heparin, as required by hospital policy, and check.	
7 Place syringes in a clinically clean receptacle on the bottom shelf of the dressing trolley, along with the receptacle containing any drug(s) to be administered.	
8 Collect the other equipment and place it on the bottom of the trolley.	
9 Place a sterile dressing pack on top of the trolley.	
10 Check that all necessary equipment is present.	To prevent delays and interruption of the procedure.
11 Wash hands thoroughly.	To maintain asepsis.

Action	Rationale
12 Proceed to the patient.	
13 Open the sterile dressing pack. Add lotion to wet the cotton wool balls.	
14 Wash hands or clean them with an alcohol-based hand wash solution.	To maintain asepsis.
15 Remove the bandage and dressing.	To observe the insertion site.
16 Inspect the insertion site of the cannula.	To detect any signs of inflammation, infiltration, etc. If present, take appropriate action.
17 Observe the infusion, if in progress, to confirm that it is running as desired. If the infusion is normal saline 0.9% with no additives, confirmation of patency and flushing with a separate syringe of normal saline are not necessary.	
18 Wash hands or clean them with an alcohol-based hand wash solution.	To maintain asepsis.
19 Place a sterile towel under the patient's arm.	To create a sterile field.
20 Clean the injection site with a swab soaked in alcohol-based solution. Allow the site to dry.	To maintain asepsis.
21 Switch off the infusion or close the fluid path of a tap or stopcock.	To prevent excessive pressure within the vein. To prevent contact with an incompatible infusion fluid. To allow the nurse to concentrate on the site of insertion and injection.
22 Inject normal saline 0.9% gently.	To confirm patency of the vein. To prevent contact with an incompatible infusion fluid.
23 Use a sterile 23 or 25G needle if the injection is made through a resealable latex site.	To enable resealing of the site at the end of the injection.
24 Change syringes and inject the drug smoothly in the direction of flow at the specified rate.	To prevent excessive pressure within the vein. To prevent speed shock.
25 Observe the insertion site of the cannula throughout.	To detect any complications at an early stage, e.g. extravasation or local allergic reaction.
26 Blood return and/or 'flashback' must be checked frequently throughout the injection.	To confirm that the device is correctly placed and that the vein remains patent.
27 Consult the patient during the injection about any discomfort, etc.	To detect any complications at an early stage, and ensure patient comfort.
28 If more than one drug is to be administered, flush with normal saline between administrations by restarting the infusion or changing syringes.	To prevent drug interactions.

29 At the end of the injection, flush with normal saline by restarting the infusion or changing syringes.

To flush any remaining irritant solution away from the cannula site.

30 Instructions in the manufacturers' literature may specifically recommend that the drug is given into the injection site of an infusion that is running rapidly.

To increase dilution and reduce venous irritation.

31 Check that the infusion fluid in progress and the drug are compatible. If not, change the fluid.

To prevent drug interaction.

32 Open the control clamp of the giving set fully. Inject the drug at a speed sufficient to slow but not stop the infusion.

To prevent a backflow of drug up the tubing.

33 Observe the insertion site of the cannula carefully.

To detect any complications at an early stage. Extra pressure within the vein caused by both fluid flow and injection of the drug may cause rupture.

34 After the final flush of normal saline adjust the infusion rate as prescribed *or* open the fluid path of the tap or stopcock *or* maintain the patency of the cannula by using heparin solution or an intravenous stylet.

35 Cover the insertion site with new sterile topical dressing and tape it in place.

To continue accurate delivery of therapy.

36 Apply a bandage.

To maintain asepsis.

37 Make sure that the patient is comfortable.

To provide support and increase the patient's comfort.

38 Record the administration on appropriate sheets.

To maintain accurate records, provide a point of reference in the event of any queries and prevent any duplication of treatment.

39 Discard waste, making sure that it is placed in the correct containers, e.g. 'sharps' into a designated receptacle.

To ensure safe disposal and avoid injury to staff. To prevent reuse of equipment.

NURSING CARE PLAN

The problems associated with injection and infusion of intravenous fluids and drugs fall into two categories:
1   local venous complications associated with the cannula insertion site;
2   systemic problems which affect the whole patient, exerting effects on vital organs and their functions.

The nurse must observe the insertion site, the infusion and the patient regularly to detect any complications at the earliest possible moment and to prevent progression to more serious conditions. Early detection also includes paying attention to the patient's comments. The patient's symptoms and physical signs both constitute reasons for a resiting of the cannula or discontinuation of the infusion. Signs and symptoms are used as problem headings.

Problem	Possible causes	Preventive nursing measures	Suggested action
Infusion slows or stops.	Change in position of the following:		
	(i) Patient.	Check the height of the fluid container if the patient is active, as all infusions run by gravity.	Adjust the height accordingly.
	(ii) Limb.	Tape, bandage or splint the limb if infusion is sited at a point of flexion.	Move the arm or hand until infusion starts again.
		Instruct the patient on the amount of movement permitted. Continued movement could result in mechanical phlebitis.	Retape, bandage or splint the limb again carefully in the desired position.
	(iii) Administration set.	Check for kinks and/or compression if the patient is active or restless.	Correct accordingly.
	(iv) Cannula.	Tape the cannula firmly to prevent movement. It may come into contact with the vein wall or a valve. Infusions sited in small veins are prone to this problem.	Remove the bandage and dressing and manoeuvre the cannula gently until the infusion starts again. Retape carefully.
	Technical problems:		
	(i) No air inlet in the rigid container.	Ensure that the container is vented.	Vent if necessary.
	(ii) Empty container.	Check fluid levels regularly.	Replace the fluid container before it runs dry.
	(iii) Venous spasm due to chemical irritation or coldness.	Dilute drugs as recommended. Remove solutions from the refrigerator a short time before use.	Apply a warm compress to soothe and dilate the vein, increase blood flow and dilute the infusion mixture.
	(iv) Injury to the vein.	Detect any injury early as it is likely to progress and cause more serious conditions (see below).	Stop the infusion and request a resiting of the cannula.
	(v) Occlusion of the cannula due to fibrin formation.	Maintain a continuous, regular fluid flow or ensure that patency is maintained by heparinization or by placement of a stylet. Instruct the patient to keep limb at waist level or below if ambulant.	Attempt to flush the cannula gently using a 1 ml syringe of normal saline. If resistance is met, stop and request a resiting of the cannula.
	(vi) The cannula has become displaced either completely or partially, i.e. it has 'tissued'.	Tape the cannula and the giving set so that no stress is placed on them. Instruct the patient on the amount of movement permitted.	Confirm that infiltration has occurred by (i) inspecting the site for leakage, swelling, etc.; (ii) testing the temperature of the skin – it will be cooler if infiltration has occurred; (iii) comparing the size of the limb with the

opposite one; (iv) applying a tourniquet above the cannula site or lower the infusion below the height of the limb.

If the vein is patent, blood will flow back into the giving set. Once infiltration has been confirmed, stop the infusion and request a resiting of the cannula. If the infusion is allowed to progress, discomfort and tissue damage will result. Apply cold or warm compresses to provide symptomatic relief. Reassure the patient by explaining what is happening.

Erythema or inflammation around the insertion site.	Phlebitis due to: (i) Sepsis	Adhere to aseptic techniques when performing all intravenous procedures.	Stop the infusion and request a resiting of the cannula. Follow hospital policy about sending equipment for bacterial analysis. Clean the area and apply a sterile dressing. Check regularly.
	(ii) Chemical irritation.	Dilute drugs according to instructions. Check compatibilities carefully to reduce the risk of particulate formation. Be aware of the factors involved, e.g. pH.	Stop the infusion and request a resiting of the cannula. If the infusion is allowed to progress, tissue damage and severe pain will result. Apply cold or warm compresses to provide symptomatic relief. Encourage movement of the limb. Reassure the patient by explaining what is happening.
	(iii) Mechanical irritation.	Tape, bandage or splint the limb if the infusion is sited at a point of flexion. Use an extension set to minimize direct handling if cannula sited in awkward position. Instruct the patient on the amount of movement permitted.	Stop the infusion and request a resiting of the cannula. Although inflammation of this type progresses more slowly, it will cause discomfort. Provide symptomatic relief as above. Encourage movement and reassure the patient by explaining what is happening. Failure to detect and act when phlebitis is at an early stage, for whatever reason, will result in painful

Problem	Possible causes	Preventive nursing measures	Suggested actions
			and incapacitating thrombophlebitis. Dislodgement of a thrombus could cause a pulmonary embolus.
	Infection with or without discharge.	Adhere to aseptic techniques when performing all intravenous procedures. Observe all recommendations for equipment changes, etc.	Stop the infusion and request a resiting of the cannula. Follow hospital policy about sending equipment for bacterial analysis. Clean the area and apply a sterile dressing. Check regularly. Observe the patient for signs of systemic infection.
	Cellulitis due to (i) Sepsis (ii) Non-specific sterile inflammation.	As above.	As above. Due to the nature of the connective tissue any infection or inflammation spreads quickly, especially if the limb is oedematous.
	Local allergic reaction.	Ask if the patient has any allergies before administration of any drugs or fluids, including sensitivities to topical solutions. Check whether the particular medication is commonly associated with local or venous flushing.	Observe the patient for systemic reaction. Treat the local area symptomatically. Reassure the patient.
Local oedema	During infusion: (i) Infiltration. (ii) Phlebitis.	Tape the cannula and giving set so that no stress is placed on the cannula. Use an extension set. Instruct the patient on the amount of movement permitted. Check regularly for swelling, e.g. tightness of bandages or a wedding ring.	Stop the infusion and request a resiting of the cannula before proceeding. Apply cold or warm compresses to provide symptomatic relief. Reassure the patient by explaining what is happening.
	During injection: (i) Extravasation of medication.	Observe the patient carefully throughout drug administration.	Stop the injection immediately extravasation is suspected. Act in accordance with hospital policy. Some drugs may cause inflammation and supportive, symptomatic relief will be required. Others may have the potential to cause necrosis of tissue and further action may be necessary.

Oedema of the limb.	Infiltration.	Tape the cannula and giving set so that no stress is placed on the cannula. Use an extension set. Instruct the patient on the amount of movement permitted. Check regularly for swelling, as above.	Stop the infusion and request a resiting of the cannula. Provide symptomatic relief and support. Reassure the patient.
	Circulatory overload.	Administer infusion fluids at the prescribed rate and do not make sudden alterations of flow. Be aware of the patient's renal and cardiac status. Monitor intake and output routinely.	Slow the infusion. Monitor vital signs for increase in blood pressure and respirations. Place the patient in an upright position and keep him/her warm to promote peripheral circulation and relieve stress on the central veins. Reassure the patient. Notify a doctor immediately.
Pain at the insertion site.	All of the previous listed conditions may be accompanied by soreness or pain.	As previously listed.	Provide local symptomatic relief as required. Administer systemic analgesia, as prescribed, if necessary.
Pyrexia, rigors, tachycardia.	Septicaemia.	Adhere to aseptic techniques when performing all intravenous procedures. Inspect all equipment, infusion fluids, etc., before use. Observe recommendations for additives, equipment changes and general management. Avoid hazardous equipment, e.g. stopcocks.	Notify a doctor immediately. Follow hospital policy about sending equipment for bacterial analysis.
Decrease in blood pressure, tachycardia, cyanosis, unconsciousness.	Embolism: (i) Air.	Check the containers and change before they run dry, especially bottles. Clear all air from tubing before commencing infusion. Check all connections regularly and make sure they are secure.	Turn the patient onto his/her left side and lower the head of the bed to prevent air from entering the pulmonary artery. Notify a doctor immediately. Reassure the patient by explaining what is happening.
	(ii) Particle	Check all infusion fluids before and after any additions have been made. Check drug compatibility and stability. Observe the solution throughout the infusion for precipitate formation.	As above, but also change the container and giving set. Replace with new equipment and normal saline 0.9% infusion from a different batch. Follow hospital policy about sending contaminated fluid

Problem	Possible causes	Preventive nursing measures	Suggested actions
			and equipment for bacterial analysis.
Itching, rash, shortness of breath.	Allergic reaction due to sensitivity to an intravenous fluid, additive or drug.	Ask the patient if he/she has any allergies *before* administration of any drugs or fluids. Check whether the particular medication is commonly associated with any allergic reactions and observe the patient more closely.	Stop drug infusion or injection and maintain the patency of the intravenous line using normal saline 0.9%. Notify a doctor immediately. Reassure the patient.
Flushed face, headache, congestion of the chest, possibly progressing to loss of consciousness	Speed shock due to too rapid administration of drugs.	Administer drugs and infusion at the correct rate. Check the flow rate frequently. Use mechanical aids if the delivery rate is crucial.	As above.

FLOW CONTROL

Definition
The delivery of intravenous fluids and medications at an appropriate rate and in a constant, accurate manner, to achieve the desired therapeutic response and to prevent complications. The nurse has a responsibility to determine the correct rate in individual circumstances and to maintain that rate throughout the infusion.

Indications
The following should be considered when a decision on flow control is to be made.
Complications associated with over-infusion include:
1 fluid overload with accompanying electrolyte imbalance;
2 metabolic disturbances during parenteral nutrition, mainly related to serum glucose levels;
3 toxic concentrations of medications, which may result in a shock-like syndrome ('speed shock');
4 air embolism, due to containers running dry before expected;
5 an increase in venous complications, e.g. chemical phlebitis, caused by reduced dilution of irritant substances.
Complications associated with under-infusion include:

1 dehydration;
2 metabolic disturbances, as above;
3 a delayed response to medications;
4 occlusion of a cannula/catheter due to slowing or cessation of flow.
Delivery of fluids and medications should be constant over a period with no major adjustments to 'catch up'. Small alterations are permissible.

REFERENCE MATERIAL
Factors affecting infusion rates
FLUID AND CONTAINER
The type of fluid, viscosity and the temperature at which it is delivered affect the rate of flow. The amount of fluid within the container exerts a pressure which falls as delivery continues. Therefore, adjustments in height may be required. The optimum height of the container above the patient is 0.9 m and consequently changes in the patient's position may mean further adjustment.

FLOW CONTROL CLAMPS
The roller clamps used to control fluid flow may slip, loosen or distort the tubing causing a phenomenon known as 'cold flow'. Any marked tension or stretching of the tubing, due to movement by the patient, can render the clamp ineffective.

CANNULA/CATHETER/INTRAVENOUS LINE
The flow rate may be affected by any of the following:
1 the condition and size of the vein;

2 the gauge of the cannula/catheter;
3 the position of the device within the vein;
4 the site of the intravenous device, e.g. it may be positional;
5 kinking or compression of the cannula/catheter;
6 occlusion of the cannula/catheter due to clot formation.

The drop calibration of the administration set limits flow rate and when slower delivery is required microdrip sets should be used.

The tubing of the administration set may become pinched or kinked causing variations in the set rate.

Inclusion of other in-line devices, e.g. filters, may also affect the flow.

THE PATIENT

Patients occasionally tamper with the control clamp or other parts of the delivery system, e.g. adjusting the height of the infusion container, thereby making flow unreliable.

Complications associated with flow control

At-risk groups include:
1 infants and young children;
2 the elderly;
3 patients with compromised cardiovascular status;
4 patients with impairment or failure of organs, e.g. kidneys;
5 patients with major sepsis;
6 patients suffering from shock, whatever the cause;
7 postoperative or post-trauma patients;
8 stressed patients, whose endocrine homeostatic controls may be affected;
9 patients receiving multiple medications, whose clinical status may change rapidly.

FLUID/ELECTROLYTE IMBALANCE

The most common disorder of fluid and electrolyte balance is circulatory overload, that is isotonic fluid expansion. It is caused by infusion of excessive quantities of isotonic fluids such as normal saline 0.9%. No flow of fluid from the extracellular to the intracellular compartment occurs and, therefore, the extracellular volume increases.

Due to electrolyte concentration, no extra water is available to enable the kidneys selectively to excrete and restore the balance. Early clinical manifestations of this condition are:
1 weight gain;
2 an increase in fluid intake over output;
3 a high pulse pressure;
4 raised central venous pressure measurements;

5 an increased peripheral hand vein emptying time (normal 3–5 seconds);
6 peripheral oedema;
7 hoarseness.

Progression will lead to dyspnoea and cyanosis, due to pulmonary oedema, and neck vein engorement.

The nurse needs to recognize the condition early so that fluid can be withheld until excesses have been excreted. Careful monitoring should continue to prevent isotonic contraction occurring.

If a patient is receiving large quantities of electrolyte free water, such as glucose 5% in water, to replace losses from gastric suction, vomit, diarrhoea, diuresis or insensible loss, hypotonic expansion may develop. This involves both extracellular and intracellular compartments.

This condition is more frequently seen in the early postoperative period and in the elderly patient. Signs which differentiate hypotonic from isotonic expansion are:
1 the pulse and blood pressure usually remain normal;
2 intracranial pressure is raised causing headache, nausea, vomiting, muscle twitching and confusion;
3 tibial oedema is present.

Fluids will be withheld and careful correction of electrolyte balance undertaken.

METABOLIC DISTURBANCE

Metabolic disturbances are related to total parenteral nutrition and most commonly to glucose intolerance. This may result in either a hyper- or hypoglycaemic state. Signs of hypoglycaemia include weakness, headache, thirst and a cold, clammy skin. Hyperglycaemia will lead rapidly to coma.

Disturbances in fat metabolism may occur if too rapid infusion takes place. These are most likely in patients with disordered liver function, major infections or other conditions which create stress.

Accurate control of flow rates of all feeding solutions is essential and the *maximum* recommended adjustment of flow is 4 drops per minute every 15 minutes.

ADMINISTRATION OF DRUGS

Rapid, uncontrolled administration of drugs will result in toxic concentrations reaching vital organs. Toxicity may be manifested by an exaggeration of the usual pharmacological actions of the drug or by signs and symptoms specific for that drug or class of drugs. The most extreme toxic response which can occur if a drug is given at a dose or rate exceeding that recommended, is the lethal response.

Signs of speed shock include:
1 flushed face;

2 headache;
3 congestion of the chest;
4 tachycardia, fall in blood pressure;
5 syncope;
6 shock;
7 cardiovascular collapse.

Administration must be slowed down or discontinued, and the medical staff notified (see p. 196).

Paediatric intravenous therapy

Paediatrics is an area where extra care is required. The heart and circulatory system are smaller, therefore fluid and electrolyte imbalance and circulatory overload can occur more rapidly. Maintenance of flow is usually achieved by the use of special sets and regular monitoring of intake and output is performed.

For example:

Intake

1 an hourly record of the amount and type of fluid;
2 a running total of the amount administered;
3 regular checks of the rate of flow;
4 recording the volume of diluent used in drug reconstitution;
5 checking the electrolyte content of drug presentations, especially sodium and potassium;
6 consideration of additional water needs due to a faster metabolic rate, and a greater loss in urine due to immature renal function.

Output

1 careful recording all output, including weighing nappies;
2 recording any other drainage, e.g. from a wound site;
3 adjustments to allow for insensible loss via a greater surface area.

Other observations include weight and general condition and behaviour, e.g. tachycardia, raised blood pressure and respirations, oedema, headache, abdominal cramps.

Dose calculations of medications should be carefully checked as micrograms are frequently used and amounts often include a decimal point.

Total parenteral nutrition in children requires extra careful delivery and monitoring.

Summary

Careful calculation and control of flow rates are essential as delivery of fluids and medications may be critical due to any of the afore-mentioned factors. There are many infusion control devices available to assist the nurse in this task, ranging from the simple to the complex. A knowledge of these systems and of their application is necessary to ensure appropriate choices are made.

References and further reading

Allwood, M.C. (1981) The control of intravenous infusions, *British Journal of Intravenous Therapy*, Vol. 2, no. 5, pp. 23–5.

British Medical Association/Pharmaceutical Society of Great Britain (1987) *British National Formulary* No. 14.

Department of Health and Social Security (1981) *Health Equipment Information Evaluation Issue* No. 96, HMSO, London.

Department of Health and Social Security (1982) *Health Equipment Information Evaluation Issue* No. 106, HMSO, London.

Department of Health and Social Security (1983) *Health Equipment Information Evaluation Issue* No. 116, HMSO, London.

Department of Health and Social Security (1984) *Health Equipment Information Evaluation Issue* No. 125, HMSO, London.

Department of Health and Social Security (1985) *Health Equipment Information Evaluation Issues* Nos. 135/ 147, HMSO, London.

Department of Health and Social Security (1986) *Health Equipment Information Evaluation Issue* No. 157, HMSO, London.

Department of Health and Social Security (1987) *Health Equipment Information Evaluation Issue* No. 175, HMSO, London.

Hudek, K. (1986) Compliance in intravenous therapy, *Journal of Canadian Intravenous Nurses Association*, Vol. 2, no. 3, pp. 7–8.

Plumer, A.L. (1987) *Principles and Practice of Intravenous Therapy*, 4th edn, Little, Brown & Co, Boston, USA.

Sager, D. and Bomar, S. (1980) *Intravenous Medications*, J.B. Lippincott, Philadelphia.

Wittig, P. and Semmler-Bertanzi, D.J. (1983) Pumps and controllers: a nurse's assessment guide, *American Journal of Nursing*, Vol. 7, pp. 1023–5.

GUIDELINES: CHOICE OF AN INFUSION CONTROL SYSTEM

Available choices
1 Gravity drip, including measured volume sets
2 In-line devices for use with gravity drip, e.g. Dial-a-flow
3 Drip rate controller
4 Volumetric controller
5 Drip rate pump
6 Volumetric pump
7 Syringe pump/driver

SIMPLE GRAVITY DRIP

Advantages	Disadvantages
Low cost.	Infusion pressure limited by height of fluid container.
Familiar to all staff.	Requires frequent observation and adjustment.
Minimal risk of extravascular infusion.	Variability of drop size influences accuracy of flow rate. Inclusion of a burette chamber increases accuracy as delivery is in millilitres/hour.
Infusion of air unlikely.	
	Infusion rates limited especially with viscous fluids and small cannula/catheters.
	Arterial infusion impossible.

Indications for use
1 Delivery of fluids without additives on the majority of peripheral lines.
2 Delivery of fluids without additives on some central venous lines.
3 Administration of fluids containing a small amount/low concentration of medication, e.g. 20 mmol KC1/litre, in the above circumstances.
4 Administration of drugs where adverse effects are not anticipated if the infusion rate varies slightly.
5 Where the patient's condition does not give cause for concern and no complications are predicted.
6 In situations where the rate of infusion is too great to be controlled by the devices available, e.g. 500 ml/hr.

Comments
Many infusions are adequately controlled using the above method. Increased accuracy can be achieved by use of burette set.

IN-LINE DEVICES

Advantages	Disadvantages
Relatively inexpensive.	Infusion pressure limited by height of fluid container.
Greater accuracy over range of flow rates due to measurement in ml/hr.	Infusion rate may relate to cannula gauge/length (specified).

Advantages	**Disadvantages**
Minimal risk of extravascular infusion.	May not be suitable, or may require recalibration, for nutrition solutions.
Infusion of air unlikely.	May not be suitable for or accurate with viscous fluids.
Less frequent adjustments required.	Margin of error increases with high flow rates.
	Methods of calibration, priming of device, etc. require training of staff and accuracy may depend on familiarization.
	Arterial infusion impossible.

Indications for use
As for simple gravity drip, where more constant rate of flow is required.

Comments
These devices are available separately or may be integral to an administration set, so reducing in-line connections. Examples are Dial-a-Flo®, Isoflux®.

DRIP RATE CONTROLLER

Advantages	**Disadvantages**
Automatic control eliminates the frequent adjustment required by the simple gravity drip.	Infusion pressure limited by height of fluid container.
Conventional low-cost administration sets usually used, dependent on tubing size.	Variability of drop size makes accurate determination of flow rate difficult.
Minimal risk of extravascular infusion.	Infusion rates limited especially with viscous fluids and small cannulae.
Infusion of air unlikely.	Not suitable for use on central lines due to increased venous pressure causing frequent alarms.
Alarms available.	Not suitable for use in blood transfusion.
	Arterial infusion impossible.

Indications for use:
Control of flow on peripheral lines when:
(a) the patient is in an 'at-risk' category;
(b) the infusion contains a large dose/high concentration of medication;
(c) accurate delivery of a drug over a long period of time, e.g. 12–24 hours, is required;
(d) the nature of the drug is such that a slight variation in delivery may alter the therapeutic response.

Comments
The maximum rate at which drip counters can be set is 99 drops/minute. This further restricts their use. Power is supplied by mains or battery. To charge the battery machines should always be stored plugged in.

VOLUMETRIC CONTROLLERS

Advantages	**Disadvantages**
Automatic control eliminates frequent adjustment required by gravity drip.	Infusion pressure limited by height of fluid container.
Greater accuracy achieved as delivery in ml/hr.	Infusion rates limited especially with viscous fluids and small cannulae.
Minimal risk of extravascular infusion.	If volume delivered is reliant on drop counting, compensation for drop size is necessary, otherwise accuracy will be variable.
Infusion of air unlikely.	May be restrictions on group of fluids it can be used with, including blood products.
Alarms available.	Higher instrument and software cost, as dedicated sets usually required.
	Not suitable for central lines (see Drip rate controllers, p. 200).
	Arterial infusion impossible.

Indications for use
As for drip rate controller, where greater accuracy is required.

Comments
The type of device is not widely available in the United Kingdom at this time and experience of its use is, therefore, limited.

DRIP RATE PUMP

Advantages	**Disadvantages**
Pressure maintains infusion rate in spite of variable resistance.	Pressure can produce extensive extravascular infusion.
Higher infusion rates with more viscous fluids.	Variability of drop size can make accurate determination of flow rate difficult.
Alarms available.	If incorrectly used can pump air.
Conventional low-cost administration sets normally used, not dependent on tubing size.	
Arterial infusion possible.	

Indications for use
1   Peripheral lines:
   (a)   an infusion sited in a lower limb, to prevent stasis;
   (b)   an infusion sited in an oedematous limb, to prevent stasis;
   (c)   an infusion sited in a precarious vein – regular flow under pressure may prolong the life of the line;

    (d) if two simultaneous infusions are in progress and one is under pressure, e.g. a syringe pump, the second may also require pressure to ensure consistent flow.

2 Central lines:
- (a) when the patient is in an 'at-risk' category;
- (b) an infusion containing a large dose/high concentration of medications;
- (c) when accurate delivery of drugs or fluids over a long period of time is required;
- (d) where the nature of the drugs is such that a slight variation in delivery may alter the therapeutic response.;
- (e) delivery of total parenteral nutrition; flow control is essential on a 3-litre bag.

3 Arterial lines.

Comments

The maximum rate at which a drip counting pump can be set is 99 drops/minute. This may restrict usage. Machines should be stored plugged in to charge the batteries for portable use. Ideally all central venous lines should have a mechanical flow control device attached.

VOLUMETRIC PUMP

Advantages	Disadvantages
Accurate control of volumetric rate in ml/hr or mg/hr.	Generally higher instrument cost.
Accurate control of volume infused.	Higher cost, special administration sets required (cost of disposables may soon exceed instrument cost if used frequently).
Pressure maintains rate in spite of variable resistance.	Pressure may produce extensive extravascular infusion.
Wide choice of infusion rates.	
Wide range of features provided, e.g. central venous pressure (CVP) monitoring.	
Arterial infusion possible.	
Alarms available, including protection against air embolism usually provided.	

Indications for use

1 Central lines:
- (a) when infusion of drugs or fluids is critical, e.g. total parenteral nutrition, high-dose chemotherapy, high-dependency situations using drugs which affect cardiovascular, respiratory or central nervous system;
- (b) where other features provided by the device are required, e.g. central venous pressure monitoring.

2 Arterial lines.

Comments

Volumetric pumps are required in critical situations and, therefore, are mainly used in specialized units.

SYRINGE PUMP/DRIVER

Advantages	Disadvantages
Accurate control of volumetric rate.	Unsuitable for large volumes.
Accurate control of volume infused.	Pressure may produce extravascular infusion.
Particularly suited for small volumes and low infusion rates.	Comprehensive alarm systems not always provided.
Pressure maintains rate in spite of variable resistance.	
Infusion of air unlikely.	
Some alarms are available.	
Some pumps are portable (battery/mains powered).	
Arterial infusion is possible.	
Generally cheaper than volumetric pumps, with low-cost disposables.	

Indications for use
Delivery of small-volume continuous infusions, e.g. insulin, heparin, analgesia, chemotherapy.

Comments
When using a syringe pump/driver on a peripheral line, it must be regularly checked to detect any extravasation at the earliest moment.

Reports that, when used on central catheters, a vacuum created by negative venous pressure may lead to rapid infusion of medications, are under investigation.

PROBLEM SOLVING
Problems are listed under general headings. The action to be taken to prevent or correct these may vary depending on the make or model of the equipment. Therefore, the most important point of reference is the manufacturer's instruction sheet or booklet, which should be read carefully prior to use.

OCCASIONAL MALFUNCTIONS, INCLUDING FALSE ALARMS
Although machines provide a valuable aid to patient care they do not replace the need for good nursing assessment and intervention. They should be checked frequently to ensure the device is functioning correctly, the flow rate is maintained and that no infiltration has occurred, if attached to a peripheral line.

INFECTION
Strict aseptic technique should be maintained when setting up or changing the pump/controller administration set. Connections must be secure, preferably Luer locks when fluid is delivered under pressure. All components of the system should be changed every 24 hours, as per hospital policy.

AIR EMBOLISM
Administration sets should be carefully primed and all air eliminated. Connections must be secure, preferably Luer locks when fluid is delivered under pressure. Pumps with a peristaltic action can pump air if it enters the tubing below the drip chamber.

FLOW RATE INACCURACIES
These may occur due to:
1   variability of drop size;
2   air trapped in the cassette chamber of volumetric sets;
3   a malposition of the drop sensor – drops may be

missed or splashes counted as drops;

4   tilting or dirt on the drip chamber may affect the sensor.

OCCLUSION

Occlusion of the tubing or kinking can cause alarms. Tubing should be looped and taped to prevent this. If maximum pressure is reached by a pump, connections may rupture and if a catheter becomes occluded the pressure may cause it to split with serious consequences for the patient. A peripheral insertion site should be checked frequently for infiltration.

CRUSHING OF THE TUBING

Crushing of the tubing of the administration set may occur resulting in malfunction. Tubing should be repositioned every few hours to prevent this if using a peristaltic mechanism. A movement of 5–7.5 cm forward or backward is sufficient.

OPAQUE FLUIDS

Fluids such as blood and fat emulsions may not be detected by some drop sensors. Manufacturers' information should be checked. Most models can pump blood without causing haemolysis but again refer to the literature.

THE ALARM

An alarm should always be turned on, and taken notice of, to be of value. It may be silenced while the problem is being assessed but should not be permanently turned off. The delivery system should be checked and the pump reset. Only after a thorough assessment should malfunction be assumed to be the cause.

DISLODGEMENT OF THE TUBING OR CASSETTE

The patient may accidentally or deliberately dislodge the tubing or cassette or manipulate flow rate setting. Adequate explanation may prevent this but in confused or restless patients restraint may be necessary.

ELECTRICAL OR MECHANICAL MALFUNCTION

Electrical or mechanical malfunction may occur due to inadequate cleaning or inexperienced handling. All equipment requires regular servicing, but simple measures – such as ensuring the drop sensor is clean and moves freely – can result in trouble-free usage.

18

Iodine 131 Protocol

Definition

Iodine 131 is an unsealed liquid radioactive source with a half-life of 8 days. It emits both gamma and beta radiation. The chief contribution to the therapeutic dose absorbed by an iodine-concentrating organ is from the beta radiation.

Indications

1   The thyroid gland concentrates iodine 131 by selective absorption, causing it to receive a large radiation dose. For thyrotoxicosis a treatment of 75–400 MBq or iodine 131 can be given.
2   iodine 131 plays an important role in the treatment of well-differentiated thyroid cancers of the papillary and follicular type.
3   By the same selective absorption process, metastases that function similarly to the thyroid tissue will also concentrate iodine 131 and be destroyed.

REFERENCE MATERIAL
Treatment programme for carcinoma of the thyroid
SURGICAL REMOVAL OF THE THYROID
Normal thyroid tissue usually concentrates iodine 131 more efficiently than the malignant tissue. Some malignant tissues only concentrate iodine 131 after normal tissues have been removed, therefore, it is normal practice to remove the thyroid surgically before administration of iodine 131.

ABLATION DOSE OF IODINE-131
Following a thyroidectomy an initial ablation dose of iodine 131 is administered. A dose of 1,100 MBq is commonly given, but up to 5,500 MBq may be given in older patients. This ablates residue thyroid tissue and/or residue tumour of the thyroid.

If the cancer is inoperable, a repeated treatment with iodine 131 is prescribed. The first treatment ablates normal functioning thyroid tissue and the second is used to treat malignant tissue.

TREATMENT COURSE
Once the thyroid gland has been ablated, the functioning metastases will concentrate the iodine 131 and be destroyed. To achieve this, repeated courses, commonly of 5,500 MBq, are given with the aim of eventually removing:
1   deposits in local lymph nodes;
2   distant metastases.

Principles of protection polices
The precautions to be observed by individual hospitals and institutions should be available in written form to hospital personnel.

FILM BADGES
Film badges should be worn at all times when on duty.

YELLOW RADIATION WARNING NOTICE BOARD
Such a warning board must be displayed at the door of the treatment room:
1   it indicates what radioactive substances have been administered;
2   the permissible time allowance indicated by the warning notice is intended as a guide. Routine nursing procedures can safely be carried out but unnecessary time must not be spent in close proximity to the patient while the warning notice is displayed;
3   the time given in the table is such that a nurse remaining at a distance of approximately 60 cm from the patient for the time indicated each day would, after 5 consecutive days, receive the maximum permissible dose for the working week.

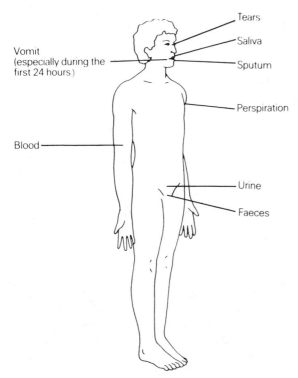

Tears

Saliva

Sputum

Vomit
(especially during the
first 24 hours)

Perspiration

Blood

Urine

Faeces

Figure 18.1   The patient's body fluids will be highly radioactive,
especially during the first few days after administration of iodine
131.

GENERAL CARE

Whenever possible, the ward manager should organize
the duties of the staff so that the nursing care of such
patients is shared. No one nurse is subjected, therefore,
to repeated exposure to radiation during the period
when the warning notice is in operation and displaying a
permissible time.

In the event of any article needing to be removed from
the patient's room, the physics department should be
informed so that its safe removal can be monitored; i.e.
there may be a need to store the article in the physics
department if levels of radioactivity are unacceptably
high.

The patient must be strictly confined to the treatment
area unless required for uptake measurements, scans or
X-rays. These should be organized by the physics
department. It is important that the patient washes,
bathes and changes into clean clothes before going to
these departments.

Iodine 131 has a relatively short half-life and its activity
decays rapidly. Following administration the patient's
body fluids will be highly radioactive, especially during
the first few days (see Figure 18.1).

The principles of
1   distance,
2   shielding, and
3   time minimization
are important in the safe use of all radioactive material.
Since iodine 131 is in an unsealed form, however, it is
important to guard against contamination both of personnel and the hospital environment by the correct use
of protective gloves, gowns and overshoes, thereby preventing the transfer of active material to the individuals
and areas outside the treatment area.

In the event of any accident involving contaminated
material, the physics department must be advised immediately, even if the incident occurs outside normal
working hours.

Contaminated bare hands must be washed thoroughly in hot, soapy, running water, special attention being
given to the areas around the fingernails, between the
fingers and the outer edges of the hands. If gross contamination of the hands is suspected, the physics department must be advised and the washing procedure continued until the arrival of the appropriate personnel.
The application of cosmetics, eating, drinking or smoking while there is any possibility that the hands are
contaminated is absolutely contraindicated.

Preparation of an iodine 131 therapy room
EQUIPMENT

Equipment should be kept to a minimum. It must be
checked to ensure that it is in working order as maintenance staff will only be allowed into the room in exceptional circumstances. Such items as disposable bed
linen, gloves, aprons, overshoes, cutlery and crockery
should be kept separate in a utility room or anteroom
along with the patient's treatment chart and a Geiger
counter.

PERSONAL ITEMS

Patients are advised not to take their personal belong-
ings into the room. These should be stored away from
the iodine 131 treatment room. Valuables should be
sent home or put in the hospital safe. If the patient
wishes to have his/her own possessions, it must be
clearly understood that they will not be allowed out of
the iodine 131 treatment room without permission.

PROTECTIVE FLOOR COVERING

Each patient is assessed individually to decide what
protective floor covering is necessary. The types available are as follows:

Absorbent paper

This is used to retain accidental urine spills or splashes.

Normally one piece is kept in place by two-sided tape immediately next to the toilet. One piece below a catheter bag is sufficient.

Polythene sheeting
If there is the likelihood of vomiting or incontinence, polythene sheeting may be placed over the floor area and kept in place with two-sided tape. This will also be put in place should the patient not be fluent in English or if the patient is incapable of understanding the instructions given.

Cleaning of an iodine 131 therapy room
During occupancy of the treatment room by the patient, cleaning of the room is kept to a minimum and should be organized by the physics department.

When the patient is discharged, decontamination of the room will be arranged by the physics department who will inform the remaining personnel when the decontamination has been completed. The domestic staff may then enter the room and clean it thoroughly.

Preparation of the patient
BEFORE ADMISSION
Twenty-one days prior to admission
Patients taking tetraiodothyronine (T4) (thyroxine) must stop taking this medication.

Ten days prior to admission
Patients taking triiodothyronine (T3) must stop taking this medication.

Three days prior to admission
Occasionally, to enhance the uptake of iodine 131, three daily injections of thyroid stimulating hormone are administered.

ON ADMISSION
Before the administration of iodine 131, any symptoms of diarrhoea or constipation must be remedied. Diarrhoea is a hazard as it can contaminate the treatment area. Constipation not only inhibits the elimination of radioactivity, but obscures any radiological investigations, e.g. scanning.

Patients and relatives must be fully acquainted with the radiation protection procedures and agree to co-operate with them.

The patient should also agree to stay in hospital until the physics department states that the radioactivity level is at a legally permissible level for discharge.

Discharge of the patient
A patient must not be discharged from hospital until the amount of iodine 131 activity present in his/her body has fallen below a certain legal requirement. The value for that level will depend on:
1   mode of transport;
2   journey time involved;
3   home circumstances.

Each patient is individually assessed, usually by the physics department, as in certain cases the biological half-life of iodine 131 is relatively long. An estimate has to be made of how long it will take for the residual activity in the patient to fall to values which will require no further precautions after the patient leaves the hospital.

Patients who are discharged with more than 138.75 MBq of iodine 131 in their bodies are given special written and verbal instructions before discharge.

Reference and further reading
The Royal Marsden Hospital (1978) *Physics Manual Protocol*, The Royal Marsden Hospital, London.

GUIDELINES: NURSING THE PATIENT BEFORE THE ADMINISTRATION OF IODINE 131

Action	Rationale
1 The patient is to be fasted for 2 hours before and after administration of a dose. Offer a light diet for the remainder of the day.	To reduce the risk of nausea and/or vomiting.
2 Administer a prophylactic anti-emetic.	
3 Check that the preparation of the room and the patient is complete.	

Action	Rationale
4 Ensure that any surplus items, e.g. water jug and glasses, have been removed.	To prevent contamination of extraneous equipment.
5 Assist the patient to remove dentures.	To prevent radioactive material being trapped in the mouth.
6 The patient drinks the dose through a straw supervised by physics department staff. These staff are usually responsible for preparing the dose prescribed by the doctor and for bringing it to the patient.	Drinking through a straw reduces the amount of radioactive material left around the mouth.
7 Offer the patient a drink of water to rinse out the mouth.	To remove any iodine 131 from inside the mouth.
8 Apply a wristband showing the radiation warning symbol to the patient's wrist.	To identify the patient as being radioactive.
9 Place a yellow radiation warning notice board at the entrance to the treatment room.	To identify the patient as radioactive.

GUIDELINES: NURSING THE PATIENT AFTER ADMINISTRATION OF IODINE 131

ENTERING THE ROOM

Action	Rationale
1 Put on disposable gloves.	To prevent contamination of the hands.
2 Put on a suitable protective gown:	
(a) plastic disposable apron, e.g. for presenting meals;	To have adequate protection for short procedures when contamination will not occur.
(b) long-sleeve cotton gown, e.g. for lifting patient;	To be protected from small amounts of contamination, e.g. from the patient's skin.
(c) disposable water-repellent gown, e.g. for dealing with vomit or incontinence.	To be protected from large amounts of contamination.
3 Work quickly and efficiently, keeping within the time allowance stated on the door.	To prevent risk of over-exposure to radiation.

MAINTAINING PATIENT COMFORT AND HYGIENE

Action	Rationale
1 Encourage the patient to bathe at least once a day.	To remove radioactive perspiration from the skin.
2 Encourage the patient to wash his/her hands thoroughly after each possible contact with body fluids, e.g. cleaning teeth, going to the toilet, etc.	To remove radioactive material from his/her hands.

3 The patient must remove and clean his/her dentures under running water regularly.	To remove radioactive saliva from around dentures.
4 The patient must remove and rinse his/her contact lenses in their usual cleaning fluid regularly.	To remove radioactive tears from lenses.
5 Encourage a good fluid intake.	To increase the urinary output and elimination of radioactivity.
6 Ensure that the patient has his/her own personal toilet facilities and flushes the toilet twice after use.	To prevent contamination of others and of the environment. Urine of patients treated with iodine 131 is highly radioactive.
7 If the patient is bedbound, catheterize him/her before the dose is given. Empty the catheter bag every 4–6 hours, or more frequently if necessary.	Catheterization reduces the nursing time spent with the patient. Frequent emptying of the bag reduces the level of radioactivity within the area.
8 If the patient requires a bedpan or urinal, this item must be kept solely for this patient's use. The bedpan or urinal must be handled carefully with gloved hands and the contents disposed of in the toilet, which is flushed twice. The bedpan or urinal may be washed in the bedpan washer. It should be sealed in a plastic bag for the journey to and from the sluice.	To prevent contamination of the environment and of other patients and staff.
9 If leakage occurs from injection sites, abdominal paracentesis sites, etc., the nurse should contact the medical staff and the physics department immediately. Any contact with the dressing should be done with long-handled forceps.	It must be remembered that all body fluids are potentially contaminated with radioactivity.
10 Gloves and a protective gown must be worn whenever handling soiled bed linen.	To prevent contamination of the nurse's hands or uniform.
11 All soiled linen must be deposited in a special container provided for this purpose.	Soiled linen must not go direct to the laundry but should be dealt with by the appropriate personnel.

VISITORS

Action	**Rationale**
1 Visiting is discouraged during the first 24 hours following administration of iodine 131.	The patient is very radioactive during this period.
2 On the second and subsequent days, visiting inside the room is allowed if the physics department staff do not advise to the contrary.	
3 Visitors must adhere to the instructions for entering a room. They must sit at least 120 cm from the patient and confine their stay to the time stated on the notice board.	To minimize the exposure of visitors to radiation.
4 Physical contact with the patient or bed linen is not allowed.	To prevent contamination of the visitors.

Action	Rationale
5 Children and pregnant women must not be allowed into the room.	Rapidly dividing cells are at greatest risk of damage from radioactivity.

ON LEAVING THE ROOM

Action	Rationale
1 Remove gloves by peeling them off the hands, taking care not to touch the outside surfaces with bare hands.	To prevent transfer of contaminated material from the gloves' outer surfaces to hands.
2 Remove overshoes and apron or gown and discard them in the bin provided.	These are removed after the gloves as they are less likely to be contamined.
3 Wash hands thoroughly.	To remove any contamination picked up from the protective clothing.
4 Using the radiation monitor or Geiger counter, monitor the activity of hands, feet and clothes. If contamination has occurred, inform the physics department immediately and continue to wash the contaminated area until only background radioactivity shows on the monitor.	To ensure that no active material is present on the nurse.

GUIDELINES: EMERGENCY PROCEDURES

INCONTINENCE AND/OR VOMITING

Action	Rationale
1 Inform the physics department immediately. Put on gloves and a gown. Remove the patient from the contaminated area.	
2 If physics department staff are not immediately available, use a Geiger counter to assess the extent of the spillage.	
3 Put some absorbent material on top of all the radioactive wet area.	To absorb contamination.
4 Leave the area until physics department staff arrive. Polythene sheets may be placed over all of the contaminated area.	

CONTAMINATION OF BARE HANDS

Action	Rationale
1 Wash hands in hot soapy water, paying special attention to the areas around the fingernails, between the fingers and on the outer edges of the hands. Continue washing until only the background radioactivity shows on the monitor.	To remove radioactive material from any areas where it might be trapped.
2 If a wound is produced in a contamination accident, wash thoroughly under running water, opening the edges of the cut. This should be continued until physics department staff can demonstrate that no residual radioactivity remains in the wound.	To stimulate bleeding and permit thorough flushing of the cut.

DEATH

Action	Rationale
1 Inform the physics department immediately.	So that the physics department staff can begin making the necessary arrangements for removal of the body to the mortuary.
2 Two nurses wearing gloves, plastic aprons, gowns and overshoes should perform last offices. All orifices must be carefully packed. Any vomit, blood, faeces or urine must be cleaned from the body.	To avoid contamination with body fluids. Minimal handling of the body reduces the risk of contamination.
3 The body should be totally enclosed in a plastic cadaver bag.	To avoid contamination of the porters and the mortuary staff.
4 Transfer of the body should be arranged with the physics department.	The physics department will supervise the transfer of the body.

CARDIAC ARREST

Action	Rationale
1 When alerting the emergency resuscitation team, the switchboard must also be told to inform the physics department.	
2 Do not use mouth-to-mouth resuscitation. All areas should be supplied with an Ambu bag for this purpose.	Mouth-to-mouth contact could seriously contaminate the resuscitator.
3 The physics department will supervise and provide shielding for the crash team.	
4 Overshoes, gloves and gowns must be put on as soon as is practicably possible.	The emergency equipment may have been contaminated by the patient.

FIRE

Action	**Rationale**
1 Every effort should be made to contact the physics department.	To help in the evacuation of the patients treated with iodine 131.
2 Following evacuation the patients treated with iodine 131 should be kept at a safe distance from the other patients and staff.	To prevent exposure of others to radiation.

19

Last Offices

When a person dies, a number of procedures are carried out under the generic term 'postmortem care'. As nursing students, we learned to wash the body carefully, protect orifices and pad certain areas to prevent bruising. The rationale for these actions was generally presented as 'showing respect for the deceased'. Respect is not the only reason for these procedures: there is a scientific rationale for them.

(Pennington, 1978)

REFERENCE MATERIAL

Little in the way of nursing reference material is available on last offices. The works listed below should be used as a basis for further reading.

References and further reading

Henley, A. (1982) *Caring for Muslims and Their Families: Religious Aspects of Care*, DHSS/King Edward's Hospital Fund for London, London.

Henley, A. (1983) *Caring for Hindus and Their Families: Religious Aspects of Care*, DHSS/King Edward's Hospital Fund for London, London.

Henley, A. (1983) *Caring for Sikhs and Their Families: Religious Aspects of Care*, DHSS/King Edward's Hospital Fund for London, London.

Lally, M.M. (1978) Last rites and funeral customs of minority groups, *Midwife Health Visitor & Community Nurse* Vol. 14, no. 7, pp. 224–5.

McGilloway, O. and Myco, F. (eds.) (1985) *Nursing and Spiritual Care*, Harper & Row, London.

Mascaro, J. (ed.) (1962) *Bhagavad Gita*, Penguin, Harmondsworth.

Neuberger, J. (1978) *Caring for Dying People of Different Faiths*, Austen Cornish Publishers in association with the Lisa Sainsbury Foundation, London.

Olivant, P. (1986) Coping with death: last offices, *Nursing Times*, Vol. 82, no. 12, pp. 32–3.

Pennington, E.A. (1978) Postmorten care: more than ritual, *American Journal of Nursing*, Vol. 78, pp. 846–7.

Royal College of Nursing of the United Kingdom (1981) *Verification of Death and Performance of Last Offices*, Typescript B5/pn, Royal College of Nursing, London.

Sampson, C. (1982) *The Neglected Ethic: Religious and Cultural Factors in the Care of Patients*, McGraw-Hill, New York.

Storr, E. (1986) The cost of dying – practical details the relatives have to face, *Geriatric Medicine*, Vol. 16, no. 16, pp. 40–4.

Thomas, C.H. (1971) Last Offices – a reassessment, *Nursing Mirror*, Vol. 132, no. 15, p. 30.

Williams, A. (1982) *Procedures following Deaths in Hospitals*, Institute of Health Services Administrators.

Useful addresses

Buddhist Society, 58 Eccleston Square, London SW1 (Tel. 01–834 5858).

Hindu Society, Unit 43, 95 Tooting High Street, London SW17 (Tel. 01–672, 1543.

Hospital Chaplaincies Committee, Church House, Deans Yard, Westminster, London SW1 (Tel. 01–222 9011).

Sextons Office of United Synagogue Burial Society, Woburn House, Upper Woburn Place, London WC1 (Tel. 01–837 7891).

GUIDELINES: LAST OFFICES

Equipment

1　Bowl, soap, disposable towel
2　Razor, comb, scissors
3　Foam sticks for oral toilet
4　Receiver
5　Identification labels
6　Any documents required by law or hospital policy, for example notification of death cards
7　Plastic or paper shroud or patient's personal clothing
8　Mortuary sheet
9　Tape or sellotape
10　Sterile dressing pack
11　Bandages
12　Valuables or property book
13　Plastic bag for waste.

Procedure

Action	**Rationale**
1 Inform appropriate medical staff.	A registered medical practitioner who has attended the deceased person during his/her last illness is required to give a medical certificate of the cause of death. The certificate requires the doctor to state the last date on which he/she saw the deceased alive and whether or not he/she has seen the body after death.
2 Inform the appropriate senior nurse and portering staff.	So that relatives may be informed if they are not in the hospital at the time of death. To alert portering staff to begin arrangements for transfer of the body to the mortuary.
3 Place the patient on his/her back. Close his/her eyelids. Remove any pillows. Support the jaw by placing the pillow on the chest underneath the jaw. Remove any mechanical aids, such as foam rings, heel pads, etc. Straighten the limbs.	Rigor mortis occurs 2–4 hours after death.
4 Wash the patient. Clean the nostrils, ears and mouth. Replace any dentures. Trim the nails. Shave male patients.	For aesthetic and hygienic reasons.
5 Drain the bladder by pressing on the lower abdomen. Pack all orifices. Use gloves.	The body continues to secrete fluids after death. Leaking orifices pose a health hazard to any staff coming into contact with the body.
6 Remove dressings, drainage tubes, etc., unless otherwise instructed. If tubes are left in position, cut them to just above skin level, cover them with a dressing pad and secure them with tape or a loose bandage.	It is unnecessary to leave these in position unless the patient has died within 24 hours of surgery or insertion of the drain or if the tube or drain is considered to have contributed to the cause of death.

7	Re-dress any wounds, secure dressings with tape or a loose bandage.	Clean dressings are reapplied to prevent any further leakage from wound sites.
8	Remove all jewellery, in the presence of another nurse, unless requested to do otherwise.	To meet with legal requirements and other relatives' wishes.
9	Put a plastic or paper shroud or personal clothing on the body unless requested to do otherwise.	For aesthetic reasons, particularly if relatives want to view the body.
10	Label one wrist and one ankle with an identification label.	To ensure correct identification of the body.
11	Complete any documents, such as notification of death cards. Copies of such cards are usually required. Tape one securely to the shroud.	To ensure identification of the body in the mortuary.
12	Wrap the body in a mortuary sheet ensuring that the face and feet are covered and that all limbs are held securely in position.	To avoid possible damage to the body.
13	Secure the sheet with tape.	Pins, although providing more security, are contraindicated. If they open, they pose a potential health hazard to staff since bacterial fermentation occurs consequent to decomposition of the body.
14	If required, tape the second notification of death card to the outside of the sheet.	For ease of identification of the body in the mortuary.
15	Check the patient's property with a second nurse. List the property in the valuables or property book. Lock the property in a safe place.	To ensure that all property can be accounted for.
16	Clear away any equipment used during this procedure.	
17	Request the portering staff to remove the body.	Decomposition occurs rapidly particularly in hot weather and in overheated rooms, and may create a bacterial hazard for those handling the body. Autolysis and growth of bacteria are delayed if the body is cooled.
18	Transfer all property, etc. to the appropriate administrative department.	The administrative department cannot begin to process the formalities such as the death certificate or the collection of property by the next-of-kin, until the required documents are in its possession.
19	Amend appropriate nursing documents.	

NURSING CARE PLAN

Problem	Suggested action
Death occurring within 24 hours of an operation.	All tubes and/or drains must be left in position. Spigot any cannulae or catheters. Treat stomas as open wounds. Leave any endotracheal or tracheostomy tubes in place. Postmortem examination will be required to establish the cause of death. Any tubes, drains, etc. may have been a major contributing factor to the death.
Unexpected death.	As above. Postmortem examination of the body will be required to establish the cause of death.
Patient with hepatitis B or who are HIV positive.	For further information see the procedures in the sections on hepatitis B (p. 23) and AIDS (p. 27).
Patient who dies after receiving systemic radioactive iodine.	For further information see the procedure on iodine 131, p. 207.
Patient who dies after insertion of gold grains or colloidal radioactive solution. Patient who dies after insertion of caesium needles or applicators or irradium wires or hair pins.	Inform the physics department as well as appropriate medical staff. Once a doctor has verified death the sources are removed and placed in a lead container. A Geiger counter is used to check that all sources have been removed. This reduced the radiation risk when completing the last offices procedure. Record the time and date of removal of the sources.
Relatives not present at the time of the patient's death.	Inform the relatives as soon as possible of the death as they may want to view the body before last offices are completed.
Relatives want to see the body after removal from the ward.	Inform the mortuary staff, in order to allow time for them to prepare the body. The body will normally be placed in the hospital's chapel of rest. Accompany the relatives to the chapel. Seeing a dead body of a loved one can be a tremendous shock and the relatives require preparation and support for this. Ask the relatives to remain outside the chapel at first. Check that all is ready before allowing the relatives to enter the chapel. Wait outside the chapel while relatives remain with the body unless asked to stay.
Relatives want the body to be placed in the hospital's chapel of rest.	Accompany the body to the chapel and remain with it or outside the chapel according to the wishes of the relatives. When the relatives have left, contact the porter, who will remove the body to the mortuary.

GUIDELINES: REQUIREMENTS FOR PEOPLE OF DIFFERENT RELIGIOUS FAITHS

Buddhism

1   A buddhist may request a Buddhist monk (bhikku) or nun (sister) to be present.
2   A buddhist may refuse analgesia as he/she believes it will cloud his/her thoughts and inhibit meditation prior to death.
3   At death, inform the buddhist priest as soon as possible. This may be done by relatives. The body should not be moved for at least 1 hour after informing the priest as prayers will need to be said. The body is also wrapped in an unmarked sheet.
4   Check all details with the family for there are many different types of Buddhism and each form may vary in its local practices.

Hinduism

1   Inform the Hindu priest. If the priest is unavailable, read from the *Bhagavad Gilta* (1962, chapters 2, 8 and 15) before or during the last offices. There may be a request to place the body on the floor near to Mother Earth before death occurs.
2   The family will usually remain with the patient. The eldest son should be present. Relatives, of the same sex as the deceased, wash the body. Nursing staff may do this if the relatives prefer.
3   Postmortems are not usually carried out since they are regarded as disrespectful to the deceased.

Islam

1   Family members stay with the dying patient and perform all rites and ceremonies. If possible the patient should face Mecca (south-east).
2   The body should be left untouched. Disposable gloves should be worn if the deceased has to be touched.
3   If necessary, the eyes should be closed and the body straightened. The head should be turned towards the right shoulder and covered with a plain sheet. The body must not be washed. The body will be taken home or to the mosque as soon as possible where it will be washed by another moslem of the same sex. Moslems are buried, never cremated, preferably within 24 hours of death. Postmortems are only allowed if required by law. Organs donation is only permitted if absolutely necessary.

Judiasm

1   Inform the Rabbi who will say special prayers with the patient.
2   Usually the eldest son or nearest relative will close the eyes and mouth, straighten the body and bandage the jaw.

ORTHODOX JEWS

1   The body is placed on the floor with the feet towards the door, covered with a sheet and a lighted candle placed by its head.
2   At Sabbath (Friday sunset – Saturday sunset) or on festivals the body must not be moved.
3   Watchers shall stay with the body until burial. It must not be left alone. Burial takes place as soon as possible, preferably within 24 hours of death. Postmortems and organ donations are only permitted under exceptional circumstances.
4   Where it is not possible to obtain the services of a Jewish chaplain, contact the Sextons Office.
5   Hospital staff should carry out the following procedures:
    (a)   close the eyes;
    (b)   tie up the jaw;
    (c)   keep the arms and hands straight and by the side of the body;
    (d)   any tubes or instruments in the body should be removed and the incision plugged unless contraindicated;

(e) the corpse should then be wrapped in a plain sheet without any religious emblems and placed in the mortuary or other specific room for Jewish bodies.

Sikhism

1 Family and friends are normally present.
2 The family may want to be responsible for carrying out the last offices. If requested by the family, close the eyes, straighten the body and wrap it in a plain sheet.
3 The family will wash and dress the body.
4 Cremation will take place as soon as possible, preferably within 24 hours of death.
5 Postmortems are only permitted if required by law.
6 Organ donation for transplants is not permitted.

20

Lifting

The aim of successful lifting is to achieve the required results with minimal effort by the lifter and minimal discomfort to the patient. By fully assessing every situation in which it is necessary to lift, both patient and staff can be protected from injury.

REFERENCE MATERIAL
Potential hazards of lifting
When a patient has to be lifted both he/she and the nurses involved are potentially at risk of injury. The patient may experience discomfort or pain due to being held or lifted in an unsuitable fashion. For example, dragging a patient up the bed causes friction against the sheets and may cause or exacerbate a sore area. Being lifted physically by others can be an unpleasant or even a frightening experience, particularly if the patient has not had the manoeuvre explained beforehand.

The occupational hazard of back pain is well known. It is estimated that 185,000 nurses (43% of the National Health Service's total nursing population of England and Wales) suffer back pain at least once a year (Nursing Practice Research Unit, 1980). Of these episodes of back pain, 44% occur while the nurse is on duty and 84% of them are attributed directly to moving or supporting a patient. Thus one out of every six nurses is likely to suffer back pain while on duty as a result of moving of lifting a patient.

As well as the personal suffering and inconvenience caused by back pain among nurses, sick leave reduces the staffing levels and patient care may be correspondingly affected. It is estimated that 764,000 nurse working days per year are lost in the National Health Service due to back pain. Stubbs *et al.* (1983, 1984) offer a comprehensive account of back pain in the nursing profession.

It is, therefore, of the utmost importance that nurses are aware of the principles of safe lifting and can employ techniques that reduce the hazard of lifting both to their patients and to themselves. Lifting a patient demands

considerable effort but the lifter will be at far less risk of strain if he/she uses skill rather than strength.

Biomechanics of lifting
The spine is capable of bearing large compression forces but is vulnerable to damage from shearing forces along the surface of the discs as well as torsional and twisting forces. Structural damage to the cartilaginous structures may occur as the result not only of one bad lifting experience, but also from continual poor posture or repeated lifting of comparatively light objects in an incorrect manner.

If the trunk is nearly erect, most of the weight of the upper body and the lifted load is directly down through the vertebral column, stabilizing it and causing some compression of the discs. If, however, the trunk is horizontal, these weights produce a shearing force, rather than compression, on the discs.

The erector spinae muscles which provide some of the tension support of the spine during lifting are able to exert greater force lifting a given weight when the spine is in the upright rather than flexed position.

It is not only safer but also more mechanically efficient to lift with a straight back, using the strong thigh and hip muscles to provide the lifting force. When lifting, therefore, the hips and knees should be bent as the quadriceps muscles can be employed to gain vertical movement with minimum reliance on the erector spinae muscles.

The stress on the spine during lifting can be reduced by standing as close as possible to the patient. A large distance of separation will increase the force on the spine and, therefore, increase stress. For the same reasons twisting and jerking should be avoided during lifting.

Factors affecting spinal stress during lifting
By using a pressure-sensitive radio pull it is possible to measure intra-abdominal pressure (IAP) during lifting

procedures. Intra-abdominal pressure may be used as an index of spinal stress as research has shown a close correlation between the magnitude of the IAP, the size of the load and the forces acting on the spinal mechanism (Davis, 1981).

THE LOAD

Studies have shown that the nurse's IAP increases when heavier patients are lifted (Hyde, 1980). Confused, unco-operative or paralysed patients produce higher pressures than others, usually because they make the lift unpredictable or impossible to carry out in a pre-arranged fashion. Patient behaviour as well as weight therefore contribute to the potential hazard of lifting. Many patients, however, can assist the nurses when being lifted, e.g. by digging their heels into the bed.

The lifting technique

The stress experienced by the spine when lifting is largely affected by the technique used. However skilful the lifter may become, he/she must always recognize his/her limitations and get further assistance when necessary.

The lifts most frequently used by nurses are now listed.

THE SHOULDER (AUSTRALIAN) LIFT (FIGURE 20.1a)

If a hoist is not available this is the lift of choice,

although it is not suitable for patients with rib or shoulder injuries. It is particularly valuable when lifting heavy patients as using the shoulders gives the lifter a mechanical advantage.

The patient sits forward and both nurses stand level with the patient's hips. The foot nearer the head of the bed points in the direction of the lift and the knees and hips are bent, keeping the back straight and the head up.

The nurses press their near shoulder against the chest wall under the axillae and, if possible, the patient rests his/her arms on the nurses' backs. One nurse grasps the other's forearm well up under the patient's thighs. The lift is then accomplished by pressing the free hand on the bed, straightening the hips and knees and transferring weight on to the forward leg.

This technique may be used for lifting the patient up and down the bed, or from the bed to the chair or commode, for example.

THE ORTHODOX LIFT

This lift in which two nurses hold each other's hands under the patient involves excessive stooping and twisting for its successful completion. *It is now not recommended as a safe manual lift* (Back Pain Association, 1987).

THE THROUGH ARM LIFT (FIGURE 20.1b)

The nurse stands behind the patient, who is in the sitting position, and places his/her arms under the patient's axillae. The nurse then grips the patient's forearms as near to the wrists as possible by placing his/her hands

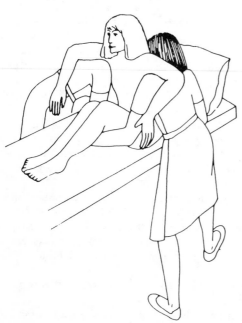

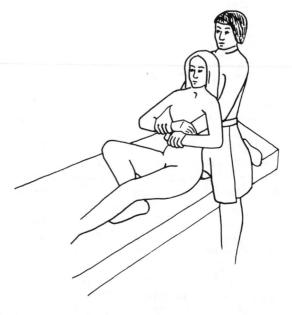

Figure 20.1   *a*, Shoulder Australian lift.   *b*, Through arm lift (second nurse not shown).

between the patient's chest and upper arms. The patient is asked to grip one of his/her own wrists firmly.

The other nurse faces the patient and puts his/her arms under the patient's thighs from opposite sides so that the nurse can grab his/her own wrist. The lift is performed by the nurses extending their hips and knees while keeping their backs straight.

This lift does put unequal strain on the nurses and the one who lifts the upper part of the patient experiences higher spinal stress. However, it is a useful procedure, for example moving a severely disabled patient from chair to bed. It may also be used to lift a patient from the floor and in this situation one nurse stops the patient's feet from slipping, while the other lifts with a through arm grip.

In comparing the afore-mentioned lifting techniques the shoulder lift has been shown to produce significantly lower intra-abdominal pressures (IAPs), and therefore less spinal stress than the other two manoeuvres. The reason for the higher IAPs of the other lifts as compared to the shoulder lift is an outcome of the initial stooped or semi-stooped starting position. The shoulder lift is, therefore, recommended whenever practically possible.

The through arm lift may also be carried out with two nurses – one on either side of the patient. The patient is 'parcelled up' more effectively by holding him/her forward in a sitting position with the through arm grip. The nurses place one knee on the bed and face the foot of the bed. With their free hands they grasp the handling sling placed under the patient's thighs and lift the patient back towards them, sitting back on their heels as they do so.

Equipment
Patients should be encouraged to move themselves whenever possible or to assist nurses to move them by using monkey poles, blocks or other suitable equipment.

References and further reading

Back Pain Association (1987) *The Handling of Patients: A Guide for Nurses*, 2nd ed, Back Pain Association in collaboration with the Royal College of Nursing of the United Kingdom, London.

Davis, P.R. (1981) The use of intra-abdominal pressure in evaluating stresses on the lumber spine, *Spine*, Vol. 6, no. 1, pp. 90–2.

Hyde, N.J. (1980) A comparative analysis of a lifting method commonly used by nurses versus a recommended method of lifting patients, using pressure sensitive radio pill methodology, BSc Thesis, Leeds Polytechnic.

Nursing Practice Research Unit (1980) *Prevention of Back Pain in Nursing*, Proceedings of the Conference held at Northwick Park Hospital, 26 September 1980, Nursing Practice Research Unit.

Rodgers, S. (1985) Shouldering the load, *Nursing Times*, Vol. 81, no. 3, pp. 24–6.

Sorenson, K.C. and Luckan, J. (1979) *Basic Nursing – A Psychophysiological Approach*, W.B. Saunders, London.

Stubbs, D.A. *et al.*, (1983) Back pain in the nursing profession – Part I. Epidemiology and pilot methodology, *Ergonomics*, Vol. 26, pp. 755–65.

Stubbs, D.A. *et al.* (1984) *Patients Handling and Back Pain in Nurses: Main Study*, Report no. JR 125/120), DHSS, London.

Swaffield, L. (1985) Out of Court, out of mind, *Nursing Times*, Vol. 91, no. 3, pp. 27–8.

GUIDELINES: LIFTING

Procedure

Action	Rationale
1 Assess the patient and the environment to establish what help or aids will be required for the lift.	To ensure that the patient is well enough to be lifted and that all necessary help and equipment can be acquired before disturbing the patient.
2 Decide how the patient is to be lifted and ensure that the other nurse(s) and the patient understand what they are going to do.	So that those involved in the lift can co-operate and co-ordinate their movements and any problems can be taken into account beforehand.

Action	**Rationale**
3 Prepare the area. Move equipment into a suitable position, put brakes on the bed and move any unnecessary equipment out of the way. Screen the area if necessary.	The environment must allow safe lifting and reduce the need for the nurse to twist or be impeded in his/her movements.
4 Adopt a suitable stance for the proposed lift as described and illustrated in the reference section, p. 219.	To ensure the lift is carried out correctly.
5 Stand as close as possible to the patient.	To reduce the spinal stress.
6 Lift the patient into the desired position. One nurse acts as leader and co-ordinates the moment of lifting.	So that effort is exerted simultaneously by those involved and unequal strain does not fall on any one person.
7 Check that the lift was comfortable for the patient and nurses, and note any points which could be improved on for future use.	

Note: If something goes wrong when lifting a patient and he/she appears to be falling, it is safest to let the patient fall in a controlled fashion, i.e. by allowing the patient to slide gently to the floor or the bed. The nurse should make the patient comfortable and get assistance to lift him/her up again.

21

Liver Biopsy

Definition
Liver biopsy is the removal of a small piece of liver tissue by percutaneous puncture using a special needle.

Indications
Liver biopsy is a procedure performed by trained medical staff to establish a diagnosis in certain liver diseases, e.g. cirrhosis, carcinoma (primary or secondary), amyloidosis, miliary tuberculosis.

Contraindications
Liver biopsy is contraindicated in patients who
1   are confused or unco-operative;
2   have a prolonged clotting time;
3   have an increased bleeding time;
4   have severe purpura;
5   have a coagulation defect;
6   are severely jaundiced;
7   are under the age of 3 years;
8   have a right lower lobe pneumonia or pleuritis.

REFERENCE MATERIAL
Needle biopsy of the liver was first used by Ehrlich in 1883. For varying reasons it fell out of favour as a diagnostic method until reintroduced in 1939 by Iversen and Roholm. It is now a widely practised technique for the diagnosis of certain liver diseases (see Figures 21.1 and 21.2). It has the advantage of being performed at the patient's bedside. No general anesthetic is required and the patient suffers significantly less pain than with open biopsy.

Anatomy and physiology
The liver is the largest organ in the body, weighing about 1.5 kg. It is highly vascular, is situated to the right upper side of the abdomen below the diaphragm and extends vertically for 15–18 cm. Laterally it measures about 20–30 cm and its anterior posterior measurement is about 10–13 cm. The lower surface is covered with peritoneum. The liver has two lobes: a large right lobe, under which the gall bladder lies and a smaller left lobe. The hepatic flexure of the colon lies underneath the liver.

The function of the liver is sevenfold:
1   to process digested food and convert it into substances which the body can use;
2   to store converted food substances until the body requires them;
3   to produce plasma proteins – albumen, globulin and fibrinogen;
4   to store vitamins A, B, D, E and K;
5   to reprocess body substances, e.g. haemoglobin and amino acids;
6   to detoxify poisons;
7   to maintain body temperature.

Investigations prior to biopsy
1   Blood is taken for:
    (a) bleeding, clotting and prothromibin times;
    (b) platelet count;
    (c) grouping and, if necessary, cross-matching.
2   A plain abdominal X-ray is taken to ensure avoidance of colonic puncture if the patient has a small liver.

Physical preparation of the patient
FASTING
Fasting is required as for preoperative cases.

SEDATION
For very nervous patients a mild tranquillizer such as diazepam may be ordered by the doctor.

Complications
HAEMORRHAGE
Haemorrhage may occur as a result of inadvertent puncture of an intra- or extrahepatic blood vessel. Signs of this will appear within 4 hours of the biopsy. (Loss of

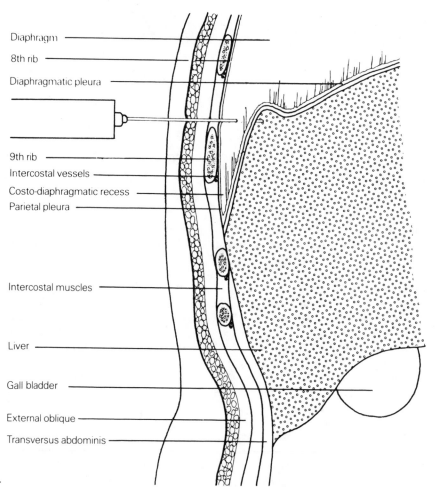

Diaphragm

8th rib

Diaphragmatic pleura

9th rib

Intercostal vessels

Costo-diaphragmatic recess

Parietal pleura

Intercostal muscles

Liver

Gall bladder

External oblique

Transversus abdominis

Figure 21.1 Anatomy of the liver.

5–10 ml of blood from the liver surface is normal following needle biopsy.)

PERITONITIS

Peritonitis may be caused by inadvertent puncture of the bile duct, resulting in bile leaking into the peritoneal cavity.

PNEUMOTHORAX

Pneumothorax may result from inadvertent puncture of the pleura.

Mortality rate

A mortality rate of 0.17% following needle biopsy was recorded by Zamcheck and Klausenstock (1953) and the incidence of complications of any significance is quoted as being below 5% (Read, 1968).

References and further reading

Abrahams, P. and Webb, P. (1975) *Clinical Anatomy of Practical Procedures*, Pitman Medical, London.

Bevan, J. (1978) *A Pictorial Handbook of Anatomy and Physiology*, Mitchell Beazley, London.

Booth, J.A. (1983) *Handbook of Investigations*, Harper & Row, London.

Deeley, T.J. (1974) *Needle Biopsy*, Butterworth, London.

Kilday, D. (1981) Assisting with liver biopsy, in J. Hirsch and I. Hancock (eds.) *Mosby's Manual of Clinical Nursing Procedures*, C.V. Mosby, St Louis.

Pagnana, K.D. and Pagnana, T.J. (1982) *Diagnostic Testing and Nursing Implications*, C.V. Mosby, St Louis.

Read, A.E. (1968) Needle biopsy of the liver, in A.E. Read (ed.) *Biopsy Procedures in Clinical Medicine*, John Wright and Sons, Bristol.

Skydell, B. and Crowder, A. (1975) *Diagnostic Procedures – A Reference for Health Practitioners and a Guide*

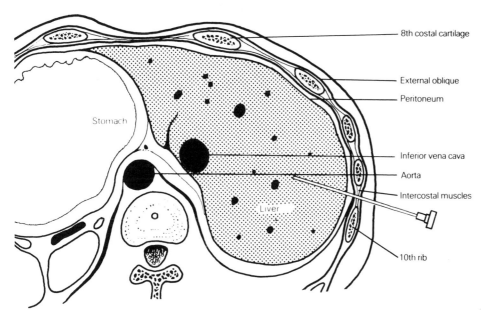

Figure 21.2
Transverse section showing liver biopsy from above.

8th costal cartilage

External oblique

Peritoneum

Inferior vena cava

Aorta

Intercostal muscles

10th rib

Stomach

Liver

for Patient Counselling, Little, Brown, Boston. Zamcheck, N. and Klausenstock, O. (1953) The risk of needle biopsy, *New England Journal of Medicine*, Vol. 249, pp. 1062–9.

GUIDELINES: LIVER BIOPSY

Equipment

1   Antiseptic skin cleansing agent
2   Syringes and needles
3   Local anaesthetic
4   Sterile normal saline
5   Disposable scalpel
6   Plaster dressing or plastic dressing spray
7   Hypo-allergenic tape
8   Liver biopsy needle, usually a Menghini or disposable Trucut needle
9   Sterile dressing pack
10 Sterile gloves
11 Normal saline.

Procedure

Action

1   Explain the procedure to the patient.

2   Demonstrate holding the breath on expiration and observe the patient practising the manoeuvre.

Rationale

To obtain the patient's consent and co-operation.

To minimize the risk of accidental puncture of lung tissue when the biopsy needle is inserted into the liver, the patient will be asked to hold his/her breath on expiration.

Action

Rationale

3 Administer a sedative at an appropriate time, if ordered.

To reduce the patient's anxiety.

4 Assist the patient to lie in supine position with his/her right side as close to the edge of the bed as possible, the left side may be supported by a pillow. His/her right hand should be placed beneath his/her head and the head turned to the left.

To allow the doctor ease of access to the eighth or ninth intercostal space.

5 Continue to observe and reassure the patient throughout the procedure.

6 Assist the doctor as required. The doctor will
  (a) clean the appropriate area with an antiseptic solution;

To maintain asepsis throughout the procedure and thus diminish the risk of infection.

  (b) give a local anaesthetic intradermally and in successive layers down to the pleura (usually 10–20 ml are required);

To minimize pain during the procedure and ensure maximum co-operation of the patient. (No further pain should be felt once the local anaesthetic has been introduced.)

  (c) make a small incision in the skin over the area to be punctured;

To allow ease of introduction of the borer (part of the biopsy set).

  (d) flush the biopsy apparatus with saline to check for patency of the needle. Some saline will be left in the syringe barrel;

To flush out the piece of liver obtained at biopsy, which will be in the core of the needle.

  (e) introduce the needle through the diaphragm and inject a little of the saline;

To remove any pieces of tissue caught in the needle during its introduction.

  (f) ask the patient to breathe in and out fully several times. The patient will then be asked to breathe out and hold his/her breath. The biopsy needle is then rapidly inserted and withdrawn from the liver.

At this stage there is minimal risk of puncturing lung tissue as the biopsy is obtained. Delay increases the risk of a liver tear.

7 Once the doctor has indicated that the biopsy has been obtained, cover the puncture site with a sterile topical swab and apply pressure for 5 minutes.

To prevent infection and stop bleeding.

8 Once bleeding is minimal or has ceased, apply a small dry dressing and secure with hypo-allergenic tape. (A plastic dressing spray may be used over the puncture site.)

9 Make the patient comfortable and position him/her on his/her right side for the next 1–2 hours.

To compress the liver capsule against the chest wall and prevent haemorrhage.

10 Observe the patient, initially, every 15–30 minutes for the next 1–2 hours, monitoring in particular:
  (a) pulse rate;
  (b) blood pressure;
  (c) respiration rate;
  (d) pain;
  (e) abdominal tenderness and/or rigidity;
  (f) leakage from the wound site;
  (g) haematoma formation.
Observations may be decreased according to the patient's condition.

To monitor any complications that may occur as a result of the procedure.

11 Remove and dispose of equipment as appropriate.

To prevent spread of infection.

12 Food and fluids may be recommenced when observations are stable.

To allow adequate time for assessment of potential complications before reintroducing diet.

13 Record necessary information in the appropriate documents and ensure that the specimen obtained is sent to the appropriate laboratory with any necessary forms and labelling.

NURSING CARE PLAN

Problem	Cause	Suggested action
Patient restless and perspiring with a low blood pressure and fast pulse rate.	Haemorrhage from biopsy site due to either a tear in the liver or inadvertent puncture of a blood vessel.	Ensure that the patient lies on his/her right side to produce pressure over puncture site for 1–2 hours. Record the patient's pulse and blood pressure every 15–30 minutes for the first 1–2 hours and decrease the frequency as the patient's condition allows. Call a doctor if there is any alteration in observations as the patient may require blood transfusion, analgesia and sedation.
Patient complains of severe pain which may be accompanied by signs of shock and collapse, with abdominal tenderness and rigidity.	Leakage of bile into the peritoneal cavity from an accidentally perforated bile duct.	Record the patient's pulse and blood pressure every 15–30 minutes for the first 1–2 hours and decrease the frequency as the patient's condition allows. Call a doctor if there is any alteration in observations as the patient may require a laparotomy to rectify biliary duct puncture.
Patient complains of dyspnoea.	Pneumothorax due to a puncture of the lung tissue caused by the patient inhaling as the biopsy needle is introduced into the liver.	Record the patient's respiration rate every 15–20 minutes for the first 1–2 hours and decrease the frequency as the patient's condition allows. Call a doctor if there is any change in observations as the patient may require intrapleural drainage and oxygen therapy.

22

Lumbar Puncture

Definition

Lumbar puncture is the withdrawal of cerebrospinal fluid by the insertion of a special needle into the lumbar subarachnoid space for diagnostic or therapeutic purposes.

Indications

Lumbar puncture is indicated for the following purposes:
1 diagnostic purposes;
2 introducing contrast media for radiological examination;
3 introducing chemotherapeutic agents, e.g. antibiotics or cytotoxics.

Contraindications

This procedure is contraindicated in the following cases:
1 *Raised intracranial pressure*. The procedure could lead to herniation of the brainstem (coning).
2 *Suspected cord compression*.
3 *Local infection*. Meningitis is a rare complication of lumbar puncture. If skin infection is present, examination should be delayed until the problem is resolved.
4 *Unco-operative patients*. Lumbar puncture is a potentially hazardous procedure which requires maximum patient co-operation.
5 *Severe degenerative spinal joint disease*. In such cases difficulty will be experienced both in positioning the patient and in access between the vertebra.

REFERENCE MATERIAL
Anatomy and physiology

The spinal cord extends from the base of the brain down into the spinal column (Figure 22.1). It is encased and protected by the vertebrae. Its width decreases as it descends and below the second lumbar vertebrae it continues as a fine thread, the filum terminale, which is attached internally to the coccyx. Like the brain, the spinal cord is covered by the meninges – the dura, arachnoid and pia mater. The dura and arachnoid mater line the spinal canal to the level of the second sacral vertebra, the pia becomes the filum terminale.

The subarachnoid space, which contains cerebrospinal fluid, is fairly narrow until the first lumbar vertebra, when it widens as the spinal cord terminates. Below the first lumbar vertebra the subarachnoid space contains cerebrospinal fluid, the filum terminale and the cauda equinae (the anterior and posterior roots of the lumbar and sacral nerves). This area is used to obtain specimens of cerebrospinal fluid by lumbar puncture as there is no danger of damage to the spinal cord (Figure 22.2).

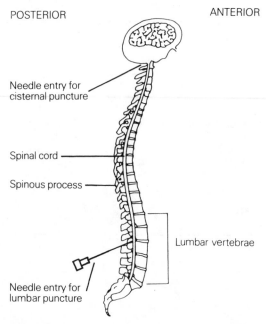

POSTERIOR   ANTERIOR

Needle entry for
cisternal puncture

Spinal cord

Spinous process

Lumbar vertebrae

Needle entry for
lumbar puncture

Figure 22.1 Lateral view of the spinal column and vertebrae showing the level at which the spinal cord ends, and the needle entry sites for lumbar and cisternal puncture.

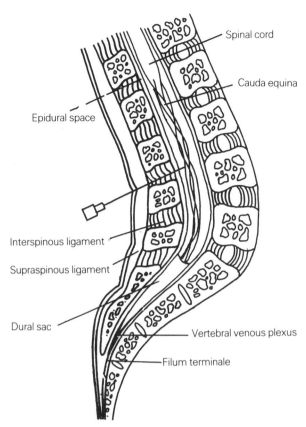

Labels on figure:
- Spinal cord
- Cauda equina
- Epidural space
- Interspinous ligament
- Supraspinous ligament
- Dural sac
- Vertebral venous plexus
- Filum terminale

Figure 22.2 Lumbar puncture. Saggital section through lumbosacral spine.

The cerebrospinal fluid is secreted by the choroid plexus which is situated in the ventricles of the brain. The fluid, which is clear and colourless, fills the ventricles of the brain and the subarachnoid space. Its functions are as follows:

1 to act as a shock absorber;
2 to carry nutrients to and remove metabolites from the brain.

At lumbar puncture, depending on the investigations required, about 5–10 ml of cerebrospinal fluid is removed for laboratory analysis.

Investigations
PRESSURE
The pressure of the cerebrospinal fluid is investigated at the time of lumbar puncture, using a manometer. Queckenstedt's test may also be performed. The latter consists of applying pressure to the jugular vein. When normal, there is a sharp rise in pressure followed by a fall as the pressure is released. Blockage of the spinal canal will result in a sluggish rise and fall or absence of response. Queckenstedt's manoeuvre is a potentially hazardous procedure if both jugular veins are compressed at the same time. Temporal lobe or brainstem herniation may occur. Normal cerebrospinal fluid pressure is approximately 60–180 mm H_2O.

COLOUR
The fluid should be clear and colourless. The first 3–4 ml may be blood-stained due to local trauma at the time of insertion of the lumbar needle. In this case the blood will usually clot. The fluid clears as the procedure continues. However, if blood-staining is due to subarachnoid haemorrhage, no clotting will occur and all samples will be blood-stained.

BLOOD
There should not be any blood in the samples. The presence of blood indicates either a traumatic puncture or subarachnoid haemorrhage.

BLOOD CELLS
There should be no blood cells, except for a few lymphocytes, in the sample. The presence of polymorphonuclear leucocytes (white cells) is indicative of meningitis or cerebral abscess. Monocytes would indicated viral or tubercular meningitis or encephalitis.

CULTURE AND SENSITIVITY
The presence of microorganisms would indicate

meningitis or cerebral absess. By isolating the specific organism the appropriate antibiotic therapy may be commenced.

PROTEIN
The total amount of the protein in the cerebrospinal fluid should be 15.45 mg/dl (= 154.5 μg/ml). Proteins are large molecules which do not readily cross the blood/brain barrier. There is normally more albumen (approximately 80% of total protein) than globulin (approximately 12–20% of total protein) in cerebrospinal fluid as albumens are smaller molecules. Raised globulin levels are indicative of multiple sclerosis, neurosyphilis, degenative cord or brain disease. Raised protein levels may indicate meningitis, encephalitis, myelitis or the presence of a tumour.

CYTOLOGY
Central nervous system tumours tend to shed cells into the cerebrospinal fluid, where they float freely. Examination of these cells after lumbar puncture will determine whether the tumour is benign or malignant.

SEROLOGY FOR SYPHILIS
If other tests are positive, the appropriate antibiotic therapy may be commenced.

Instillation of chemotherapy
Lumbar puncture may be used as a means of introduc-ing drugs into the central nervous system which do not cross the blood/brain barrier. This is done to treat specific infections and malignant diseases such as leukaemia, to prevent recurrence in the central nervous system when remission has been attained.

References and further reading
Abrahms, P. and Webb, P. (1975) *Clinical Anatomy of Practical Procedures*, Pitman Medical, London.

Bevan, J. (1978) *A Pictorial Handbook of Anatomy and Physiology*, Mitchell Beazley, London.

Booth, J.A. (1983) *Handbook of Investigations,* Harper and Row, London.

Brunner, L.S. and Suddarth, D.S. (1982) *The Lippincott Manual of Medical-Surgical Nursing*, Harper and Row, London, Vol. 3.

Clough, C. and Pearce, J.M.S. (1980) Lumbar puncture, *British Medical Journal*, Vol. 280, 297–9.

Pagana, K.D. and Pagana, T.J. (1986) *Diagnostic Testing and Nursing Implications*, 2nd edn, C.V. Mosby, St. Louis.

Skydell, B. Crowder, A.S. (1975) *Diagnostic Procedures – A Reference for Health Practitioners and a Guide for Patient Counselling*, Little & Co., Brown, Boston.

Vannini, V. and Pogliani, G. (1980) *The New Atlas of the Human Body*, Corgi, London.

GUIDELINES: LUMBAR PUNCTURE

Equipment
1 Antiseptic skin-cleansing agent
2 Selection of needles and syringes
3 Local anaesthetic
4 Sterile gloves
5 Sterile dressing pack
6 Lumbar puncture needles of assorted sizes
7 Disposable manometer
8 Three sterile specimen bottles. (These should be labelled 1, 2 and 3. The first specimen, which may be blood-stained due to needle trauma, should go into bottle 1. This will assist the laboratory to differentiate between blood due to procedure trauma and that due to subarachnoid haemorrhage.)
9 Plaster dressing or plastic dressing spray

Procedure

Action	Rationale
1 Explain the procedure to the patient.	To obtain patient's consent and co-operation.

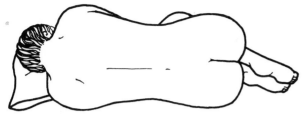

Figure 22.3   Position for lumbar puncture. Head is flexed onto chest and knees are drawn up.

2   Assist the patient into the required position:
   (a) Lying (Figure 22.3):
      (i) One pillow under the patient's head.
      (ii) Firm surface.
      (iii) On side with knees drawn up to the abdomen and clasped by the hands.
      (iv) Support patient in this position by holding him/her behind the knees and neck.

To ensure maximum widening of the intervertebral spaces and thus easier access to the subarachnoid space.

To avoid sudden movement by the patient which would produce blood-stained fluid.

   (b) Sitting:
      (i) Patient straddles a straight-backed chair so that his/her back is facing the doctor.
      (ii) Patient folds his/her arms on the back of the chair and rests his/her head on them.

This position may be used for those patients unable to maintain the lying position. It allows more accurate identification of the spinous processes and thus the intervertebral spaces.

3   Continue to support, encourage and observe the patient throughout the procedure.

4   Assist the doctor as required. The doctor will proceed as follows:
   (a) Clean the skin with the antiseptic cleansing agent.

To maintain sterility throughout.

   (b) Identify the area to be punctured and infiltrate the skin and subcutaneous layers with local anasthetic.
   (c) Introduce a spinal puncture needle between the 3rd and 4th or 4th and 5th lumbar vertebrae and into the subarachnoid space.

This is below the level of the spinal cord but still within the subarachnoid space.

   (d) Ensure that the subarachnoid space has been entered and probably attach the manometer to the spinal needle.

To obtain a cerebrospinal fluid pressure reading (normal pressure is 60–180 mm H_2O).

   (e) Decide whether Queckensteadt's manoeuvre may be performed (Figure 22.4).

To check for obstruction to cerebrospinal fluid flow in the spinal column. (Usually obstruction is caused by a tumour.)

   (f) The appropriate specimens of cerebrospinal fluid about 10 ml in total) are obtained for analysis.
   (g) Once all specimens have been obtained and the appropriate pressure measurements made the spinal needle is withdrawn.

5   When the needle is withdrawn, apply pressure over the lumbar puncture site using a sterile topical swab.

To maintain asepsis and to stop blood and cerebrospinal fluid flow.

6   When all leakage from the puncture site has ceased, apply a plaster dressing or plastic dressing spray.

To prevent secondary infection.

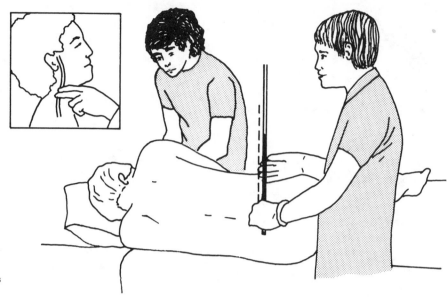

Figure 22.4 Queckenstedt's manoeuvre.

7 Make the patient comfortable. He/she should lie flat or the head should be tilted slightly downwards for a period of up to 24 hours (according to the doctor's instructions).

To avoid headache and decrease the possibility of brainstem herniation (coning) due to a reduction in cerebrospinal fluid pressure.

8 Observe patient for the next 24 hours for the following:
(a) Leakage from the puncture site.

There may be a small amount of blood-stained oozing. The presence of clear fluid should be reported immediately to the doctor, especially if accompanied by fluctuation of other observations, as it may be a cerebrospinal fluid leak.

(b) Headache.

Not unusual following lumbar puncture. Usually relieved by lying flat and, if ordered by the doctor, a mild analgesic.

(c) Backache.

As above.

(d) Neurological observations/vital signs.

These may indicate signs of a change in intracranial pressure. (For further information on neurological observations and the vital signs, see pp. 252–77.)

9 Encourage a fluid intake of 2–3 litres in 24 hours.

To replace lost fluid and assist the patient to micturate, which may be difficult due to the supine position.

10 Remove equipment and dispose of as appropriate.

To prevent the spread of infection.

11 Record the procedure in the appropriate documents.

12 Ensure that specimens are appropriately labelled and sent with the correct forms to the laboratory.

NURSING CARE PLAN

Problem	Cause	Suggested action
Pain down one leg during the procedure.	A dorsal nerve root may have been touched by the spinal needle.	Inform the doctor, who will probably move the needle. Reassure the patient that no permanent damage has occurred.
Headache following procedure (may persist for up to a week).	Removal of the sample of cerebrospinal fluid.	Reassure the patient that it is a transient symptom. Ensure that he/she lies flat for the specified period of time. Encourage a high fluid intake to replace fluid lost during the procedure. Administer an analgesic as ordered. If the headache is severe and increasing, inform a doctor – there is a possibility of rising intracranial pressure.
Backache following procedure.	(a) Removal of the sample of cerebrospinal fluid. (b) Position required for puncture.	Reassure the patient that it is a transient symptom. Ensure that he/she lies flat for the appropriate period of time. Administer an analgesic as ordered.
Fluctuation of neurological observations, i.e. level of consciousness, pulse, respirations, blood pressure or pupillary reaction.	Herniation (coning) of the brainstem due to the sudden decrease of intracranial pressure. (*Raised intracranial pressure is a contraindication to lumbar puncture.*)	Observe the patient every 30 minutes for the first 2 hours for signs of alteration in intracranial pressure. The frequency may be diminished to 4-hourly as the patient's condition allows. Report any fluctuations in these observations to a doctor immediately.
Leakage from the puncture site.	(a) Resolution of bleeding. (b) Leakage of cerebrospinal fluid.	(a) No further action required. (b) Report immediately to a doctor, especially if accompanied by fluctuation in neurological observations.

23

Mouth Care

Definition

Mouth care is the process of cleaning the contents of the buccal cavity.

Indications

1 To achieve and maintain oral cleanliness.
2 To prevent plaque, dental decay and infections.
3 To stimulate oral tissues.
4 To keep oral mucosa moist.
5 To promote patient comfort.

These aims are interrelated as healthy oral tissues are dependent on the mouth remaining clean, moist and free from infection.

The only effective way to achieve this is to ensure that the patient is hydrated adequately and that the correct tools, solutions and mouth cleaning methods are used.

Patients most at risk of developing mouth problems are those who become unable to maintain good oral hygiene themselves. Predisposing factors to poor oral health are:

1 the inability to take adequate fluids;
2 poor nutritional status;
3 insufficient saliva production leading to dry mouth, collection of debris and possible infection;
4 major intervention altering oral status – surgery, radiotherapy or chemotherapy;
5 lack of knowledge or motivation towards maintaining correct oral hygiene.

REFERENCE MATERIAL
Agents used for mouth care

The choice of agents used for mouth care is determined by the individual needs of the patient together with a detailed nursing assessment of the oral cavity. The most commonly used agents are evaluated below.

SALINE

This solution is made up as required by dissolving salt in water. An isotonic solution is recommended for mouth care, i.e. 4.5 g of salt to 500 ml of water (4.5 g of salt are equivalent to 1 level teaspoonful). Stronger solutions may be irritating to the mucosa and will be unpleasant to the taste. Sterile sachets of normal saline are available for immunosuppressed patients. Saline is thought to aid the formation of granulation tissue and promote healing. No damaging effects are known at concentrations that are isotonic or below and the solution is cheap and easy to use. Normal saline is ineffective for removing hardened mucus, debris or crusts.

SODIUM BICARBONATE

This solution is prepared as required by diluting approximately 1 teaspoonful of sodium bicarbonate in 500 ml of warm water. It has a good cleaning effect and is suitable for dissolving mucin and loosening debris. If the solution is made too concentrated, it will taste unpleasant and may damage the mucosa. It is recommended that sodium bicarbonate is only used in mouth care when tenacious mucous is present. There is evidence, however, to support the view that it is not suitable for removing long-standing or hardened debris from the tongue and surrounding tissues (Hallett, 1984).

HYDROGEN PEROXIDE

This mouthwash solution is made up immediately prior to use by diluting the preparation in the strength advised by the hospital pharmacist. Hydrogen peroxide is decomposed to water and oxygen on contact with the enzyme catalase present in blood and tissues. The vigorous release of oxygen bubbles during this reaction acts as a mechanical cleaning agent and is, therefore, useful for loosening necrotic ulcers, crusting and debris. This may also result in the breakdown of new tissue in fresh granulation surfaces. The increased oxygen concentration created by the reaction does inhibit the growth of anaerobic organisms but the foaming effect within the mouth is potentially dangerous if the cough reflex is impaired in any way. Suction should be available if this is the case. Hydrogen peroxide may act as an irritant to the tongue and buccal mucosa, especially where stomatitis is present. It is advisable, therefore, to clean the mouth after its use with warm or normal saline.

BOCASAN

This product is presented in individual sachets containing sodium perborate and sodium hydrogen tartrate. The sachet contents are dissolved in 30 ml of water prior to use and, when rinsed around the mouth, they react to release bubbles of oxygen. This product compares with hydrogen peroxide in that cleaning is achieved by the mechanical action of the bubbles released and by the increased oxygen environment incompatible with anaerobic growth. The mouth should not be rinsed with anything else for half an hour after using this agent.

The effectiveness of Bocasan against hydrogen peroxide has not been evaluated but the taste is considered unpleasant and it is comparatively expensive. Because of the risk of toxicity from boric acid accumulation, the use of Bocasan is contraindicated for patients with renal insufficiency. It would appear that hydrogen peroxide should be the agent of choice here. The precautions for use include the availability of suction when the cough reflex is impaired due to the frothing action.

CHLORHEXIDINE

An aqueous solution of chlorhexidine 0.1–0.2% is sometimes prescribed as a mouthwash. It has a disinfectant action on Gram-positive and Gram-negative bacteria and is useful in preventing the accumulation of plaque and the development of gingivitis when brushing is contraindicated. It does, however, have an unpleasant taste. An alcoholic solution of chlorhexidine may be used for soaking dentures in patients with oral infections of Candida species.

If patients are unable to use a mouthwash, chlorhexidine gel that may be applied directly to teeth and gums is available. Chlorhexidine may stain teeth if used over long periods.

THYMOL

Thymol is the main component of the majority of mouthwash tablets in current use. The solution has a mild disinfectant action and is easy to use, cheap and has a pleasant refreshing taste. It should be used with caution in patients with gastrointestinal disorders or impaired kidney function due to the absorption of thymol during mouth care procedures. It is not suitable for long-term use and has no part to play in cleaning the oral cavity.

MILTON

This product may be used as a mouthwash when diluted in the ratio 2–5 ml Milton: 100 ml water. The main advantage of this agent over others is its antiviral action and it should be used whenever viral invasion of the mouth is suspected.

COMMERCIALLY AVAILABLE MOUTHWASHES

Most commercially available mouthwashes, such as Listerine, are acidic in nature and may have a high alcohol content that patients with an impaired oral mucosa may find painful. Their beneficial action extends little beyond creating a pleasant taste for a short time. The long-term use of some commercial mouthwashes can be detrimental to oral tissues.

LEMON AND GLYCERINE SWABS

Large oral swabs impregnated with a lemon and glycerine solution may be used for a short period (24–48 hours). These swabs are useful in stimulating salivary flow. However, long-term use may cause reflex exhaustion of the salivary glands leading to less saliva being produced.

LEMON JUICE

Lemon juice is an effective salivary stimulant used in several mouth care preparations. Its effectiveness as a salivary stimulant may be counter-productive if the patient is unable to swallow all the saliva produced or if this stimulation leads to exhaustion of the saliva reflex resulting in severe drying of the soft tissues. Lemon juice can also decalcify the teeth and may cause pain when applied to broken or irritated mucosa such as when stomatitis or oral lesions are present.

GLYCERINE

Glycerine has a characteristic ability to bring relative humidities into equilibrium because of its mode of osmotic action. This means that when applied undiluted or in a strong solution to the skin or mucous membranes, it absorbs moisture from them and may lead to dehydration. If glycerine is required to moisten the mouth, it must be used in a diluted form, less than 40% concentration, so that moisture is drawn from the diluent towards the tissues.

SYNTHETIC SALIVA

This product was designed for use by astronauts unable to produce saliva in a low-gravity environment. The constituents resemble those of natural saliva and may be used as often as required for dry mouths without any detrimental effect. This is particularly useful for patients with impaired saliva production.

VASELINE

Vaseline may be used sparingly on the lips to create an occlusive oil film that prevents the loss of moisture by evaporation. Mineral oils are not recommended for this purpose due to the small risk of aspiration pneumonia.

A water soluble lubricating agent, such as petroleum jelly, is preferably for intraoral use.

Instruments used in mouth care

The most commonly used instruments in mouth care are evaluated below.

SWABBING WITH A GLOVED FINGER OR WITH A TOPICAL SWAB AND FORCEPS

This is a useful method of cleaning debris from the soft tissue of the mouth, especially in edentulous patients. Swabbing will not remove debris from the teeth, where it is most likely to accumulate. A gloved finger can be useful for cleaning sore mouths as many nurses feel this is more sensitive than using other instruments. A topical swab wrapped around the end of a pair of forceps is not generally recommended as it is more time consuming than other methods and clumsy to use. There is also a greater risk of trauma to the gums from the pointed end of the forceps.

FOAM STICKS

Foam sticks are useful for cleaning oral mucosa but will not remove debris between or from the surface of the teeth. They are easy to use and there is little risk of mechanical trauma from them. The stick should be rotated gently over the mucosa so that all of the foam surface is utilized.

TOOTHBRUSHES

Research indicates that a toothbrush is the best way of cleaning teeth as the fine hairs loosen the debris trapped between the teeth and remove plaque from the tooth surface: 'The present evidence in favour of the use of a toothbrush for the care of teeth is so outstanding that it would seem to remove all question that this is the method of choice for teeth cleaning' (Howarth, 1977).

Most patients are familiar with toothbrushing and it would seem sensible for this practice to be encouraged. Brushing the teeth, gums and oral tissues with a toothbrush not only removes debris and keeps the mouth fresh and clean but also stimulates tissues thus promoting good oral health.

A small toothbrush with soft bristles that the patient can keep throughout his/her stay in hospital is recommended. There is some evidence for advocating the use of automatic toothbrushes, especially for patients who are unable to use an ordinary toothbrush correctly. The type with an oscillating movement is favoured as those with a purely rotational movement may damage the gums. Teeth should be brushed with firm individual strokes so that any loosened debris is directed away from the gums. The toothbrush should be rinsed and dried after use.

Frequency of mouth care

The frequency of mouth care depends entirely on patient assessment and varies with the particular circumstances of the individual. Dental decay will not take place until plaque and debris have been in place for 24 hours or more. Brushing the teeth after each meal should minimize this risk. Certain factors act as stressors to the state of the oral mucosa. These include the following:

1   mouth breathing;
2   continuous oxygen therapy;
3   intermittent suction;
4   no oral intake.

After experiencing all the above for only 1 hour, a healthy young adult developed dryness of the lips and mouth together with colour changes in the oral mucosa (DeWalt and Haines, 1969). It is reasonable to expect more rapid changes in a more debilitated individual. Normally the saliva lubricates and cleans the mouth and reduces the need for frequent mouth care. For patients who complain of a dry mouth, saliva production may be stimulated by the use of chewing gum or an artificial saliva preparation. Patients with poor appetites should be offered mouth care before and after a meal as a dirty mouth may inhibit the appetite.

References and further reading

Bersan, I.G. and Carl, W. (1983) Oral care for cancer patients, *American Journal of Nursing*, Vol. 83, pp. 533–6.

Bruya, M.A. and Madeira, N.P. (1975) Stomatitis after chemotherapy, *American Journal of Nursing*, Vol. 75, pp. 1349–52.

Campbell, D.G. (1980) Prevention of infection in extended care facilities, *Nursing Clinics of North America*, Vol. 15, pp. 857–68.

Daeffler, R. (1980) Oral hygiene measures for patients with cancer I–II, *Cancer Nursing*, Vol. 3, pp. 347–56, 427–32.

Daeffler, R. (1981) Oral hygiene measures for patients with cancer III, *Cancer Nursing*, Vol. 4, pp. 29–35.

De Walt, E.M. and Haines, A.K. (1969) The effects of specific stressors on healthy oral mucosa, *Nursing Research*, Vol. 18, no. 1, pp. 22–7.

Gibbons, D.E. (1983) Mouth care procedures, *Nursing Times*, Vol. 79, p. 30.

Hallett, N. (1984) Mouth care, *Nursing Times*, Vol. 159, pp. 31–3.

Harris, M.D. (1980) Tools for mouth care, *Nursing*

Times, Vol. 76, pp. 340–2.

Hilton, D. (1980) Oral hygiene and infection, *Nursing Times*, Vol. 76, pp. 1270–2.

Howarth, H. (1977) Mouth care procedures for the very ill, *Nursing Times*, Vol. 73, pp. 354–5.

Lane, B. and Forgay, M. (1981) Upgrading your oral hygiene protocol for the patient with cancer, *Canadian Nurse*, Vol. 77, pp. 27–9.

Lewis, I.A. (1984) Developing a research based curriculum: an exercise in relation to oral care, *Nurse Education Today*, Vol. 3, pp. 143–4.

Macmillan, K. (1981) New goals for oral hygiene, *Cancer Nursing*, Vol. 77, pp. 40–2.

Maurer, J. (1977) Providing optimal oral health, *Nursing Clinics of North America*, Vol. 12, pp. 671–85.

Munday, P. and Geilbier, S. (1984) Provision of dental health education in nurse training, *Nurse Education*

Today, Vol. 3, pp. 124–5.

Nally, F.F. (1977) Infection of the mouth, *Nursing Times*, Vol. 73, pp. 1275–8.

Ostchega, Y. (1980) Preventing and treating cancer chemotherapy's oral complications, *Nursing* (US), Vol. 10, no. 8, pp. 47–52.

Schweiger, T.L. *et al*. (1980) Oral assessment – how to do it, *American Journal of Nursing*, Vol. 80, pp. 654–7.

Todd, B. (1982) Drugs and the elderly – dry mouth causes and cures, *Geriatric Nursing*, Vol. 3, no. 2, pp. 22–3.

Trowbridge, T.E. and Carl, W. (1975) Oral care of the patient having head and neck irradiation, *American Journal of Nursing*, Vol. 75, pp. 921–22.

Wallace, T. and Freeman, P.A. (1978) Mouth care in patients with blood dyscrasias, *Nursing Times*, Vol. 74, pp. 921–2.

GUIDELINES: MOUTH CARE

Equipment

1 Clinically clean tray
2 Gallipots or plastic cups
3 Mouthwash or clean solutions
4 Foam sticks
5 Clean receiver or bowl
6 Paper tissues
7 Topical swabs
8 Wooden spatulae
9 Small soft toothbrush
10 Toothpaste
11 Disposable gloves
12 Denture pot.

All the above items may be left on the patient's locker when appropriate and should be cleaned, renewed or replenished daily.

13 Small torch.

Procedure

Action	Rationale
1 Explain the procedure to the patient.	To obtain the patient's consent and co-operation.
2 Wash and dry hands.	To reduce the risk of cross-infection.
3 Prepare the solutions required.	Solutions must always be prepared immediately prior to use to maximize their efficacy and minimize the risk of microbial contamination.

Action	Rationale
4 Remove the patient's dentures if necessary, using paper tissues or topical swabs, and place them in a denture pot.	Removal of dentures is necessary for cleaning of underlying tissues. A tissue or topical swab provides a firmer grip of the dentures and prevents contact with patient's saliva.
5 Inspect the patient's mouth with the aid of a torch and spatula.	The mouth is examined for changes in condition with respect to moisture, cleanliness, infected or bleeding areas, ulcers, etc.
6 Using a small toothbrush and toothpaste, brush the patient's natural teeth, gums and tongue.	To remove adherent materials from the teeth, tongue and gum surfaces. Brushing stimulates gingival tissues to maintain tone and prevent circulatory stasis.
7 Brush the inner and outer aspects of the teeth with firm individual strokes directed outwards from the gums.	Brushing loosens and removes debris trapped on and between the teeth and gums. This reduces growth medium for pathogenic organisms and minimizes the risk of plaque formation and dental caries. Foam sticks are ineffective for this.
8 Give a beaker of water or mouthwash to the patient. Encourage him/her to rinse his/her mouth vigorously then void contents into a receiver. Paper tissues should be to hand.	Rinsing removes loosened debris and toothpaste and makes the mouth taste fresher. The glycerine content of toothpaste will have a drying effect if left in the mouth.
9 If the patient is unable to rinse and void, use a rinsed toothbrush to clean the teeth and moistened foam sticks to wipe the gums and oral mucosa. Foam sticks should be used with a rotating action so that most of the surface is utilized.	
10 Apply artificial saliva to the tongue if appropriate and/or suitable lubricant to dry lips.	To increase the patient's feeling of comfort and well-being.
11 Clean the patient's dentures on all surfaces with a denture brush or toothbrush. Rinse them well and return them to the patient.	Cleaning dentures removes accumulated food debris which could be broken down by salivary enzymes to products which irritate and cause inflammation of the adjacent mucosal tissue. Commercial denture cleaners, such as Steradent, may have an abrasive effect on the denture surface. This then attracts plaque and encourages bacterial growth.
12 Dentures should be soaked in chlorhexidine in spirit for 10 minutes if oral Candida species are present.	Soaking in chlorhexidine reduces the risk of reinfecting the mouth with dirty dentures.
13 Discard remaining mouthwash solutions	To prevent the risk of contamination.
14 Wash and dry hands.	To minimize the risk of cross-infection.

NURSING CARE PLAN

Problem	Cause	Suggested action
Dry mouth.	Inadequate hydration.	Monitor the fluid balance and increase the fluid intake where necessary.
	Impaired production of saliva, e.g. as a consequence of radiotherapy.	Apply artificial saliva to the oral cavity as required. Give the patient ice cubes to suck.
	Presence of specific stressors, e.g. mouth breathing, oxygen therapy, no oral intake, intermittent oral suction.	Inspect the mouth frequently, e.g. half-hourly. Swab mucosa with water.
Dry lips.	As above.	Smear a thin layer of appropriate lubricant.
Thick mucus.	Postoperative closure of a tracheostomy. Radiotherapy. Poor swallowing mechanism.	Use sodium bicarbonate solution in the mouth care procedure. Rinse the mouth afterwards with water or saline.
Patient unable to tolerate toothbrush.	Pain, e.g. postoperatively; stomatitis.	Use foam sticks or a swab on a gloved finger to clean the patient's gums and mucosa. Saline is advisable. For severe pain use an anaesthetic mouth spray or mouthwash prior to giving mouth care.
Toothbrush inappropriate or ineffective.	Infected stomatitis. Accumulation of dried mucus, blood or debris.	Take a swab of any new lesions for culture prior to giving mouth care. Use a mechanical cleaning agent, e.g. hydrogen peroxide or Bocasan, for swabbing or rinsing around the mouth. Rinse with water or saline after using peroide but not after using Bocasan. Hydrogen dioxide or Bocasan should not be used on granulating tissues, e.g. following intraoral grafts. A warm saline solution may help to remove debris immediately after surgery.
Patient at risk of developing systemic or widespread infection from oral invasion of pathogens.	Immunosuppressive or neutropenic states.	Use sterile water and or sterile saline for mouthwashing and dilution of agents.

24

Nasogastric Feeding and Nutritional Assessment

NASOGASTRIC FEEDING

Definition

Enteral feeding refers to any method of nutrient ingestion involving the gastrointestinal tract and includes oral and tube feeding. Tube feeding may include gastrostomy or jejunostomy, but more commonly nasogastric feeding. Nasogastric feeding can be a very useful method of providing a complete liquid diet to patients.

Indications

Patients to be considered are those who cannot or will not eat food in adequate amounts to meet their nutritional requirements. They may:

1 be unable to eat, e.g. following oral surgery or because of an oesophageal fistula;
2 be unable to eat adequately, e.g. because of swallowing difficulties or a painful mouth;
3 require higher than normal amounts of calories and protein.

All patients, however, must have a normal gastrointestinal anatomy or have partial digestive and absorptive function of some small bowel.

REFERENCE MATERIAL

Nasogastric feeding can be a very successful method of nutrition for the patient. It is less costly and potentially less hazardous than intravenous feeding. If it is to be successfully implemented, however, it is important to understand the principles involved in administering nutrition by this method.

Types of patient suitable for nasogastric feeding

As mentioned above, it is essential that the patient has an intact gastrointestinal tract. Given this requirement, patients with the following problems are normally suitable for nasogastric feeding:

1 compromised access to the normal gastrointestinal tract, e.g. facial and jaw injuries, carcinoma of the mouth and hypopharynx, oesophageal surgery, radiotherapy, chemotherapy;
2 functional abnormalities of the gastrointestinal tract, e.g. fistulae or short bowel syndrome;
3 metabolic abnormalities of the gastrointestinal tract, e.g. malabsorption, pancreatitis, radiation enteritis;
4 hypercatabolic states, e.g. burns, major sepsis, major trauma, surgery.

Assessment

Prior to initiation of nasogastric feeding, the patient must be assessed. This is vital for the subsequent selection of suitable equipment and type and quantity of food and will act as a baseline for monitoring the patient's progress. If there is a nutrition team in the hospital, members should be involved in the assessment and in the development of any care plans.

INITIAL ASSESSMENT OF THE PATIENT

This should include a record of the following:

1 age, sex, height and weight;
2 nutritional history, e.g. any recent weight loss;
3 presenting medical, surgical and psychiatric problems.

FURTHER ASSESSMENT

The gathering of anthropometric, biochemical and immunological material should be carried out, preferably by a member of the nutrition team.

ESTIMATION OF THE PATIENT'S PROTEIN CALORIE REQUIREMENT

If nutrition team support is unavailable in the hospital,

Table 24.1   Guidelines for Estimation of Patient's Protein Calorie Requirement (Modified from Elwyn, 1980)

	Normal	Intermediate	Severely hypermetabolic
Energy per kg body weight	30 kcal	35–40 kcal	40– 60 kcal
Protein per kg body weight	1 g	1.3–1.9 g	1.9–3.1 g

Table 24.1 is offered as a guideline for estimating a patient's protein calorie requirement.

OTHER REQUIREMENTS

It is also important to estimate the patient's electrolyte and fluid requirements and to ensure that these will be met by the feed. If long-term feeding is necessary, the patient's mineral and vitamin requirements must be assessed.

Types of nasogastric feed

Many different feeds have been developed over the years. These range from liquidized hospital food to commercially prepared feeds that are ready for use. The latter are those most commonly used in hospitals in the United Kingdom. The advantages of such feeds are that they:

1 are of known nutrient content;
2 flow easily through the nasogastric tube;
3 are easy to prepare and are sterile.

The fixed composition of ready-to-use feeds may at times limit them in conditions that require modification of a particular nutrient or electrolyte. In these instances it might be more appropriate to use a hospital-prepared feed as the composition may be altered more easily to meet the requirements of the patient. These are several specialized feeds available which are designed to meet the needs of patients with unusual requirements.

Equipment

TUBES

A variety of nasogastric tubes are available. They vary in the material from which they are made, the internal diameter and the length. Soft plastic tubes with a narrow bore are the most suitable as they are more comfortable than the large, stiff tubes and are less likely to cause ulceration. Silicone tubes are even softer but are expensive. PVC tubes are also suitable for short-term use.

RESERVOIR

Two types of reservoir are available:
1 PVC bags with a capacity of 500–1500 ml;
2 rigid glass or plastic bottles.

Bags have an advantage in that they require less storage space. Among their disadvantages are that filling the bags and using the calibrations may be difficult because of their flexible nature. Bottles require the use of an airway and larger storage space. They are easier to fill and calculation of fluid content is more accurate. Reservoirs should be discarded after 24 hours.

Administration of the feed

TEMPERATURE

The temperatures at which tube feeds are administered range from cold to hot. The reasons for administration at a particular temperature are various. Using cold tube feeds has been associated with diarrhoea (Gormican, 1970) but Holt et al. (1962) reported no such difficulty in giving cold formula to infants. Fason (1967) found no ill effects after giving feeds from the refrigerator. A study on primates (Williams and Walike, 1975) showed that cold tube feeds had only a minimal effect on gastric emptying and motility. In view of this and the fact that pathogens multiply more rapidly in warm conditions it is suggested that nasogastric and nasojejunal feeds be given as cool as possible. If a bolus method is used food should be at approximately 37 °C, i.e. body temperature.

RATE

The feed must be given over a period of time that suits the patient. In normal subjects, forced or rapid feedings were related to an increased incidence of accelerated heart rate, nausea, gagging and regurgitation (Hanson et al., 1975). Gregg and Rees (1970) recommend that rapid administration is avoided to prevent distension and nausea. For adults feeds may be introduced at a rate of 25 or 50 ml per hour by continuous drip and gradually increased to the desired rate according to the volume required in 24 hours.

QUANTITY

The volume of feed given will depend on the patient's daily nutrient requirements. Most commercially prepared feeds provide one kilocalorie (Kcal) per millilitre.

The majority of patients will therefore require between 1,500 and 3,000 ml per day depending on age, sex, body weight and medical condition.

FREQUENCY

The ideal way to feed a patient by the nasogastric route is to administer the feed continuously, thereby minimizing undesirable side-effects and maximizing the absorption. This can be achieved by using a pump that regulates the flow of the feed and reduces the danger of the tube becoming blocked. Some patients, however, find 24-hour feeding too restricting, especially if they are mobile. In such cases feeds can be given intermittently.

The frequency of intermittent feeding is usually determined by the total daily intake, duration and volume of each feed. Feeds are usually administered every 2–4 hours and the duration is normally 1–2 hours, depending on volume and the individual patient's tolerance. Some patients may prefer to have the feed during the night, especially if they cannot tolerate the entire prescribed feed during the day.

PATIENT MONITORING

Several complications affecting the fluid and electrolyte balance of the body and associated with tube feeding have been identified. These occur particularly in unconscious patients or in those who cannot communicate or alleviate their thirst. Hypernatraemia, uraemia and dehydration are potential complications, especially when fluid losses are increased as in the presence of diarrhoea. Day and Buckell (1977) and Ohlson (1982) advise monitoring the patient's urine solute concentration, blood urea, electrolytes and haemoglobin. It is also advisable to monitor blood glucose. These parameters should be recorded daily until the patient's condition is stable and feeding has been established.

Nursing care should include accurate records of fluid balance including the exact volume of feed given so that nutrient intake can be calculated.

The patient's weight should be recorded twice weekly. Fine-bore nasogastric tubes should be flushed with 10–20 ml of water after each feed to prevent blockage.

Attitudes to tube feeding

Eating is not only a physiological necessity but also a social and emotional experience. Nasogastric feeding dramatically alters the patient's attitude to food. The nurse plays a vital role in helping patients to understand and accept this method of feeding. The nurse can make it pleasant and relaxed or it can become a distressing affair, guaranteed to destroy the patient's confidence. The outcome is, therefore, dependent on the nurse's attitude and clinical knowledge.

References and further reading

Day, S. and Buckell, M. (1977) Feeding the unconscious patient, *Proceedings of the Nutrition Society*, Vol. 30, pp. 184–90.

Elwyn, D.H. (1980) Nutritional requirements of adult surgical patients, *Critical Care Medicine*, Vol. 8, pp. 9–20.

Fason, M.F. (1967) Controlling bacterial growth in tube feeding, *American Journal of Nursing*, Vol. 67, pp. 1246–47.

Gault, H.M. *et al*. (1968) Hypernatraemia azotaemia and dehydration due to high protein tube feeding, *Annals of Internal Medicine*, Vol. 68, pp. 778–91.

Gormican, A. (1970) Prepackaged tube feedings, *Hospital* Vol. 44, pp. 58–60.

Gregg, S.H. and Rees, O.M. (1970) *Scientific Principles in Nursing*, C.V. Mosby, St Louis.

Hanson, R.L. (1973) Effects of administration of cold and warmed tube feedings, in M.V. Batey (ed.) *Communicating Nursing Research* 6, WICHE, pp. 136–40.

Hanson, R.L. *et al*. (1975) Patient responses and problems associated with tube feeding, *Washington State Journal of Nursing*, Vol. 47, No. 1, pp. 9–13.

Holt, E. *et al*. (1962) A study of premature infants fed cold formulas, *Journal of Paediatrics*, Vol. 61, pp. 556–61.

Lee, H.A. (1979) Why enteral nutrition? *Research and Clinical Forums*, Vol. 1, no. 1, pp. 15–24.

Mitchell, H.S. *et al*. (1968) *Cooper's Nutrition in Health and Disease*, 15 ed, J.B. Lippincott, Philadelphia.

Ohlson, M. (1982) *Handbook of Experimental and Therapeutic Diets*, Burgess, Philadelphia.

Pareina, M.D. (1959) *Therapeutic Nutrition with Tube Feeding*, Charles C. Thomas, Chicago, Illinois.

Walike, B.C. *et al*. (1975) Patient problems related to tube feeding, in M.V. Batey (ed.) *Communicating Nursing Research 7*, WICHE, pp. 89–112.

White, D.T. *et al*. (1972) *Fundamentals: The Foundation of Nursing*, Prentice Hall, Englewood Cliffs, NJ.

Williams, K.R. and Walike, B.C. (1975) Effect of temperature of tube feeding on gastric motility of monkeys, *Nursing Research*, Vol. 24, pp. 4–9.

GUIDELINES: NASOGASTRIC INTUBATION WITH TUBES USING A GUIDEWIRE

Equipment

1   Clinically clean tray
2   Clinifeed tube
3   Guidewire for tube
4   Sterile receiver
5   Sterile water or normal saline
6   Hypo-allergenic tape
7   Adhesive patch if available
8   Glass of water.

Procedure

Action	Rationale
1 Explain the procedure to the patient.	To obtain the patient's consent and co-operation.
2 Arrange a signal by which the patient can communicate if he/she wants the nurse to stop, e.g. by raising his/her hand.	The patient is often less frightened if he/she feels able to have some control over the procedure.
3 Assist the patient to sit in a semi-upright position in the bed or chair. Support the patient's head with pillows. *Note:* the head should not be tilted backwards or forwards.	To allow for easy passage of the tube. This position enables easy swallowing and ensures that the epiglottis is not obstructing the oesophagus.
4 Select the appropriate distance mark on the tube by measuring the distance on the tube from the patient's ear lobe to the bridge of the nose plus the distance from the bridge of the nose to the bottom of the xiphisternum.	To ensure that the appropriate length of tube is passed into the stomach.
5 *Either:* (a) Wash hands and assemble the equipment needed. Pour normal saline into the receiver and check that the guidewire is free from kinks. Pass the wire through the normal saline and insert it into the tube as fast as the plastic safety stopper will allow (see Figure 24.1).	Lubrication of the wire promotes easy insertion and removal of the wire from the tube. The safety stopper prevents protrusion of the wire from the tube end, a potential source of trauma to the nasopharynx and oesophagus.

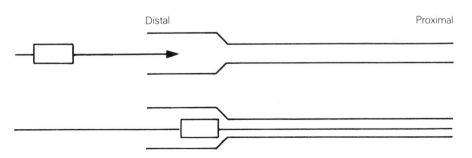

Figure 24.1   Passing a nasogastric tube.

Action	Rationale
or.	
(b) Wash hands and assemble the equipment needed. For 'silk' nasogastric tube and others with guidewire packaged inside the tube: ensure wire is firmly anchored inside the tube. Flush tube with 10 ml of water. Dip proximal end of tube in water to activate hydrometer coat.	Contact with water activates hydromer coating inside tube and on the tip. This lubricates the tube assisting its passage through the nasopharynx and allowing easy withdrawal of the guidewire.
6 Check that the nostrils are patent by asking the patient to sniff with one nostril closed. Repeat with the other nostril.	To identify any obstructions liable to prevent intubation.
7 Insert the proximal end of the tube into the clearest nostril and slide it backwards and inwards along the floor of the nose to the nasopharynx. If any obstruction is felt, withdraw the tube and try again in a slightly different direction or use the other nostril.	To facilitate the passage of the tube by following the natural anatomy of the nose.
8 As the tube passes down into the nasopharynx, ask the patient to start swallowing and sipping water.	To focus the patient's attention on something other than the tube. A swallowing action closes the glottis, enabling the tube to pass into the oesophagus.
9 Advance the tube through the pharynx as the patient swallows until the predetermined mark has been reached.	
10 Remove the guidewire by using gentle traction. If the wire is difficult to remove, then remove the tube as well. Do not discard the wire.	If the wire sticks in the tube, it may be indicative that the tube is in the bronchus. After use the guidewire should be cleaned carefully with an antiseptic solution, such as Savlodil, and dried thoroughly. Each wire may be used up to a maximum of five times.
11 Check the position of the tube to confirm that it is in the stomach by: (a) Aspirating 2–3 ml of gastric fluid through the tube and test with litmus paper (blue turns red). *or* (b) Introduce 2–5 ml air into the stomach via the tube and check for bubbling sounds using a stethoscope placed over the epigastrium. *or* (c) X-ray of chest and upper abdomen.	The acid nature of stomach contents verifies the position of the tube. Air can be detected by a 'whoosing' sound when entering the stomach. Radio-opaque tube shows up on the X-ray.
12 Secure the tube to the nostril with hypo-allergenic tape and to the cheek with an adhesive patch (if available).	To main the tube in place. To ensure patient comfort. Feeding via the tube must not begin until the correct position of the tube has been confirmed by one of the above methods.

GUIDELINES: NASOGASTRIC INTUBATION WITH TUBES WITHOUT A GUIDEWIRE

Equipment

1   Clinically clean tray
2   Nasogastric tube that has been stored in a deep freeze for at least half an hour before the procedure is to begin, to ensure a rigid tube that will allow for easy passage
3   Topical gauze
4   Lubricating jelly
5   Hypo-allergenic tape
6   20-ml syringe
7   Blue litmus paper
8   Receiver
9   Spigot
10   Glass of water
11   Stethoscope.

Procedure

Action	Rationale
1 Explain the procedure to the patient.	To obtain the patient's consent and co-operation.
2 Arrange a signal by which the patient can communicate if he/she wants the nurse to stop, e.g. by raising his/her hand.	The patient is often less frightened if he/she feels able to have some control over the procedure.
3 Assist the patient to sit in a semi-upright positions in the bed or chair. Support the patient's head with pillows.	To allow for easy passage of the tube. This position enables easy swallowing and ensures that the epiglottis is not obstructing the oesophagus.
4 Mark the distance which the tube is to be passed by measuring the distance on the tube from the patient's ear lobe to the bridge of the nose plus the distance from the bridge of the nose to the bottom of the xiphisternum. Mark this distance with tape.	To indicate the length of tube required for entry into the stomach.
5 Wash hands and assemble the equipment needed.	
6 Check that the patient's nostrils are patent by asking him/her to sniff with one nostril closed. Repeat with the other nostril.	To identify any obstructions liable to prevent intubation.
7 Lubricate the tube for about 15–20 cm with a thin coat of lubricating jelly that has been placed on a topical swab.	To reduce the friction between the mucous membranes and the tube.
8 Insert the proximal end of the tube into the clearest nostril and slide it backwards and inwards along the floor of the nose to the nasopharyns. If an obstruction is felt, withdraw the tube and try again in a slightly different direction or use the other nostril.	To facilitate the passage of the tube by following the natural anatomy of the nose.
9 As the tube passes down into the nasopharynx, ask the patient to start swallowing and sipping water.	To focus the patient's attention on something other than the tube. The swallowing action closes the glottis, enabling the tube to pass into the oesophagus.

Action	Rationale
10 Advance the tube through the pharynx as the patient swallows until the tape-marked tube reaches the point of entry into the external nares. If the patient shows signs of distress, e.g. gasping or cyanosis, remove the tube immediately.	Distress may indicate that the tube is in the bronchus.
11 Ascertain whether the tube is in the stomach by: (a) Aspirating the contents of the stomach with a syringe. The aspirate should turn blue litmus paper red. (b) Placing a stethoscope over the epigastrium and injecting 2–3 ml of air into the tube.	The acid nature of the stomach contents verifies the position of the tube. Air can be detected by a 'whoosing' sound when entering the stomach.
12 Tape the tube to the patient's nose and secure the distal end in a suitable position. Spigot the tube.	To maintain the tube in place. To ensure patient comfort.

GUIDELINES: ADMINISTRATION OF A NASOGASTRIC FEED

Two methods are available:
1   intermittent feeding;
2   continuous feeding.
Continuous feeding has two main advantages:
   (a)   it saves nursing time;
   (b)   it reduces the risk of gastrointestinal problems.
Its disadvantages is that mobile patients may feel restricted.

Equipment
1   Prescribed feed*
2   Reservoir* and airway**
3   Giving set
4   Suitable connection or Clinifeed comfort clip
5   Three-way tap, if required
6   2- and 10-ml syringes
7   Stethoscope
8   10-ml water in a syringe
9   Clean jug
10   Suitable stand for holding reservoir.
Note: The reservoir and airway, giving sets and connections should be kept in a tank of Milton solution by the patient's bedside.
*   These may come as one unit.
**   This may be an integral part of the giving set.

Procedure

INTERMITTENT FEEDING

Action	Rationale
1 Explain the procedure to the patient.	To obtain the patient's consent and co-operation.
2 Wash hands.	To minimize cross-infection

3 Take the feed and necessary equipment to the patient's bedside. If the patient is capable of doing so, he/she should assist in the procedure.

To encourage feelings of independence.

4 Remove the reservoir from the tank and drain the fluid back into the tank. Do not rinse before use.

Rinsing may introduce infection and counteracts the cleansing effect of a solution such as Milton.

5 *Remove the cap of the reservoir, and pour the prescribed feed into it.

6 Replace the cap and insert the giving set. Close the airway. Hang the reservoir on the stand beside the patient. Run the feed through to the end of the tubing, collecting the waste Milton solution in a jug if necessary. Clamp the tubing firmly.

To prevent the feed escaping from the reservoir via the airway.

Running the feed through the tubing removes excess solutions, such as Milton, and any air bubbles from the system and prevents them from reaching the stomach.

7 Check the position of the nasogastric tube by auscultation or aspiration (for intubation with tubes without a guidewire, using 50-ml syringe, see p. 245).

To ensure that the tube is in the stomach before feeding begins.

8 Connect the giving set to the nasogastric tube using a three-way tap or an appropriate connector if required.

The three-way tap allows the addition of drugs or water for flushing without having to disconnect the system.

9 Open the airway and set the flow of feed at the prescribed rate. Pumps are commercially available for administering feeds at a constant rate.

The rate of feed must be regulated to meet the patient's need. If possible, the patient should control his/her own feeding rate.

10 Return periodically to check the patient's comfort and the rate of flow of the feed.

The rate of flow of the feed may alter suddenly, especially if the patient is mobile.

11 On completion of a feed, disconnect the giving set from the distal end of the nasogastric tube and flush the tube with 10 ml of water.

To remove particles of feed likely to block the tube.

12 Wash the reservoir and the giving set in hot water and a suitable detergent. Rinse well.

Washing with detergent removes any feed left in the equipment. Thorough rinsing is required to prevent inactivation of Milton by the detergent.

13 Submerge the syringes, giving set and reservoir in a solution such as Milton in a suitable tank. Leave them submerged until the next feed.

To sterilize this equipment. The Milton solution and equipment should be discarded every 24 hours.

After completing step 11 the procedure begins again at step 1. The empty reservoir or bottle is discarded.

* Step 5 may be omitted if a prepacked bottled feed or a prefilled reservoir from the pharmacy or catering department is used.

CONTINUOUS FEEDING

Follow the above procedure for Intermittent Feeding, omitting steps 4, 12 and 13.

Note: With both the continuous and intermittent methods of nasogastric feeding, the giving set should be discarded after 24 hours.

NURSING CARE PLAN

Problem	Cause	Suggested action
Abdominal distension, nausea or diarrhoea.	Feed given too rapidly.	Reduce the rate of feed.
	Oral antibiotics.	Administer any medication prescribed for nausea or diarrhoea.
	Malabsorption due to enzyme depletion, villous atrophy following periods of starvation or inadequate nutrition.	Dilute the feed or decrease the rate of feed. Inform the nutrition team.
	Hyperosmolar feeds.	As above.
	Lactose intolerance, especially in patients of African and Asian origin or severely debilitated patients.	Use a lactose-free feed.
	Contaminated feed and/or equipment.	Obtain a stool for bacteriological investigation. Take swabs from the equipment and any solutions used.
Weight gain is unsatisfactory and/or urea output high.	Inadequate nutrition for patient's needs.	Inform the nutrition team.
Dehydration.	Inadequate water intake to meet patient's needs.	Offer fluids. Inform the nutrition team.

APPENDIX: SUGGESTED MANAGEMENT OF A NASOGASTRIC FEEDING REGIMEN

Starting the regime

This will vary depending on the following:
1. nutritional requirements of patient;
2. condition of the patient, e.g. has the patient been starved prior to starting the regime?;
3. type of feed being used.

Action	Rationale
1 Gradual build up, over 4–5 days, of volume and rate of feed to meet nutritional requirements.	Gradual increase in regimen allows the gastrointestinal tract to adjust to a liquid diet, thus reducing the risk of intolerance.

Timing of the feed

Action	Rationale
1 Preferably as a continuous drip feed over 24 hours.	Patients may find this restricting but it has the advantage of allowing a large volume of feed to be dripped in slowly over a long period of time, thus giving a high level of nutrition while keeping the osmotic load low.
2 Alternatively, four or five feeds daily. Timing determined by convenience to patient and staff.	Patients may prefer intermittent feeds given throughout the day.

Duration of the feed

Action

1   Depends on volume of feed required and drip rate used.

Rationale

The number of feeds and the drip rate should be decided in the light of patient requirements, condition and personal preference. Too rapid an administration may lead to nausea, distension and diarrhoea.

Monitoring the patient

	Action	Rationale
1 Fluid balance.	Measure daily input and output.	To monitor state of hydration.
2 Weight.	Weigh twice weekly (in same clothing and at same time of day).	To monitor weight changes which may be associated with a tube-feeding regimen.
3 Urine.	Daily urine analysis for glucose during first week of feeding. If glucose detected, check the urine throughout the whole period of tube feeding.	To ensure that the urine glucose levels relates to the feed just given.
4 Bowels.	Check daily, by observation or by asking the patient about the frequency and nature of stools.	To detect and combat diarrhoea or constipation related to tube feeding.
5 Haematological investigations.	Test for urea and electrolytes and glucose levels once or twice weekly.	To monitor the patient's state of hydration. Nitrogen balance may be of value in some patients.
6 General condition.	Observe daily for thirst, lethargy, glycosuria and polyuria – all symptoms of dehydration.	To prevent the complication of end-state dehydration.

NUTRITIONAL ASSESSMENT

Definition

Nutritional assessment involves the recording of specific parameters in order to obtain a profile of an individual's nutritional status and nutrient intake.

Indications

Nutritional assessment may be used to:

1   identify individuals who require nutrition education or special nutritional support;

2   monitor changes in the nutritional status of an individual over time;

3   assess the nutritional status of a population.

All patients should have a basic assessment of their nutritional status as part of the initial nursing assessment on admission to hospital. This will reveal whether referral to the dietitian is necessary.

REFERENCE MATERIAL
Methods of nutritional assessment

The principal methods of nutritional assessment are:

1   dietary history;

2   anthropometry;

3   laboratory investigations;

4   immunological methods.

DIETARY HISTORY

Useful information about an individual's nutritional status can be obtained by asking questions about food preferences, appetite and eating patterns.

The 24-hour dietary recall of food intake was recommended by Burke in 1974 and is still a valuable tool. It involves asking an individual to describe his/her food and fluid intake during the previous 24 hours in terms of the amount and kind of items consumed. This will usually reveal any potential inadequacies in the diet which can then be investigated further.

ANTHROPOMETRY

This term refers to the scientific measurement of the human body (Gk: *anthropos* = human being; *metron* = a measure).

The parameters pertinent to the assement of nutritional status are as follows:

1   height (or length in infants);
2   weight;
3   mid upper arm muscle circumference (non-dominant arm – calculated from mid upper arm circumference and triceps skinfold thickness):
    AMC (cm) = AC (cm) − 0.314 × TST (mm);
4   skinfold thickness at five recognized sites:
    (a) biceps;
    (b) triceps;
    (c) subscapular;
    (d) supra-iliac;
    (e) mid-calf.

The measurement of skinfold thickness gives an indication of the size of subcutaneous adipose tissue stores. This is directly related to nutritional status. Measurements can be compared with standard tables of data and serial measurements show individual progress.

The measurements should be made using specialized skinfold calipers (e.g. Harpenden or Holtein calipers). There is a strict and recognized technique for performing such measurements which must be adhered to for worthwhile results to be obtained. The operator should be well practised in the use of skinfold calipers before undertaking serious measurements. Since there is a degree of intra-observer error even with experienced operators, one individual should be responsible for all measurements.

LABORATORY INVESTIGATIONS

Biochemical tests may be carried out on samples of blood or urine to determine the levels of the following:

1   blood proteins, e.g.
    (a) haemoglobin
    (b) total protein
    (c) serum albumin (half-life 20 days)
    (d) prealbumin (half-life 2 days)
    (e) transferrin (half-life 8–10 days)
    (f) retional binding protein (half-life 10 hours).
2   urine:
    (a) nitrogen
    (b) urea
    (c) creatinine.

Blood proteins are related to nutritional status. Their value as indications of changes in nutritional status varies depending on their rate of turnover in the blood. Generally the long half-life proteins are measured routinely (albumin, haemoglobin, total protein) but they are not as sensitive to day-to-day changes in feeding as prealbumin, transferrin and retinol binding protein.

The levels of all these proteins can also be affected by intravenous infusions and by surgery. This must be borne in mind when interpreting results.

Urine urea and creatinine levels indicate the amount of muscle catabolism and protein breakdown. The creatinine/height index can be used to assess nutritional status by measuring an individual's creatinine excretion in a 24-hour urine collection, dividing by his/her height and comparing the results with standard tables.

Urine urea nitrogen can be used for calculating nitrogen balance (in combination with data for nitrogen intake). Negative nitrogen balance indicates that protein catabolism is occurring. For growth and healing to take place the body should be in positive balance (intake exceeds output).

IMMUNOLOGICAL METHODS

Changes in immune status may be related to nutritional status. This relationship is sometimes used to assess nutritional status.

Immune status is most commonly assessed by testing the patient's capacity to mount a cellular response to recall antigens (i.e. substances they are likely to have encountered before).

Minute amounts of each substance (e.g. tuberculin, *Candida albicans*, mumps and varidase) are injected intradermally and the appearance of each site noted 24–72 hours afterwards.

A raised red indurated area is taken as a positive response, indicating that the patient is able to amount an immune response.

Summary

Ideally a combination of several of the above parameters should be chosen in order to assess nutritional status.

From the nurse's point of view, the following are the most simple, and reliable:

1   height;
2   weight;

3 recent change in weight (previous 6 months) (as a percentage of previous weight*);
4 24-hour dietary recall;
5 observation of food intake.

* Unintentional weight loss of 5% body weight in 3 months or 10% in 6 months signifies possible malnutrition.

If it is suspected that an individual is malnourished, the dietitian should be contacted so that a more detailed assessment can be made.

References and further reading

Burke, B.S. (1974) The dietary history as a tool in research, *Journal of American Dietetic Association*, Vol. 23, pp. 1041–6.

Goode, A.W. *et al.* (1985) Nutritional management of the compromised patient, in *Clinical Nutrition and Dietetics for Nurses*, Hodder & Stoughton, London.

Jenson, T.G. *et al.* (1983) Nutritional Assessment – A Manual for Practitioners, Appleton, Century Crofts, New York.

Kettlewell, M. (1982) Meeting the patients' needs (assessment of nutritional status), in A. Grant and E. Todd (eds.) *Enteral and Parenteral Nutrition*, Blackwell Scientific Publications, Oxford.

Moghissi, K. and Boore, J. (1983) Nutritional assessment, in *Parenteral and Enteral Nutrition for Nurses*, Heinemann Medical Books, London.

Pittam, M. (1982) Nutritional assessment, *Nursing* (Second Series), Vol. 4, pp. 94–8.

25

Neurological Observations

Definition

Neurological observations relate to the evaluation of the integrity of an individual's nervous system by obtaining specific information about it.

Indications

Neurological observations are required to monitor and evaluate changes in the nervous system by indicating trends, thus aiding diagnosis and treatment, which in turn may affect prognosis and rehabilitation.

REFERENCE MATERIAL

The main emphasis is on assessing five critical areas:
1 level of consciousness;
2 pupillary activity;
3 motor function;
4 sensory function;
5 vital signs.

Level of consciousness

Level of consciousness is the single most important indicator of a patient's brain function. It ranges from alert wakefulness to deep coma with no apparent responsiveness. Categories of impaired consciousness, in order of deteriorating condition, include the following:
1 *Full consciousness*: the patient is fully aware of his/her surroundings and is orientated to time, place and person. The patient responds appropriately to auditory, visual and somatosensory stimuli.
2 *Lethargy*: the patient is inactive and indifferent. The patient responds slowly or incompletely to stimuli. Although capable of verbal responses, the patient may ignore some stimuli completely.
3 *Obtundation*: the patient is very drowsy and indifferent, although capable of remaining awake.
4 *Confusion and delerium*: thinking and behaviour aberrations occur due to cortex dysfunction. The confused patient is disorientated and appears

dazed. The delirious patient is unco-operative and easily agitated.
5 *Stupor*: the patient can be aroused only by painful stimuli.
6 *Coma*: response to painful stimuli may be rudimentary or absent.

Specific diseases and injuries can impair level of consciousness since they depress or destroy the brain-stem's reticular activating and mechanism or the conduction pathways leading to and from the cerebral cortex.

Assessment of level of consciousness involves two phases:
1 evaluation of verbal responses;
2 evaluation of motor responses.

Changes in blood pressure and pulse normally occur late, after the patient's level of consciousness had begun to deteriorate. Call for medical assistance at the first sign of neurological deterioration.

VERBAL RESPONSES

Assess the ability of the patient to respond verbally and note any evidence of disorientation as to time, place and person. Note also the clarity with which the patient responds.

MOTOR RESPONSES

In the first instance these should be elicited by noting whether the patient responds to simple verbal commands, e.g. 'Open your eyes', 'Squeeze and release my fingers'. Test both sides of the patient's body.

PAINFUL STIMULI

Painful stimuli should only be employed if the patient does not respond to commands. Use the least amount of pressure to elicit a response. For suggested methods see p. 255. As the ability to localize pain is lost, various responses may be observed when painful stimuli are applied:

1 *Decorticate posturing*: one or both arms are in full flexion on the chest. The legs may be stiffly extended.
2 *Decerebrate posturing*: one or both arms are stiffly extended. There is possible extension of the legs. The head may also be arched backwards.
3 *Flaccid*: no motor response is observed in any extremity.

Pupillary activity

Pupillary constriction and dilation are controlled by the third cranial nerve (oculomotor). Any changes may indicate third cranial nerve involvement and/or brainstem damage. (Note that pupillary changes may also be the result of drug treatment or trauma to the eye.)

Assessment of the pupils must include an evaluation of size, shape, whether or not they are equal and their reaction to light.

Motor function

Damage to any part of the motor nervous system can affect the ability to move. Motor function assessment involves evaluation of the following:
1 muscle strength;
2 muscle tone;
3 posture;
4 muscle co-ordination;
5 reflexes;
6 abnormal movements.

MUSCLE STRENGTH

This involves testing the patient's muscle strength against one's own muscle resistance and then against the pull of gravity.

MUSCLE TONE

This involves flexing and extending the patient's limbs on both sides and noting how well such movements are resisted. Increased resistance would denote increased muscle tone and vice versa.

POSTURE

The posture of a patient is frequently an ominous sign and may occur spontaneously or in response to painful stimuli. Some such postures have been outlined above.

CO-ORDINATION

Any disease or injury that involves the cerebellum or basal ganglia will affect co-ordination. Assessment of hand and arm and leg co-ordination can be achieved by testing the rapidity and rhythm of alternating movements and of point-to-point movements. For such tests see p. 255.

REFLEXES

Among the four most important reflexes are the following: blink, gag and swallow, plantar and oculocephalic, the latter being a reflect ocular movement that occurs only in patients with a severely decreased level of consciousness. When the reflex is present the patient's eyes will move in the opposite direction from the side to which his/her head is turned. If the reflex is impaired, the eyes may not move at all or only one eye may move. Blink and gag and swallow are protective reflexes. Fifth and seventh cranial nerve involvement will affect the blink reflex. Ninth and tenth cranial nerve involvement may affect the gag reflex. Plantar and oculocephalic reflexes help to determine the site of a lesion.

ABNORMAL MOVEMENTS

When carrying out neurological observations any abnormal movements, e.g. seizures and tremors, must be noted.

Sensory function

Constant sensory input enables an individual to alter his/her responses and behaviour to suit his/her environment. When disease or injury damages the sensory pathways, the sensory responses are always affected. Any assessment of sensory function should include evaluation of the following:
1 central and peripheral vision;
2 hearing and ability to understand verbal communication;
3 superficial sensations (light, touch, pain) and deep sensations (muscles and joint pain, muscle and joint position).

Vital signs

It is recommended that assessments of vital signs should be made in the following order:
1 respirations;
2 temperature;
3 blood pressure;
4 pulse.

RESPIRATIONS

Of these four vital signs, respiratory patterns give the clearest indication of how the brain is functioning since respirations are controlled by different areas of the brain. Any disease or injury that affects these areas may produce respiratory changes. The rate, quality and pattern of a patient's respirations must be noted. Abnormal respiratory patterns are listed in Table 25.1.

TEMPERATURE

Damage to the hypothalamus, the temperature-regulating centre, may result in grossly fluctuating temperatures.

Table 25.1   Abnormal Respiratory Patterns

Type	Pattern	Significance
Cheyne–Stokes	Rhythmic waxing and waning of both rate and depth of respirations, alternating regularly with briefer periods of apnoea.	May indicate deep cerebral or cerebellar lesions, usually bilateral. May occur with upper brainstem involvement.
Central neurogenic hyperventilation	Sustained, regular, rapid respirations, with forced inspiration and expiration.	May indicate a lesion of the low mid-brain, or upper pons areas of the brainstem.
Apnoeustic	Prolonged inspiratory cramp with a pause at full inspiration. There may also be expiratory pauses.	May indicate a lesion of the low pons or upper medulla.
Cluster breathing	Clusters of irregular respiratons alternating with longer periods of apnoea.	May indicate a lesion of low pons or upper medulla.
Ataxic breathing	A completely irregular pattern with random deep and shallow respirations. Irregular pauses may also appear.	May indicate a lesion of the medulla.

BLOOD PRESSURE AND PULSE

Observations of blood pressure and pulse will provide evidence of increased intracranial pressure. Hypertension together with bradycardia need to be monitored closely. Abnormalities of blood pressure and pulse usually occur late, after the patient's level of consciousness has begun to deteriorate.

Recording observations

There is no universally accepted method for recording nursing neurological observations. The Glasgow Coma Scale attempts to assess the integrity of the central nervous system on the basis of behavioural responses that denote the patient's motor activity, verbal performance and eye-opening ability. Useful summaries of this scale may be found in Abelson (1982) and Jones (1979).

References and further reading

Abelson, M.M. (1982) Observations of the neurosurgical patient, *Curationis*, Vol. 5, no. 3, pp. 27–32.

Erickson, R. (1980) Neurological checkpoints, in *Assessing Vital Functions Accurately*, Intermed Communications, pp. 131–42.

Jones, C. (1979) Glasgow Coma Scale, *American Journal of Nursing*, Vol. 79, no. 9, pp. 1551–3.

Ricci, M.M. (1979) Neurological assessment: keeping it ongoing, in *Coping with Neurological Problems Proficiently*, Intermed Communications, pp. 30–49.

Walleck, C.A. (1982) A neurological procedure that won't make you nervous, *Nursing Times*, Vol. 12, no. 12, pp. 50–7.

GUIDELINES: NEUROLOGICAL OBSERVATIONS

Equipment

1   Pencil torch
2   Thermometer
3   Sphygmomanometer
4   Tongue depressor
5   Cotton wool balls

6 Patella hammer
7 Safety pin
8 Two test tubes.

Procedure

Action	**Rationale**
1 Inform the patient, whether conscious or not, and explain the observations.	Sense of hearing is frequently unimpaired even in unconscious patients. To ensure, as far as is possible, that the patient consents to and understand the procedure.
2 Talk to the patient. Note whether he/she is alert and is giving full attention or whether he/she is restless or lethargic and drowsy. Ask the patient who he/she is, the correct day, month and year, where he/she is, and to give details about his/her family.	To establish whether the patient's level of consciousness is deteriorating. If the patient is becoming disorientated, changes will occur in this order: (a) Disorientation as to time (b) Disorientation as to place (c) Disorientation as to person.
3 Ask the patient to squeeze and release your fingers and then to stick out his/her tongue. (Include both sides of the body.)	To evaluate motor responses.
4 If the patient does not respond, apply painful stimuli. Suggested methods are as follows: (a) Exerting pressure on the patient's fingernail bed with a pen or pencil (b) Applying pressure to the ridge under the eyebrow (the supraorbital notch).	Responses grow less purposeful as the patient's level of consciousness deteriorates. As the condition worsens, the patient may no longer localize pain and respond to it in a purposeful way.
5 Record, precisely, the findings. Write exactly what stimulus was used, where it was applied, how much pressure was needed to elicit a response, and how the patient responded.	Vague terms, e.g. semicomatose, can be easily misinterpreted.
6 Hold the eyelids open and note the size, shape and equality of the pupils.	To assess the size, shape and equality of the pupils as an indication of brain damage. Normal pupils are spherical, usually at mid-position and have a diameter ranging from 1.5 to 6 mm.
7 Darken the room.	To enable a better view of the eye.
8 Hold each eyelid open in turn. Move a pupil torch towards the patient from the side. Shine it directly into the eye. This should cause the pupil to constrict promptly.	To assess the reaction of the pupils to light. Indicates no lesions in the area of the brain stem regulating pupil constriction.
9 Hold both eyelids open but shine the light into one eye only. The eye into which the light is not shone should also constrict.	To assess consenual light reflex. Prompt constriction indicates intact connections between the brainstem areas regulating pupil constriction.
10 Record unusual eye movements.	To assess cranial nerve damage.

Action	**Rationale**
11 Extend your hands and ask the patient to squeeze your fingers as hard as possible. Compare grip and strength.	To test grip.
12 Ask the patient to close his/her eyes and hold his/her arms straight out in front of him/her, with palms upwards, for 20–30 seconds.	
13 Stand in front of the patient and extend your hands. Ask the patient to push and pull against your hands. Ask the patient to lie on his/her back in bed. Place the patient's leg with knee flexed and foot resting on the bed. Instruct the patient to keep his/her foot down as you attempt to extend his/her leg. Flex the knee and place your hand in the flexion. Instruct the patient to straighten his/her leg while you offer resistance. *Note:* If a patient cannot follow the instruction due to a language barrier or unconsciousness, observe spontaneous movements and note how strong they appear. Then, if necessary, apply painful stimuli.	To test arm strength. If one arm drifts downwards or turns inwards, it may indicate hemipharesis. To test flexion and extension strength in the patient's extremities by having him/her push and pull against your resistance.
14 Flex and extend all the patient's limbs. Note how well he/she resists the movements.	To test muscle tone.
15 Ask the patient to pat his/her thigh as fast as possible. Note whether the movements seem slow or clumsy. Ask the patient to turn his/her hand over and back several times in succession. Evaluate his/her co-ordination. Ask the patient to touch the back of his/her fingers with his/her thumb in sequence rapidly.	To assess hand and arm co-ordination. The dominant hand should perform better.
16 Extend one of your hands towards the patient. Ask the patient to touch your index finger, then his/her nose, several times in succession. Repeat the test with the patient's eyes closed.	
17 Ask the patient to place a heel on his/her opposite knee and slide it down his/her shin to his/her foot. Check each leg separately.	To assess leg co-ordination.
18 Ask the patient to look up or hold his/her eyelid open. With your hand, approach his/her eye unexpectedly or brush his/her eyelashes.	To test the blink reflex.
19 Ask the patient to open his/her mouth and hold down his/her tongue with a tongue depressor. Touch the back of the pharynx, on each side, with a cotton wool swab.	To test the gag reflex.
20 Ask the patient to lie on his/her back in bed. Place your hand under his/her knee. raise and flex it. Tap the patellar tendon. Note whether the leg responds.	To assess the deep tendon reflex.

21	Stroke the lateral aspect of the sole of the patient's foot. If the response is abnormal (Babinski response), the big toe will dorsiflex and the remaining toes will fan out.	To assess for upper motor neurone lesion.
22	Ask the patient to read something aloud. Check each eye separately. If vision is so poor that the patient is unable to read, ask the patient to count your upraised fingers or distinguish light from dark.	To test the visual activity.
23	Occlude the ear with a cotton wool swab. Stand a short way from the patient. Whisper numbers into the open ear. Ask for feedback. Repeat for both ears.	To test aural activity and comprehension.
24	Ask the patient to close his/her eyes. Using the point of an open safety pin, stroke his/her skin. Use the blunt end occasionally. Ask him/her to tell you what he/she feels. See if the patient can distinguish between sharp and dull sensations.	To test superficial sensations to pain.
25	Ask the patient to close his/her eyes. Fill two test tubes with water: one warm, one cold. Touch the patient's skin with each test tube and ask him/her to distinguish between them.	To test superficial sensations to temperature.
26	Stroke a cotton wool swab lightly over the patient's skin. Ask the patient to say what he/she feels.	To test superficial sensations to touch.
27	Ask the patient to close his/her eyes. Hold the tip of one of the patient's fingers between your thumb and index finger. Move it up and down and ask the patient to say in which direction it is moving. Repeat with the other hand. For the legs, hold the big toe.	To test proprioception.
28	Note the rate, quality and pattern of the patient's respirations.	Respirations are controlled by different areas of the brain. When disease or injury affects these areas, respiratory changes may occur.
29	Take and record the patient's temperature at specified intervals.	Damage to the hypothalamus, the temperature-regulating centre in the brain, will be reflected in grossly abnormal temperatures.
30	Take and record the patient's blood pressure and pulse at specified intervals.	To monitor signs of increased intracranial pressure. Hypertension and bradycardia usually occur late, after the patient's level of consciousness has begun to deteriorate. Call for medical assistance as soon as it is evident that there is a deterioration in the patient's level of consciousness.

NURSING CARE PLAN

Category	Frequency	Rationale
All patients diagnosed as suffering from neurological or neurosurgical conditions.	At least 4-hourly. Frequency is affected by the patient's condition.	To monitor the condition of the patient so that any necessary action can be instigated.
Unconscious patients (including ventilated and anaesthetized patients).	At least half-hourly; quarter-hourly if the condition is critical.	To monitor the condition closely and to detect trends so that appropriate action may be taken.

26

Observations

BLOOD PRESSURE

Definition

Blood pressure may be defined as the force which the blood exerts on the walls of the vessels in which it is contained. This may be represented as an equation:

blood pressure = cardiac output × peripheral resistance.

Indications

Blood pressure is measured for one of two reasons:

1   to establish a baseline in blood pressure;
2   to monitor fluctuations in blood pressure.

REFERENCE MATERIAL

Blood flows from the heart, to arteries, to capillaries and to veins, as a result of differences in their internal pressure, pressure being least in the veins. These vascular pressures are controlled by the vasomoter centre in the medulla oblongata.

Normal blood pressure is maintained by reflex arcs derived from stretch receptors found in the wall of the proximal arterial tree, especially in the region of the aortic arch and carotid sinuses. When arterial pressure rises, there is increased stimulation of these nerve endings. The increased number of impulses along the vagus and glossopharyngeal nerves leads to reflex vagal slowing of the heart and reflex release of vasoconstrictor tone in the peripheral blood vessels. The resulting fall in cardiac output and the reduction of peripheral resistance tend to restore the blood pressure to the normal value. A fall in the arterial pressure decreases the stimulation of the arterial stretch receptors. The reflex tachycardia and vasoconstriction that ensue tend to raise the blood pressure to its normal value.

A fall in renal flow, due to a fall in arterial pressure,

results in chemical changes which lead to stimulation of the suprarenal glands, leading in turn to salt and water retention. Such retention and vasoconstriction tend to raise arterial pressure.

Blood pressure varies, not only from moment to moment, but also with condition. It is lowest in neonates and increases with age, with weight gain and with stress and anxiety. Shock, myocardial infarction and haemorrhage are among the things that cause a fall in blood pressure as they reduce cardiac output and peripheral vessel resistance or they diminish venous return after fluid loss.

The conditions of hypertension (high blood pressure) and hypotension (low blood pressure) are defined by the following equations:

hypertension = increased cardiac output × greater total peripheral resistance

hypotension = lessened cardiac output × lesser total peripheral resistance.

Normal blood pressure

Normal blood pressure is generally held to range from 100/60 to 140/90 mmHg.

Systolic pressure

The systolic pressure is the maximum pressure of the blood against the wall of the vessel following ventricular contraction and is taken as an indication of the integrity of the heart, arteries and arterioles.

Diastolic pressure

The diastolic pressure is the minimum pressure of the blood against the wall of the vessel following closure of the aortic valve and is taken as a direct indication of blood vessel resistance.

Pulse pressure

The pulse pressure is the difference between systolic and diastolic readings.

Mean arterial pressure

The mean arterial pressure is the average pressure attempting to push blood through the circulatory system. This can be determined electronically or mathematically as well as by using an intra-arterial catheter and mercury manometer, e.g.

mean arterial pressure (mathematically) =
$\frac{1}{3}$ systolic + $\frac{2}{3}$ diastolic
pressure   pressure.

A blood pressure of 130/85 mmHg gives a mean arterial pressure of 100 mmHg.

Basal blood pressure

The basal blood pressure is the lowest blood pressure taken in a supine position after several days in hospital without treatment.

Factors affecting blood pressure

1 Circulating blood volume.
2 Elastic recoil of the arteries.
3 Blood viscosity.
4 Cardiac output.
5 Neurogenic factors.

Methods of recording and equipment

There are two main categories of method for recording the blood pressure: direct and indirect.

Direct methods are highly developed and of precise accuracy. The ideal direct method of measuring blood pressure involves the insertion of a minute pressure transducer unit into an artery for transmission of a waveform or digital display on a monitor. The most commonly used techniques involve placing a cannula in an artery and attaching a pressure-sensitive device to the external end.

The *indirect* method is the one most suitable for the nurse's purpose. All indirect methods are based upon the occluding devised by Riva-Rocci at the end of the last century and Korotkoff at the beginning of this century.

THE SPHYGMOMANOMETER

The sphygmomanometer (see Figure 26.1) consists of a compression bag enclosed in an unyielding cuff, an inflating bulb, pump or other device by which the pressure is increased, a manometer from which the applied pressure is read, and a control valve to deflate the system.

Manometer

Mercury sphygmomanometers are reliable, on the whole, and easily maintained. Care should be taken to avoid loss of mercury. Substantial errors may occur if the manometer is not kept vertical during the measurement. The air vent at the top of the manometer must be kept patent. Aneroid sphygmomanometers are generally less accurate than mercury ones.

Cuff

The cuff is an inelastic cloth that encircles the arm and encloses the inflatable rubber bladder. It is secured around the arm or leg by wrapping its tapering end to the encircling material, by Velcro surfaces or by hooks.

Inflatable bladder

A bladder that is too short and/or too narrow will give falsely high pressures. One that is too wide and/or too long will give falsely low pressures. O'Brien and O'Malley (1979) recommended a bladder that is 20% greater than (1.2 times) the diameter of the extremity of the limb that is being used.

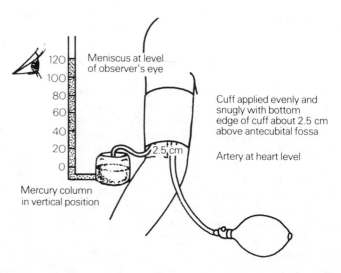

Figure 26.1   Principles of a sphygmomanometer.

Control valve, pump and rubber tubing

The control valve is a common source of error. It should allow the passage of air without excessive pressure needing to be applied on the pump. When the valve is closed it should hold the mercury at a constant level and, when released, it should allow a controlled fall in the level of mercury. The rubber tubing should be long (approximately 80 cm) and with airtight connections that can easily be separated.

It is essential that the sphygmomanometer be kept in good working order. Conceicao *et al.* (1976) and North (1979) have shown that as many as 50% of the sphygmomanometers used in the hospitals they studied were inaccurate.

THE STETHOSCOPE

The stethoscope must be of a standard variety and in good working order.

Using the stethoscope, it is possible to identify a series of five phases as blood pressure falls from the systolic to the diastolic. These phases are known as Korotkoff's sounds (see Figure 26.2):

1   the appearance of faint, clear tapping sounds which gradually increase in intensity;

2   the softening of sounds, which may become swishing;

3   the return of sharper sounds which become crisper but never fully regain the intensity of the phase 1 sounds;

4   the distinct muffling sounds which become soft and blowing;

5   the point at which all sound ceases.

The choice of phase 4 or phase 5 as the tone diastolic pressure is a controversial one, as can be seen from Burton (1967). It is recommended that both pressures should be recorded, e.g. 142/78/78 (if the levels are identical) or 142/82/78 (for different levels). If this practice is not followed, all nurses should agree on a pre-determined diastolic end-point.

Some additional information

Much recent research has focused on the faulty techniques employed when nurses take blood pressures. Maxwell (1982) has shown that the number of obese patients diagnosed as hypertensive may be grossly overestimated due to the use of cuffs of the incorrect size. Thompson (1981) discussed, analysed and evaluated the methodology of blood pressure recording. Poor technique and observer bias as potential sources of error were also examined. He concluded that many nurses are often inadequately trained in blood pressure measurement and that, with increasing reliance on the nurse for recording vital signs, more attention needs to be paid to this area.

References and further reading

Bell, G.H. *et al.* (1980) *Textbook of Physiology and Biochemistry*, Churchill Livingstone, Edinburgh.

Brunner, L.S. and Suddarth, D.S. (1982) *The Lippincott Manual of Medical-Surgical Nursing* Volume 2, Harper & Row, London.

Burton, C.A. (1967) The criterion for diastolic pressure and revolution and counter-revolution, *Circulation*, Vol. 36, pp. 805–9.

Conceicao, S. *et al.* (1976) Defects in sphygmomanometers, *British Medical Journal*, Vol. 2, pp. 886–8.

Jarvis, C.M. (1980) Vital signs: a preview of problems, in *Assessing Vital Functions Accurately*, Intermed Communications.

Kilgour, D. and Speedie, G. (1985) Taking the pressure off, *Nursing Mirror*, Vol. 160, pp. 39–40.

Korotkoff, M.S. (1905) On the subject of methods of measuring blood pressure, *Bulletin of the Imperial Medical Academy of St Petersburg*, Vol. 11, pp. 365–7.

Maxwell, M.H. (1982) Error in blood pressure measurement due to incorrect cuff size in obese patients, *Lancet*, Vol. ii, pp. 33–6.

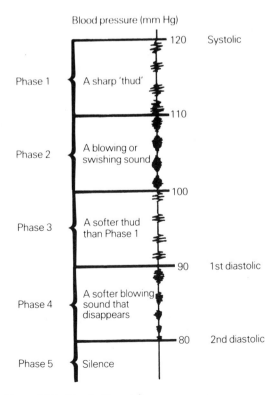

Blood pressure (mm Hg)

	120	Systolic
Phase 1	A sharp 'thud'	
	110	
Phase 2	A blowing or swishing sound	
	100	
Phase 3	A softer thud than Phase 1	
	90	1st diastolic
Phase 4	A softer blowing sound that disappears	
	80	2nd diastolic
Phase 5	Silence	

Figure 26.2   Korotkoff's sounds.

North, L.W. (1979) Accuracy of sphygmomanometers, *Association of Operating Room Nurses Journal*, Vol. 30, pp. 996–1000.

O'Brien, E.T. and O'Malley, K. (1979) ABC of blood pressure measurement: sphygmomanometer, *British Medical Journal*, Vol. 2, pp. 851–3.

Petrie, J.C. *et al.* (1986) Recommendations on blood pressure measurement, *British Medical Journal*, Vol. 293, pp. 611–5.

Rebenson-Piano, M. *et al.* (1987) An examination of the differences that occur between direct and indirect blood pressure measurement, *Heart and Lung*, Vol. 16, no. 3, pp. 285–94.

Thompson, D.R. (1981) Recording patients' blood pressure: blood pressure: a review, *Journal of Advanced Nursing*, Vol. 6, no. 4, pp. 283–90.

Wieck, L. *et al.* (1986) *Illustrated Manual of Nursing Techniques*, 3rd edn, J.B. Lippincott, Philadelphia.

GUIDELINES: BLOOD PRESSURE

Equipment
1 Sphygmomanometer
2 Stethoscope.

Procedure

Action

1 Explain to the patient that his/her blood pressure is going to be taken.

2 Measure the blood pressure under the same conditions each time.

3 Ensure that the patient is in the desired position – lying, standing or sitting.

4 Use the correct size of blood pressure cuff.

5 Apply the cuff of the sphygmomanometer to the arm above the antecubital fossa or to the leg above the popliteal fossa. The extremity should be positioned for maximum patient comfort and examiner accessibility. The leg should only be used if both arms are inacessible.

6 Place the bell of the stethoscope over the artery.

7 Inflate the cuff to a point approximately 20–30 mmHg above the last recorded reading or until the pulse can no longer be heard or palpated. Release the pressure valve on the cuff slowly.

Rationale

To obtain the consent and co-operation of the patient.

To ensure continuity and consistency in recording.

To obtain the required reading.

To obtain the correct reading.

The brachial and popliteal arteries are superficial in the antecubital and popliteal fossae.

When the bell of the stethoscope is placed over the artery, the sound will be heard with little distortion. The artery must be located by palpating with the fingertips.

Pressure exerted by the inflated cuff prevents blood from flowing through the artery. The systolic pressure is the point at which blood in the artery is first able to force its way through against the pressure exerted by the inflated cuff. It is found by slowly releasing the pressure valve. The point at which the first beat is heard is the systolic reading. The diastolic pressure is the point at which blood flows freely in the artery and is equivalent to the amount of pressure normally exerted on the wall of the arteries when the heart is at rest. While continuing to release the cuff pressure, a point is reached where the last distinct sound will be heard. The point at which the last beat is heard is the diastolic reading.

8   Record the systolic and diastolic pressures and compare the present reading with previous readings.

To monitor differences and detect trends. Any irregularities should be brought to the attention of the appropriate personnel.

9   Remove the equipment and clean it after use. The earpieces of the stethoscope should be wiped with a disinfectant solution that will not harm the arm.

To prevent the spread of infection.

NURSING CARE PLAN

Category	Frequency	Rationale
All new admissions.	Once only, preferably when the patient has settled in.	To provide a baseline.
Hypertensive patient.	Four-hourly until condition is stable.	To monitor the condition of the patient so that any necessary action can be taken.
Postoperative patient.	Half-hourly, depending on the patient's condition, then 4-hourly until condition is stable.	To detect postoperative hypo- or hypertension.
Critically ill patient, e.g. unconscious patient.	As often as determined by condition.	To monitor blood pressure closely.
Pregnant client.	Daily.	To detect hypo- or hypertension.
Patient receiving a blood transfusion.	When unit is put up. Observe the patient at 5-minute intervals for the first 15–20 minutes and take again 1 hour later if condition warrants it. If blood pressure fluctuates or the patient shows other signs of reaction, record again and as demanded by condition.	To record a baseline blood pressure and monitory any reaction to the transfusion.
Patient receiving intravenous infusion.	Four-hourly.	To monitor circulatory overload.
Patient with local or systemic infection.	Four-hourly until condition is stable.	To detect any signs or symptoms of shock.
Patient receiving any drug known to cause fluctuations in blood pressure.	Twice daily.	To monitor reaction to the drug.
Patient with prolonged or profound neutropenia.	Four-hourly until neutrophil count rises.	To detect septicaemic shock that may not manifest itself in pyrexia or signs of local infection.

Category	Frequency	Rationale
Patient not feeling well or nurse concerned about patient.	Once. If outside the normal ranges, check again 2–3 hours later and take appropriate action.	To reassure the patient and nurse and to ensure that appropriate action is taken if blood pressure is remarkable.

Problem	Cause	Suggested action
Falsely elevated blood pressure.	Using too narrow a cuff. The cuff bladder should be 20% wider than the diameter of the extremity in use.	Use the correct size cuff.
	Wrapping the cuff too loosely.	Wrap the cuff firmly but not tightly.
	Deflating the cuff too slowly. Venous congestion in the extremity will give a falsely high reading.	Release the pressure valve methodically.
	Tilting the mercury column away from the vertical.	Maintain the sphygmomanometer in the vertical position.
	Having the mercury column above eye level.	Place the sphygmomanometer at eye level.
Falsely low blood pressure.	Taking the blood pressure when the patient is upset, has just eaten, has just finished a cigarette or has been walking.	Ensure that the patient has been relaxed for at least half an hour before taking the blood pressure.
	Patient's arm above the level of his heart.	Ensure that the arm is below the level of the heart.
	Having the mercury column below eye level.	Place the sphygmomanometer at eye level.
	Failure to notice an 'auscultatory gap', i.e. the sound, after fading out for about 10–15 mm Hg, returns.	Palpate the radial artery as the cuff is inflated.
	Inability to hear feeble sounds.	Ask the patient to raise his/her arm before you inflate the cuff again. This decreases the venous pressure and should make the sounds louder. Then lower the arm, deflate the cuff, and listen. If the sounds are still feeble, chart the preparatory systolic pressure. Inform the medical staff.

PULSE

Definition

The pulse is a rhythmic throbbing caused by regular expansion and contraction of an artery as blood is forced into it by the contraction of the left ventricle of the heart.

Indications

The pulse is taken for the following reasons:

1 to establish a baseline pulse;
2 to monitory fluctuations in pulse.

REFERENCE MATERIAL

The pulse is measured at the following sites (Figure 26.3)

1   temporal;
2   carotid;
3   brachial;
4   radial;
5   ulnar;
6   femoral;
7   popliteal;
8   tibial;
9   pedal.

The heart beats about 70 times every minute normally

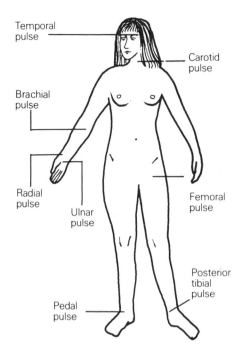

Temporal pulse

Carotid pulse

Brachial pulse

Radial pulse

Ulnar pulse

Femoral pulse

Posterior tibial pulse

Pedal pulse

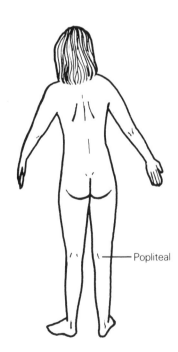

Popliteal

Figure 26.3 Pulse sites.

in the adult, sending 5 litres of blood through the body. This cardiac content equals the volume of blood in each systole (the stroke volume) times the rate per minute. This may be represented as an equation:

Cardiac output = Stroke volume × Rate.

When the stroke volume decreases, as in shock, the rate increases, maintaining a constant cardiac output.

The pulse is palpated to note the following:

1 rate;
2 rhythm;
3 force of amplitude;
4 quality;
5 elasticity.

Rate

The rate is what is palpated at some peripheral artery as the pulse count. The resting adult will normally have a pulse of between 60 and 100 beats per minute. It is slightly faster in women than men and even more rapid in infants and children. There is also a mild increase in old age.

Tachycardia (rapid pulse rate) occurs as a consequence of:

1 pain;   5 anaemia;
2 anger, fear, anxiety; 6 hypoxia;
3 exercise;   7 shock;
4 fever;   8 congestive cardiac failure.

Pain, anger, fear and anxiety all stimulate the sympathetic nervous system. Congestive cardiac failure, anaemia, exercise and fever all require greater oxygenation and, therefore, greater cardiac output.

Bradycardia (slow pulse rate) occurs in all conditions that cause stimulation of the functional parasympathetic nervous system. It is also found in fit athletes.

Rhythm

The rhythm should be regular. There are two normal exceptions:

SINUS ARRHYTHMIA

Sinus arrhythmia is an irregular pulse that increases at the peak of inspiration and decreases on expiration. It is common in children and young adults.

PREMATURE BEAT OR BIGEMINAL PULSE

This condition occurs occasionally when some other pacemaker fires ahead of the sinoatrial node. Doing so prematurely, it causes an early systole. Because of the reduced filling time, the stroke volume is decreased enough for a pause in rhythm to be felt. Frequent premature ventricular contractions may indicate cardiac irritability, hypoxia, digitalis overdose, potassium imbalance, or are signs of more serious dysrhythmias.

Force or amplitude

The pulse pressure is the difference between systolic and diastolic pressure. Amplitude is a reflection of pulse strength. A full, throbbing pulse may indicate such conditions as complete heart block, anaemia or heart failure. Anxiety, alcohol or exercise may produce the same result.

Quality

The character of the pulse may be noted on a scale such as the following:

    3+   bounding pulse;
    2+   normal pulse;
    1+   weak, thready pulse;
    0   absent pulse.

Paradoxical pulse is a pulse that markedly decreases in size during inspiration. On inspiration more blood is pooled in the lungs and so decreases the return to the left side of the heart; this affects the consequent stroke volume. A paradoxical pulse is usually regarded as normal, although in conjunction with such features as hypotension and dyspnoea it may indicate cardiac tamponade.

Elasticity

This refers to the elastic recoil of the arterial wall. The flexibility of the artery should be noted. The supple artery of the young adult feels very different from the hard artery of the patient suffering from arteriosclerosis.

Assessing gross pulse irregularity

When there is gross pulse irregularity, it may be useful to use a stethoscope to assess the apical heart beat. This is done by placing the bell of the stethoscope over the apex of the heart and counting the beats for 60 seconds. A second nurse should record, for example, the radial pulse at the same time. The deficit between the two should be noted using, for example, different colours on the patient's chart to indicate the apex and radial rates.

References and further reading

Birdsall, C. (1985) How do you interpret pulses, *American Journal of Nursing*, Vol. 85, no. 7, pp. 785–6.

Jarvis, C.M. (1980) Vital signs: a preview of problems, in *Assessing Vital Functions Accurately*, Intermed Communications.

Wieck, L. *et al.* (1986) *Illustrated Manual of Nursing Techniques*, 3rd edn, J.B. Lippincott, Philadelphia.

GUIDELINES: PULSE

Procedure

Action	Rationale
1 Explain the procedure to the patient.	To obtain the patient's consent and co-operation.
2 Ensure that the patient is in a comfortable, but also the required position.	To ensure that the patient is comfortable and relaxed. To ensure an accurate reading.
3 Palpate whichever peripheral artery is being used to record the pulse.	For routine signs the radial artery is usually used as being the most readily available.
4 Place the second or third fingers along the appropriate artery and press gently.	The fingertips are sensitive to touch. The thumb and forefinger have pulses of their own that may be mistaken for the patient's pulse.
5 The pulse should be counted for 60 seconds.	Sufficient time is required to detect irregularities or other defects. The normal ranges are: (a) about 72 beats per minute for men; (b) 72–84 beats per minute for women.

5 Record the pulse rate.	To monitor differences and detect trends. Any irregularities should be brought to the attention of the appropriate personnel.

NURSING CARE PLAN

Category	Frequency	Rationale
On admission.	Once only, preferably when patient is settled in.	To provide an accurate baseline.
Preoperative *or* preinvestigative.	Once only.	To provide an accurate baseline and to check that the patient's pulse is not irregular.
Patients receiving blood transfusion.	When unit is put up. Observe the patient at 5-minute intervals for the first 15–20 minutes and take again 1 hour later if condition warrants it. If pulse rate rises, record again and then as often as situation demands.	To record a baseline pulse and to detect any indication of reaction to the blood transfusion.

Postoperatively:
  Minor surgery
  Major surgery.
	On return from theatre only.
	On return from theatre, then 4–6-hourly. Continue at discretion depending on nature of surgery.
		To detect any cardiovascular changes and to monitor the patient's condition.

Patient with a central venous line.	Four-hourly.	To monitor the patient's cardiac function.
Patients with thyrotoxicosis, myxoedema.	Four-hourly plus sleeping pulse.	To monitor the patient's cardiac function.
Patients diagnosed as having cardiovascular problems.	Depends on the condition.	To monitor the patient's cardiac function.
Patients with signs or symptoms of local or systemic infection.	Six-hourly until six normal recordings obtained.	To monitor the development or course of the infection.

RESPIRATIONS

Definition

Respiration is the diffusion of gases between the air in the alveoli of the lungs and the blood in the alveolar capillaries.

Indications

The respiration rate is evaluated
1   to establish a baseline for respirations;
2   to monitor fluctuations in respirations.

REFERENCE MATERIAL

The movements of respiration are essential in keeping the alveolar air constant and their observation is an important contribution to the general assessment of the patient.

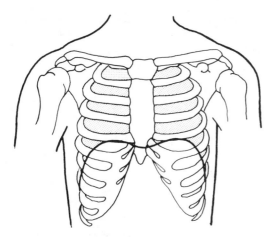

Figure 26.4   The lungs in the thorax. Note how high the diaphragm extends at the front of the chest.

Ventilation

Ventilation results from pressure changes transmitted from the thoracic cavity to the lungs. Inspiration is initiated by contraction of the diaphragm and external intercostal muscles so that the thoracic cavity expands both outwards and downwards (Figures 26.4 and 26.5).

The thoracic cavity and lungs are joined by a thin serous membrane, the pleura, which lines the ribs (parietal layer) and folds back on itself to cover the lungs (visceral layer) (Figure 26.6). As a result of this connection, the decreased intrathoracic pressure from the chest wall expansion is relayed to the intrapleural space and then to the lungs themselves. In response to a decrease in alveolar pressure, air rushes in. Expiration is a passive process by which stored energy is released and the lungs return to a resting state.

The degree to which the lungs stretch and fill during inspiration and return to their normal slight stretch during expiration is explained by the terms 'compliance' and 'elastance'.

Compliance is defined as the change in volume that occurs for a given change in pressure and varies according to lung size.

Elastance refers to the extent to which the lungs are able to return to their barely stretched position. Lung recoil is enhanced by the elastic properties of the lung tissue itself.

Resistance within the airways affects ventilation. Normally airway resistance is slight, so that minimal opposition to airflow occurs. To overcome the various resistances, the respiratory muscles must function.

Volume of air breathed (Figure 26.7)

TIDAL VOLUME

The tidal volume is the volume of air inspired or expired in a single breath (about 500 ml).

RESIDUAL VOLUME

The residual volume is the volume of air in the lungs at the end of maximum expiration (about 1200 ml).

EXPIRATORY RESERVE VOLUME

The expiratory reserve volume is the maximum volume that can be expired from a resting expiratory level (about 1200 ml).

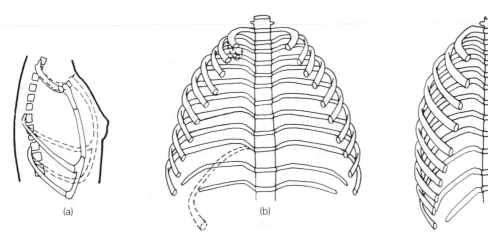

(a)   (b)   (c)

Figure 26.5   The movements of the rib cage in external respiration. *a*, The solid outline shows the ribs in expiration, and the interrupted outline shows the position of the same ribs in inspiration. *b*, The ribs seen from the front in inspiration, showing that the side diameter in the lower part of the chest is increased. *c*, The ribs seen from the front in expiration.

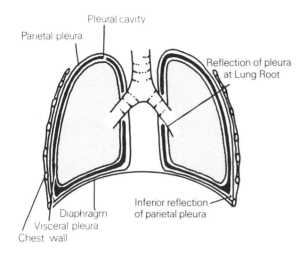

Figure 26.6 Diagram to show the relations of the pleura.

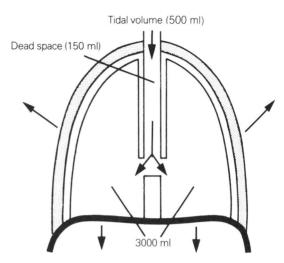

Figure 26.7 Inspiratory capacity.

TOTAL LUNG CAPACITY
The total lung capacity is the volume of air in the lungs at the end of a maximum inspiration (about 600 ml).

VITAL CAPACITY
The vital capacity is the maximum volume of air that can be expired after a maximum inspiration (about 3800 ml).

INSPIRATORY CAPACITY
The inspiratory capacity is the maximum volume of air that can be inspired from a resting expiratory level (about 2500 ml).

Composition of inspired and expired air
INSPIRED AIR
Oxygen	20%
Carbon dioxide	0.04%
Nitrogen	80%

EXPIRED AIR
Oxygen	16%
Carbon dioxide	4%
Nitrogen	80%

ALVEOLAR AIR
Oxygen	14%
Carbon dioxide	5.5–6%
Nitrogen	80%

Exchange of gases
The purpose of ventilation is to transport air to and from the alveoli (Figure 26.8). Adjacent to the alveoli is a dense vascular network.

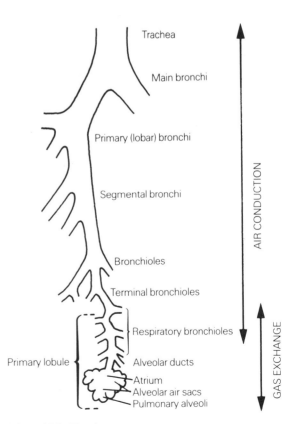

Figure 26.8 The air passages.

Movement of gas from alveolus to capillary and from capillary to alveolus occurs by simple diffusion. Oxygen moves into the alveolar capillaries and carbon dioxide moves out (Figure 26.9). Exchanges of gases is measured by investigating the levels of the arterial blood gases.

Respiratory centre

The respiratory centre in the brain comprises groups of nerve cells in the reticular formation of the medulla oblongata. Regular impulses are sent by these cells to the motor neurones in the anterior horn of the spinal cord which supply the intercostal muscles and the diaphragm. When the motor neurones are stimulated the muscles contract and inspiration occurs. When the neurones are inhibited, the muscles relax and expiration follows.

Respiratory centre activity is regulated in two ways, as described below (Figure 26.10).

CHEMICAL CONTROL

An increase in the amount of carbon dioxide in the blood supplying the respiratory centre stimulates the respiratory centre and breathing becomes faster and deeper.

During exercise, carbon dioxide is produced in the muscles by the oxidation of carbohydrate. The amount of carbon dioxide in the blood increases and this stimulates the respiratory centre, producing an increase in depth and rate of respiration. More oxygen is made available in the alveoli for the blood to transport to the muscles, at the same time eliminating more carbon dioxide.

As well as carbon dioxide, any substance that lowers the pH of the blood will stimulate the respiratory centre.

NERVOUS CONTROL

Lung tissue is stretched on inspiration and this stimulates afferent fibres in the vagus nerve. These impulses cause inspiration to cease and expiration occurs.

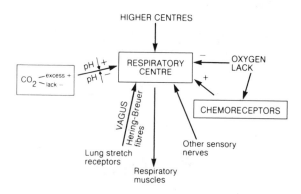

Figure 26.10   Factors controlling respiration.

Emotion, pain and new sensations also cause an increased respiratory rate.

Lung defence mechanisms

The upper airway is designed to warm, humidify and filter inspired air. The nasal passages absorb noxious gases and trap inhaled particles. Smaller particles are removed by the cough reflex.

Observation of respiration

Respirations should be observed for quality, rate, depth and pattern.

QUALITY

Normal relaxed breathing is effortless, automatic, regular and almost silent.

RATE

Rate and depth determine the type of respiration. The normal rate at rest is 12–18 breaths per minute in adults. It is faster in infants and children. The ratio of pulse rate to respiration rate is approximately 5 : 1.

DEPTH

The depth of respiration is the volume of air moving in and out with each respiration. This tidal volume is normally about 500 ml in an adult and should be constant with each breath. A spirometer is used to measure the precise amount.

PATTERN

Changes in the pattern of respiratory rate may be defined as follows:

Tachypnoea

Tachypnoea is an increased respiratory rate, seen in fever, for example as the body tries to rid itself of excess heat. Respirations increase by about 7 breaths a minute

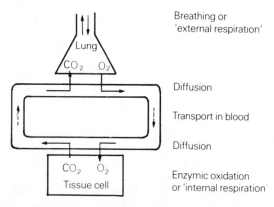

Figure 26.9   Respiratory processes.

for every 1 °C rise in temperature above normal. They also increase with pneumonia, other obstructive airway diseases, respiratory insufficiency, and lesions in the pons of the brainstem.

Bradypnoea

Bradypnoea is a decreased but regular respiratory rate, such as that caused by the depression of the respiratory centre in the medulla by opiate narcotics or a brain tumour.

Apnoea

Apnoea is the total absence of breathing; it may be periodic.

Hypernoea

Hypernoea is an increased rate of respiration.

Hypoventilation

Hypoventilation is an alteration in the pattern of respiration, which becomes irregular or slow, and the depth, which becomes shallow. This is caused by drugs, carbon dioxide narcosis and anaesthetics.

Hyperventilation

Hyperventilation is an increase in both the rate and depth of respiration. This follows extreme exertion, fear and anxiety, fever, hepatic coma, mid-brain lesions of the brainstem, and acid-base imbalance such as diabetic ketoacidosis (Kussmaul's respiration) or salicylate overdose (in both these, compensation for the metabolic acidosis is attempted through respiratory alkalosis), as well as an alteration in blood gas concentration (either increased carbon dioxide or decreased oxygen). The breathing pattern is normally regular and consists of inspiration, pause, longer expiration and another pause. But this may be altered by some defects and diseases. In adults, more than 20 breaths per minute is considered moderate, more than 30 severe.

Cheyne-Stokes respiration

This is a cycle in which respirations gradually increase in rate and depth and then decrease over a cycle of 30–45 seconds. Periods of apnoea (20 seconds) alternate with the cycles. Caused by increased intracranial pressure, severe congestive heart failure, renal failure, meningitis and drug overdose. This type of breathing is also associated with the dying patient.

Biot's respiration

This is an interrupted breathing pattern, like Cheyne–Stokes respiration, except that each breath is of the same depth. It may be seen with spinal meningitis or other central nervous system conditions.

Kussmaul's respiration

This is a breathing pattern characterized by increased rate (more than 20 per minute) and increased depth, a panting, laboured kind of respiration seen in metabolic acidosis or renal failure.

Apnoeustic respiration

This is a pattern of prolonged, gasping inspiration, followed by extremely short, inefficient expiration, seen in lesions of the pons in the mid-brain.

References and further reading

Bell, G.H. *et al.* (1980) *Textbook of Physiology and Biochemistry*, 10th edn, Churchill Livingstone, Edinburgh.

Boylan, A. and Brown, P. (1985) Respirations, *Nursing Times*, Vol. 81, pp. 35–8.

Glennister, T.W.A. and Ross, R.W. (1980) *Anatomy and Physiology for Nurses*, 3rd edn, William Heinemann Medical Books, London.

Green, J.H. (1979) *Basic Clinical Physiology*, 3rd edn, Oxford University Press.

Jarvis, C.M. (1980) Vital signs: a preview of problems, in *Assessing Vital Functions Accurately*, Intermed Communications.

Roberts, A. (1980) Systems and signs. Respiration 1, 2, *Nursing Times 76*, Systems of life nos. 71, 72, p. 8.

Rokosky, J.S. (1981) Assessment of the individual with altered respiratory function, *Nursing Clinics of North America*, Vol. 16, no. 2, pp. 195–9.

GUIDELINES: RESPIRATIONS

Procedure

Action

1 Do not explain the procedure to the patient. Attempt to count the respirations when the patient is at rest. This may be done while you are still appearing to record the pulse.

Rationale

Awareness of the patient's part of the procedure often produces changes in the respiratory rate.

Action	Rationale
2 Ensure that the patient is in a comfortable, but also the required position.	To ensure that the patient is comfortable and relaxed. To ensure accurate observations.
3 Observe the movements of the chest wall.	To detect any respiratory obstruction. To assess excessive use of the intercostal and accessory muscles of respiration. To observe for dyspnoea.
4 Evaluate the sounds made when the patient breathes.	To detect respiratory obstruction and to assess whether suction or deep breathing exercises are required.
5 Count the chest movements for 60 seconds. One inhalation and one exhalation together count as one respiration.	To allow sufficient time to detect irregularities or other defects.
6 Record the number of respiration.	To monitor differences and to detect trends. Any irregularities should be brought to the attention of the appropriate personnel.

NURSING CARE PLAN

Category	Frequency	Rationale
On admission.	Once only, preferably when patient settled in.	To provide an accurate baseline.
Preoperative or preinvestigative.	Once only.	To provide an accurate baseline.
Patients diagnosed as suffering from diseases of the respiratory and cardiovascular system.	Affected by the nature and course of the disease.	To monitor the condition of the patient so that necessary action can be instigated.
Patients receiving blood transfusions.	When the unit is put up observe the patient at 5-minute intervals for the first 15–20 minutes and again 1 hour later if the condition warrants it. If the patient shows signs of reaction to the transfusion, record again and then as often as the situation demands.	To record baseline respirations and to detect any indication of reaction to the blood transfusion.
Patients receiving oxygen inhalation therapy.	Affected by the reasons for therapy.	To monitor the patient's reaction to the therapy.
Postoperative (minor). Postoperative (major).	On return from theatre only. On return from theatre, then 4–6-hourly. Continue at discretion depending on the nature of the surgery.	To assess the return of normal respiratory function.
Patients with a central venous line.	Four-hourly.	To identify respiratory complications as a result of the catheterization.

Patients prescribed any drugs that may affect respiratory system, e.g. opiates.	Depends on the prescribed drugs and its known side-effects.	To monitor the patient's respiratory function.
Patients receiving artificial ventilation; unconscious patients; patients suffering trauma to head and/or the thoracic region.	Depends on the condition of the patient.	To monitor the patient's respiratory function.
Pyrexial patients.	At least 6-hourly; more frequently if temperature grossly abnormal.	To monitor the condition of the patient so that any necessary action can be instigated.
Asthmatic patients.	Depends on the condition of the patient.	To monitor the patient's respiratory function. Asthmatic patients experience difficulty in expiration due to the spasm of smooth muscle in the bronchi and bronchioles, which narrows the lumen of the air passages. Sitting the patient in an upright position with his/her limbs supported on a table will enable the accessory muscles of expiration, i.e. the anterior abdominal wall and latissimus dorsi muscles, to function.
Patients suffering from chronic obstructive airways disease.	Depends on the condition of the patient.	To monitor the patient's respiratory function. Positioning of the patient as above will allow the accessory muscles of respiration to function.

TEMPERATURE

Definition
Body temperature represents the balance between heat gain and heat loss as measured by a thermometer.

Indications
Measurement of body temperature is carried out for two reasons:
1   to establish a baseline temperature;
2   to monitor fluctuations in temperature.

REFERENCE MATERIAL
Temperature recording site
ORAL
The pocket of tissue at the base of the tongue lies immediately above the sublingual artery. The proximity of this artery to the external carotid artery means that changes in core temperature are quickly reflected here.

Oral temperatures are affected by the temperatures of ingested foods and fluids and by the muscular activity of chewing. Smoking will also affect the thermometer reading. It is recommended that the nurse waits 15 minutes following any of these activities before inserting the thermometer to allow the temperature to return to baseline level.

It is important that the thermometer is placed in the sublingual pocket and not in the area under the front of the tongue as there may be a temperature difference of up to 1.7 °C between these areas. The sublingual pockets are more protected from the air currents which cool the frontal areas and would result in a false low reading of a thermometer placed there.

RECTAL
The rectal temperature is often higher than the oral temperature because this site is more sheltered from the external environment. However, this does not necessarily imply an increase in accuracy as the rectum is far from the central circulation and is inferior to the oral site

Table 26.1   A Comparison of Mercury in Glass and Electronic Thermometers

Mercury in glass thermometer	Electronic thermometer
Accuracy	
Accuracy of reading varies with the time the thermometer is left in the mouth. Premature removal, i.e. less than 2 minutes, may give a false, low result.	Audible tone and a display light become apparent when the body temperature is reached – which reduces the risk of premature removal.
Reading on the scale must be interpreted by the nurse.	Digital readout minimizes the risk of interpretation error.
Instrument becomes increasingly likely to lose accuracy and be less reliable after use and/or storage (Abbey *et al.*, 1978).	Little research is available on long-term accuracy, but a comparative accuracy study by Moorat (1976) showed that this type of thermometer demonstrated less fluctuation by comparison with mercury in glass or disposable types.
Hygiene	
Thermometers should be wiped clean after each use with a new swab saturated with isopropyl alcohol 70% and left dry. Wet or dirty thermometers support bacterial growth. Wool swabs in thermometer holders are not recommended for this reason.	Disposable cover slip over probe should be discarded after a single use. The nurse should keep the instrument around his/her neck and the patient must be discouraged from holding the end of the thermometer because of the risk of cross-infection.
Cost	
Materials are less expensive but temperature taking involves more time. The nursing time for trained staff increases the cost above that of electronic thermometers (Stronge, 1980).	Materials are more expensive but the time factor is greatly reduced. Moorat (1976) suggested that a cost reduction of 300% could be achieved by utilizing this type of instrument.

in reflecting changes in temperature in the vital central organs. The presence of soft stool may separate the thermometer from the bowel wall and give a false reading, especially if the central temperature is changing rapidly. In infants this method is not recommended as it provides a risk of rectal ulceration or perforation.

A rectal thermometer should be inserted at least 4 cm in an adult to obtain the most accurate reading.

AXILLA

The axilla is considered a less desirable site than the others since it is not close to major vessels and skin surface temperatures vary more with changes in temperature of the environment. It is a convenient site for patients who are unsuitable for, or who cannot tolerate, oral thermometers, e.g. after general anaesthetic.

To take an axillary temperature reading the thermometer should be placed in the centre of the armpit, with the patient's arm firmly against the side of the chest. The thermometer will take longer to register than when in the oral site.

Note: Whatever site is chosen for temperature measurement, it is important that this is then used consistently as switching between sites can produce a record that is misleading or difficult to interpret.

Time for recording temperatures

The average person experience circadian rhythms which make their highest body temperature occur in the late afternoon or early evening, i.e. between 4 p.m. and 8 p.m. The most sensitive time for detecting pyrexias appears to be between 7 p.m. and 8 p.m. (Angerami, 1980). This should be considered when interpreting variations in 4-hourly or 6-hourly observations and when taking once-daily temperatures.

Instruments used for recording temperatures

The most commonly used instruments are mercury in glass thermometers and electronic thermometers. A comparison of the use and effectiveness of these thermometers is made in Table 26.1.

References and further reading

Abbey, J.C. *et al.* (1978) How long is that thermometer accurate? *American Journal of Nursing*, Vol. 78, pp. 1375–6.

Angerami, E.L.S. (1980) Epidemiological study of body temperature in patients in a teaching hospital, *International Journal of Nursing Studies*, Vol. 17, pp. 91–99.

Blainey, C.G. (1974) Site selection in taking body temperatures, *American Journal of Nursing*, Vol. 74, pp. 1859–61.

Boylan, A. and Brown, P. (1985) Temperature, *Nursing Times*, Vol. 81, pp. 36–40.

Campbell, K. (1983) Taking temperature, *Nursing Times*, Vol. 79, pp. 63–5.

Davies, S.P. *et al.* (1986) A comparison of mercury and digital clinical thermometers, *Journal of Advanced Nursing*, Vol. 11, no. 5, pp. 535–43.

Gooch, J. (1986) Taking temperature, *Professional Nurse*, Vol. 1, no. 10, pp. 273–4.

Litsky, B.Y. (1976) A study of temperature taking systems, *Supervisor Nurse*, Vol. 7, pp. 48–53.

Moorat, D.S. (1976) The cost of taking temperatures, *Nursing Times* Vol. 72, pp. 767–70.

Stronge, J.L. (1980) Electronic thermometers: a costly rise in efficiency? *Nursing Mirror*, Vol. 151, no. 8, pp. 29.

GUIDELINES: TEMPERATURE

Equipment

1 Electronic thermometer and oral probe
2 Disposable probe covers.
   The blue probe is for oral and axillar procedures; the red probe is for rectal procedures.

Procedure

Before use, remove the thermometer from its base unit; a neck strap is provided for convenience and its use is recommended.

Action	Rationale
1 Explain the procedure to the patient.	To obtain the patient's consent and co-operation.
2 Remove the probe from the stored position in the face of the thermometer and check that the reading is 34 °C.	If the readout does not register 34 °C the machine is faulty and should not be used.
3 Push the probe firmly into the probe cover.	The cover protects the tip of the probe and is necessary for correct functioning of the instrument.
4 Ask the patient to open his/her mouth and insert the probe under the tongue into the 'heat pocket' at the posterior base of the tongue.	The highest oral temperature reading is at the posterior base of tongue, which is least affected by environmental conditions.
5 Ask the patient to close his/her mouth.	To increase the patient's comfort and to minimize the risk of temperature lowering by the external environment.
6 Hold the thermometer in place until an audible tone is heard and the red light comes on.	Tissue contact must be maintained for an accurate reading to be obtained.

Action	Rationale
7 If figures on the display stop rising without an audible tone, tissue contact has been lost. Regain tissue contact and continue.	The probe must be supported outside the mouth as its top heavy shape tends to move the sensitive tip out of the heat pocket. The nurse should hold the probe in place as the patient may introduce cross-infection.
8 Remove the probe from the patient's mouth and note the temperature displayed.	An audible tone and a red light indicate that the patient's temperature is as displayed by the machine.
9 Discard the probe cover into a waste bag by pressing the probe top with the thumb.	Probe covers are for single-use only. The discard mechanism prevents transfer of the patient's saliva to the nurse's hands.
10 Return the probe to its storage position in the face of the thermometer, cancelling the temperature reading.	The probe is best protected from damage in this storage position.
11 Return the thermometer to its base unit and ensure that the charge light is on.	The thermometer should be left charged and ready for its next use.

NURSING CARE PLAN

Category	Frequency	Rationale
On admission.	Once only, preferably when the patient has settled in.	To provide an accurate baseline.
Preoperative or preinvestigative.	Once only.	To provide an accurate baseline and to check that the patient is not pyrexial.
Pyrexial patients.	At least 6-hourly; possibly hourly. Frequency is affected by direction of temperature movement, e.g. rising, falling or static.	To monitor the condition of the patient so that any necessary action can be instigated. *Note:* Patients receiving steroids may show only very slight rises in temperature even when suffering from severe infection.
Patients receiving blood transfusions.	When the unit is put up, observe the patient at 5-minute intervals for the first 15–20 minutes and again 1 hour later if the patient's condition warrants it. If the patient's pulse rate rises or the patient shows other signs of reaction, record again, and then as often as the situation demands.	To record a baseline temperature and to monitor any reaction to the transfusion.
Postoperative (minor surgery).	On return from the theatre only.	To detect postoperative hypothermia.
Postoperative (major surgery).	On return from the theatre, then 4- to 6-hourly. Continue at your discretion, depending on the nature of the surgery.	To detect postoperative hypothermia and to monitor any pyrexia, e.g. due to infection.

Patient receiving steroids.	Four-hourly.	A very slight rise in temperature may be indicative of severe infection.
Patients receiving cytotoxic chemotherapy or antibiotics.	Daily.	To detect any development of infection or drug reaction.
Patients receiving radiotherapy.	As necessary, depending on area and dose.	To detect developing infections when defence mechanisms are lowered by the nature of the treatment.
Patients with radioactive caesium implants.	Every 2 hours.	Frequent monitoring is required to detect development of pelvic cellulitis due to a proflavin pack or postoperative complications, e.g. urinary tract infection or chest infection.
Patients with a central venous line.	Every 4 hours.	To identify any infection introduced by the central venous catheter as soon as possible.
Patients with a white blood cell count of less than 1000 cells/mm^3.	Every 4–6 hours.	To detect any developing infection as soon as possible so that appropriate therapy can be given.
Patients with a falling white blood cell count but having more than 1000 cells/mm^3.	Daily.	A falling white blood cell count increases the likelihood of infection.
Patients in close contact with a known source of infection.	Daily.	To check that infection has not been transmitted.
Patient with signs and/or symptoms of systemic or local infection.	Every 6 hours until six normal recordings are obtained.	To monitor the development of regression of infection.
Patient not feeling well or nurse concerned about patient.	Once. However, if the temperature is elevated, check again 2–3 hours later and take appropriate action.	To reassure the patient and the nurse. To check whether the patient is pyrexial and if so ensure that appropriate action is taken.
Continuing care patients.	Daily.	Mainly because patients expect their temperatures to be taken. This is therefore omitted or increased at the nurse's discretion.

27

Oxygen Therapy

Definition

Oxygen therapy is the provision of an atmosphere of increased oxygenation and humidity by the use of specialized equipment.

Indications

The absolute indication for supplementary inspired oxygen is inadequate tissue oxygenation. Clinical signs such as cyanosis are imprecise and misleading. The only accurate assessment of respiratory failure is the measurement of blood gases and pH. Oxygen therapy is generally indicated in the following cases:

1 acute lower respiratory infections;
2 acute pulmonary oedema;
3 asthma;
4 carbon monoxide poisoning;
5 long-term therapy in chronic obstructive pulmonary disease. *The Lancet* (1981) has a useful reappraisal of the acute use of oxygen therapy in this instance.

REFERENCE MATERIAL

The modern concept of oxygen therapy began during World War I, when it was used to treat soldiers suffering from respiratory failure due to exposure to poisonous gas.

Physiology

The amount of oxygen entering the blood from the lungs depends, among other things, on its pressure in the alveoli. In turn, this depends on the percentage of oxygen in the alveoli and on the atmospheric pressure. There is approximately 21% oxygen in inspired air and at sea level the pressure is about 150 mm Hg (20 kPa), whereas in the alveoli it is about 100 mm Hg (13.3 kPa). If the atmospheric pressure is reduced, the oxygen pressure in the alveoli will be reduced. Oxygen diffuses through the alveolar membrane and capillary wall, dissolves in the blood plasma and combines with haemoglobin in the red cells to form oxyhaemoglobin. The oxygen is transported from the pulmonary capillaries through the arterial system to the tissues. The amount of oxygen combined with haemoglobin varies – the oxyhaemoglobin dissociation curve. Ata a pO_2 of 100 mm Hg blood is 97% satuarated. At lower pressures, e.g. 80 mm Hg, the saturation has scarcely altered. Between 0 and 40 mm Hg, the saturation falls rapidly. This mechanism provides a safety margin in the early stages of a fall in arterial p O_2 caused by disease, but where pO_2 is initially low, as in chronic pulmonary disease, a further fall could cause a dangerous drop in arterial pO_2. Among the causes of a low arterial pO_2 are the following:

1 *Ventilatory failure*: when an inadequate volume of air is breathed in a given time.
2 *Impairment of diffusion/gas transfer.*
3 *Ventilation perfusion imbalance*: some alveoli receive insufficient oxygen and carbon dioxide from the air and blood respectively, with the result that the blood entering the arteries from these alveoli contains too much carbon dioxide and too little oxygen.
4 *Shunting of blood*: the passage of blood from the right side of the heart to the left without an opportunity for exchange of gases in the alveoli.
5 *Carbon dioxide narcosis*: in patients with chronic respiratory diseases much of the respiratory centre's stimulus comes from lack of oxygen. If hypoxia is relieved by administering oxygen, the main stimulus to breathing is lost. The patient hypoventilates and the pCO_2 rises to anything from 80 to 100 mm Hg. This has a toxic effect on the brain resulting in stupor or coma.

General considerations

1 Oxygen is an odourless, tasteless, colourless, transparent gas that is slightly heavier than air.
2 Oxygen supports combustion, so there is always a danger of fire when oxygen is being used. It is

necessary, therefore, to:

(a) Avoid using oil or grease around oxygen connections.

(b) Eliminate antiseptic tinctures, alcohol and ether in the immediate oxygen environment.

(c) Prohibit the use of any electrical device in or near an oxygen tent.

(d) Keep any oxygen cylinders secured in an upright position away from heat.

(e) Place a NO SMOKING sign on the patient's door and in view of other patients and the patient's visitors

(f) Have fire extinguishers available.

3   Oxygen is dispensed from a cylinder or piped system and requires:

(a) A reduction gauge to reduce the pressure to that of the atmosphere.

(b) A flow meter to regulate the control of oxygen in litres per minute.

4   Oxygen is given to relieve hypoxia, either locally or generalized.

Hypoxia is a state in which there is an insufficient amount of oxygen available in the tissue cells to meet the requirements of an organ or tissue at that moment. The aim of oxygen administration is to treat the hypoxia while decreasing the work of breathing and stress on the myocardium.

Supply of oxygen

The British Oxygen Company (BOC) has a monopoly in the supply of 100% oxygen in the United Kingdom. It is available in compressed form in cylinders and as liquid oxygen. In hospitals it is available to the patient either piped from a central supply or direct from a cylinder by the patient's bedside. There are six cylinder capacities. The most popular sizes for hospital use are G and F. G is for static use at the bedside. At a flow rate of 4 litres per minute, this cylinder will empty in about 14 hours. F is used on wheeled stands for mobility and is convenient for emergency use. Oxygen cylinders are black with white shoulders and upper part. They are marked with the symbol O_2 and/or the word OXYGEN.

Oxygen giving sets

The equipment used to convey oxygen from the cylinder head or pipeline to the patient consists of a pressure gauge, regulator (optional), flow meter, tubing, mask or nasal cannulae and humidifier, if required. The pressure gauge indicates how much gas is in the cylinder and the regulator is used to reduce gas pressure in tubing and equipment distally to 60 lbf/in² (414 kPa). A regulator also ensures a steady flow rate until the cylinder is nearly empty. The flow meter indicates the oxygen flow rate in liters per minute. The majority of regulators are light

bobbins or spheres that ride up and down in the bore of a transparent vertical graduated tube. As the tube is tapered and wider above, the bobbin rises to a level corresponding to the flow rate.

Methods of administration

VENTURI MASKS

In Venturi masks, e.g. the Mixomask (Figure 27.1) and the Ventimask (Figure 27.2), oxygen is blown under pressure into the mask at a given flow rate, indicated by the flow meter. Oxygen is forced through a small hole in the nozzle and comes out at high speed. This high-speed jet sucks in surrounding air that travels along the wide tube towards the face mask. Provided that this type of mask is fed with oxygen at the required flow rate, only the stated percentage of oxygen will be available for the patient to breathe.

MC MASKS

Masks of this type (Figure 27.3) may be used when high concentrations of oxygen are required but when the

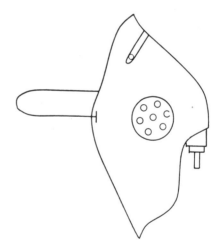

Figure 27.1   Mixomask.

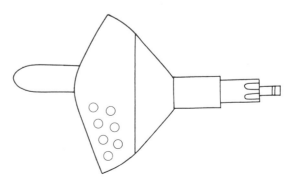

Figure 27.2   Ventimask.

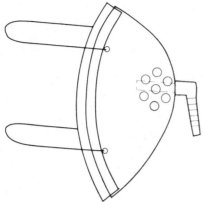

Figure 27.3 MC mask.

actual percentage is not critical. Oxygen concentrations vary from 24 to 81% depending on the flow rate (1–10 litres per minute) and tidal volume. The mask consists of a soft plastic facepiece with a large central bore tube connected directly to the oxygen supply. Vent holes are provided to allow clearance of expired air and escape of unused high-pressure gas. If a patient breathes at an inspiration rate of 10 litres per minute and 100% oxygen is being supplied at a rate of 2 litres per minute, then the inspired mixture comprises 8 litres of air containing 21% oxygen and 2 litres of 100% oxygen. Thus 20% of the inspired gas is pure oxygen and the remaining 80% already contains 21% oxygen. After mixing, the patient will be receiving:

$$\left[\frac{80}{100}\times\right]20 \ + 20 = 16.8 + 20 = 36.8\% \text{ oxygen.}$$

This demonstrates that the actual percentage delivered will not be obvious simply by regarding the flow meter on the supply. If the patient's inspiration rate alters, the delivered percentage of oxygen will also change.

NASAL CANNULAE

Nasal cannulae consist of a pair of tubes about 2 cm long, each projecting into the nostril and stemming from a tube which encircles the head and which is thus self-retaining (see Figure 27.4). Oxygen is delivered in a similar way as when given via an MC mask. Cannulae have the advantage of not interfering with feeding and are not as inconvenient as masks during coughing and sneezing. Oxygen needs to be humidified if cannulae are used as dry gas impinges directly on the nasal mucosa which may become damaged.

AMBU BAG

An Ambu bag is a self-inflating rubber bag, one end of which is fitted with a one-way air valve and gas supply tube, while the other end is connected directly to a sterile tube in the trachea or to a face mask. This bag is usually used during cardiopulmonary resuscitation procedures when oxygen is fed into the supply tube. The percentage of oxygen delivered into the trachea will depend on the rate of pumping of the bag, the bag volume and also the flow rate of oxygen from the supply.

MECHANICAL VENTILATION

Here the amount of oxygen delivered is directly controlled by a ventilator. Ventilators vary in their methods of oxygen delivery, but the same basic principles apply as in the above-mentioned types. The input oxygen is mixed with a quantity of air drawn in before or during each respiratory phase, the total volume then being delivered into the trachea.

OXYGEN TENT

Oxygen tents have almost entirely been superceded in the treatment of adults by masks and cannulae (Freedman, 1978). However, they are still useful when oxygen needs to be administered to restless and confused patients and children.

Hyperbaric oxygen therapy

Hyperbaric oxygen therapy is the administration of 100% oxygen at greater than normal atmospheric pressure. It is adminstered in a hyperbaric chamber. It can be used effectively in the primary treatment of acute carbon monoxide poisoning, acute gas embolism and decompression sickness. It is used as adjunctive treatment for

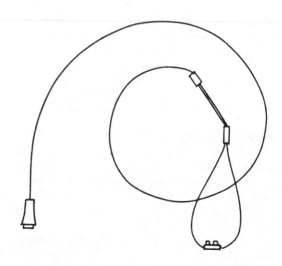

Figure 27.4 Nasal cannulae.

compromised skin grafts, gas gangrene, acute cyanide poisoning and ulcers caused by microaerophilic streptococci. Evidence is also accumulating to support its use in the treatment of osteomyelitis, osteoadiponecrosis, soft tissue injury and multiple sclerosis. It may be used to administer high concentrations of oxygen systemically or locally, to promote neovascularization and to produce vasoconstriction with subsequent reduction in oedema. Increasing oxygen concentration to 100% is one method of increasing arterial oxygen content. Further increases may be achieved by increasing barometric pressure. The greater the pressure at which a gas is administered, the denser the gas and the greater the number of molecules of gas that can be delivered for a set volume. With hyperbaric oxygenation, sufficient oxygen can be dissolved in the plasma to maintain life. Applied topically, oxygen acts to increase superficial oxygen tension sufficiently to prevent tissue death from anoxia and inhibit the growth of superficial aerobic organisms.

Two types of chambers are commonly in use:

1 *Monoplace chambers*: the patient is placed in an individual capsule with a transparent canopy.
2 *Multiplace chambers*: a large, airtight chamber constructed to accommodate either an operating team and/or a multiplicity of patients.

Treatments are carried out over a period of days or weeks.

Humidification

Oxygen supplied from cylinders or piped sources is dry. It has a potential, therefore, for drying mucous membranes of the air passages. Ambient air, which mixes with the oxygen during inspiration, contains enough water vapour to prevent drying of the air passages in most circumstances. Humidification is essential when oxygen is adminstered via a tracheostomy and desirable when nasal cannulae are used.

References and further reading

Bolton, M.E. (1981) Hyperbaric oxygen therapy, *American Journal of Nursing*, Vol. 81, pp. 1199–201.

Coady, T.J. and Bennett, A. (1978) Technology in nursing. Respiratory function 1. Oxygen administration, *Nursing Times*, Vol. 74, Scan 1–4.

Freedman, B.J. (1978) Oxygen therapy in hospital practice. The indications for oxygen therapy and its safe application. *Nursing Times*, Vol. 74, pp. 2072–6.

Lancet (1981) Acute oxygen therapy, *Lancet*, Vol. i, pp. 980–1.

Scottish Health Services Council Standing Medical Advisory Committee (1969) *Uses and Dangers of Oxygen Therapy*, Report of a Subcommittee, HMSO, London.

GUIDELINES: ADMINISTRATION OF OXYGEN BY VENTURI MASK

Equipment

1 Oxygen source
2 Mask
3 Flow meter
4 Connecting tubing
5 'No Smoking' sign.

Procedure

Action	Rationale
1 Place the NO SMOKING sign on the patient's door and in view of other patients and visitors.	Oxygen supports combustion.
2 Explain the procedure to the patient.	To obtain the patient's consent and co-operation.
3 Connect the mask, disposable tubing and flow meter to the oxygen.	To ensure that equipment functions as intended.
4 Turn on the oxygen to the prescribed rate of flow.	To check that oxygen is flowing out of the vent holes in the flexible face mask.

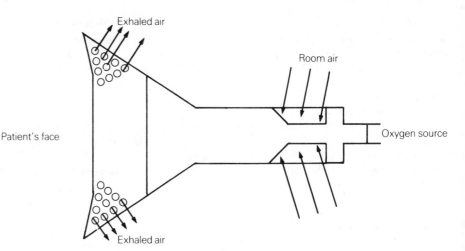

Figure 27.5
Administraton of
oxygen via a Venturi
mask.

Action	Rationale
5 Place the Venturi mask over the patient's nose and mouth and under his/her chin. Mould the mask to fit the patient's face (Figure 27.5).	To ensure that oxygen is delivered as prescribed. A correctly fitting mask is more comfortable.
6 Adjust the elastic strap around the patient's head and position the strap below the ears and around the neck.	Prevents leakage of oxygen. If oxygen leaks into the patient's eyes it causes extreme distress.
7 If high humidity is used, attach large-bore tubing to a nebulizer and connect it to the fitting for high humidity at the base of the Venturi mask.	
8 Assess the patient's condition at frequent intervals.	
9 Change the mask and tubing daily.	Contaminated equipment may cause virulent infections in debilitated patients.

GUIDELINES: ADMINISTRATION OF OXYGEN BY MC MASK

Equipment
1 Oxygen source
2 Mask
3 Large-bore connection tubing
4 'No Smoking' sign.

Procedure

Action	Rationale
1 Place the NO SMOKING sign on the patient's door and in view of other patients and visitors.	Oxygen supports combustion.
2 Explain the procedure to the patient.	To obtain the patient's consent and co-operation.

3	Attach the large-bore tubing to the mask and oxygen flow meter. Set the oxygen flow at the desired level.	To ensure that oxygen will be delivered as prescribed.
4	Place the mask to the patient's face and adjust the straps so that the mask fits securely and there are no leaks.	If the mask is comfortable, the patient is more likely to tolerate it.
5	Change the mask and tubing daily.	Contaminated equipment may cause virulent infections in debilitated patients.

GUIDELINES: ADMINISTRATION OF OXYGEN BY NASAL CANNULAE

Equipment

1   Oxygen source
2   Plastic nasal cannulae
3   Disposable connecting tubing
4   Humidifier filled with sterile distilled water to indicated level
5   Flow meter
6   'No Smoking' sign.

Procedure

Action	**Rationale**
1 Place the NO SMOKING sign on the patient's door in view of other patients and visitors.	Oxygen supports combustion.
2 Show the patient the nasal cannulae and explain the procedure.	To obtain the patient's consent and co-operation.
3 Prepare the nasal cannulae, connecting tubing, humidifier and flow meter to the oxygen source.	To ensure that oxygen is administered as prescribed.
4 Turn on the oxygen.	To determine whether oxygen is flowing through the nasal tips of the cannulae.
5 Turn off the oxygen.	Usually the patient accepts cannulae better if they are fitted with the oxygen turned off.
6 Position the tips of the cannulae in the patient's nose so that the tips do not extend more than 2.5 cm into the nares.	Over-long tubing is uncomfortable, which may make the patient reject the procedure. Sore nasal mucosa can result from pressure or friction of tubing that is too long.
7 Adjust the oxygen flow to the prescribed rate.	Inadequate flow rates may result in administration of an inaccurate oxygen concentration to the patient.
8 Fasten tubing securely.	Correctly secured tubing is comfortable and prevents displacement of cannulae.
9 Assess the patient's condition and the functioning of the equipment at regular intervals.	To ensure that oxygen is being administered as prescribed.
10 Change cannulae and humidifier tubing daily.	Contaminated equipment may cause virulent infections in debilitated patients.

NURSING CARE PLAN

OXYGEN DELIVERY BY FACE MASK

Problem	Cause	Suggested action
Noise.	The constant oxygen flow, particularly if a nebulizer is incorporated in the system, can be irritating.	Give further explanation to the patient.
Difficulty in talking.	Mask restricts talking.	Conversation should be reduced to a minimum. A paper and pencil will prove useful.
Difficulty in eating and drinking.	Impossible to eat or drink with mask in position.	Highly nourishing soft foods should be offered, which reduces the time the mask is not in position.
Feeling of claustrophobia.	Tight fitting mask.	Refit the mask.
Dry, sore mouth.	Insufficient fluid intake; oxygen has a drying effect.	Offer oral toilet frequently. Encourage the patient to take fluids.

OXYGEN DELIVERY BY NASAL CANNULAE

Problem	Cause	Suggested action
Humidifier water overflowing into gauge.	Overfilled humidifier.	Only fill the humidifier to the required level.
Air swallowing.	Excessive flow of oxygen.	Reduce the rate of oxygen delivery.
Irritation of nasal and pharyngeal mucosa.	Excessive flow of oxygen.	Reduce the rate of oxygen delivery.
Changes in patient's mental state, disturbed consciousness, abnormal colour of perspiration.	Excessive or inadequate flow of oxygen.	Check that the equipment and the rate of flow of oxygen are satisfactory.
Changes in blood pressure increasing heart and respiratory rates.		Seek medical advice.

28

Pain Assessment

Definition

Pain is not a simple sensation but a complex phenomenon having both a cognitive (physical) and an affective (emotional) component. The aim of pain assessment, therefore, is to identify *all* the factors – physical and non-physical – which affect the patient's perception of pain.

REFERENCE MATERIAL

Melzack and Dennis (1980) have distinguished three forms of pain:

1 phasic pain;
2 acute pain;
3 chronic pain.

PHASIC PAIN

This is pain of short duration which occurs at the onset of injury.

ACUTE PAIN

This is provoked by tissue damage which comprises both phasic pain and a tonic stage which persists for variable periods of time until healing takes place.

CHRONIC PAIN

This is pain which persists beyond the period of time required for healing.

Although distinct affective states appear to be associated with each form of pain, chronic pain has the greatest potential for impact on the psychological well-being of the patient.

Thus, while the principles underlying pain assessment will often be applicable to all forms of pain, it is inevitable that in the case of chronic pain, with its greater propensity for physical, psychological and social dysfunction, their application becomes more complex. It is intended, therefore, that pain assessment be seen for the purpose of this procedure in the context of the management of chronic pain.

Factors affecting pain assessment

Patients with chronic, particularly cancer, pain rarely present with this one symptom. For example, around two-thirds of advanced cancer patients will also complain of anorexia, one-half will have a symptomatic dry mouth and constipation and one-third nausea, vomiting, insomnia, dyspnoea, cough or oedema. It will be clear from these figures that pain assessment cannot be seen in isolation; identification of all related symptoms is of equal importance as they will contribute to a lowered pain threshold and impaired pain tolerance.

Furthermore, it has been shown that fewer than 20% of advanced cancer patients will have a single site of pain and that around one-half of patients will have three or more individual pains (Twycross and Fairfield, 1982). Each separate pain needs to be identified as each may have a different cause which will demand a different intervention.

The perception of painful stimuli will always be modulated by the emotional response to that perception. Changes in mood may alter considerably the experience of pain. Pain assessment needs to acknowledge this fact, and particular attention must be paid to factors such as anger, depression, anxiety and fear which will modulate pain sensitivity.

Need for assessment tools

Accurate pain assessment is a prerequisite of effective control and is an essential component of nursing care. Objective pain assessment is difficult to achieve. For example, the tendency suggested by both research and clinical practice is for the patient not to report his/her pain or to do so inadequately or inaccurately, minimizing the pain experience (McCaffery, 1983).

Hunt *et al.* (1977) found that nurses tended to overestimate the pain relief obtained from analgesia and underestimate the level of patients' pain.

Pain charts have been considered as useful tools for assisting nurses to assess pain and plan nursing care.

THE ROYAL MARSDEN HOSPITAL

PAIN ASSESSMENT CHART

SURNAME: HOSPITAL NO.

FIRST NAME: DATE:

INITIAL ASSESSMENT

Patient's own description of the pain(s):

What helps relieve the pain?

What makes the pain worse?

Do you have pain

i)   at night?   Yes/No (comment if required).

ii)   at rest?   Yes/No (comment if required).

iii)   on movement?   Yes/No (comment if required).

PAIN SITES

Please draw on the body outlines below to show where you feel pain.
Label each site of pain with a letter A.B.C. etc.

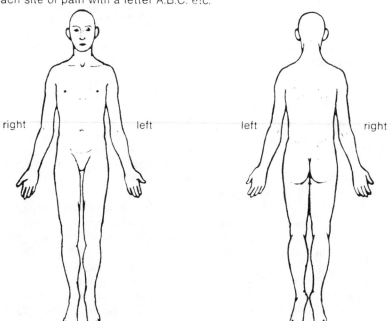

Figure 28.1   The Royal Marsden Hospital pain assessment chart.

PAIN ASSESSMENT CHART

CONTINUATION NO: _____

KEY TO PAIN INTENSITY:

0 = no pain   4 = very severe pain
1 = mild pain   5 = intolerable/overwhelming pain
2 = moderate pain
3 = severe pain   s = sleeping

It may be easier to determine the intensity of pain by looking at the pain scale below.

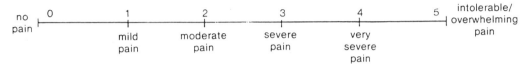

DATE	TIMES	PAIN SITES								ANALGESIA NAME, ROUTE & DOSE	PATIENT ACTIVITY AND COMMENTS
		A	B	C	D	E	F	G	H		

Raiman (1986) found that the use of a chart improved communication between staff and patients. Walker *et al.* (1987) found that the specific advantages of using a chart lie in promoting greater objectivity in both the initial assessment of pain and in its monitoring. It was also found that the involvement of many patients in their pain management helped to increase their confidence in it.

Introduction to use of assessment tools

The published literature indicates that pain assessment charts can be used successfully to assess and monitor pain. Some degree of caution, however, must be exercised in their use. The nurse must be careful to select the tool which is most appropriate for a particular type of pain experience. For example, it would not be appropriate to use a pain assessment chart which had been designed for use with patients with chronic pain to assess postoperative pain. Furthermore, pain charts should not be used totally indiscriminately. Walker *et al* (1987) found that charts appeared to have little value in cases of unresolved or intractable pain.

The Royal Marsden Hospital Pain Assessment Chart

A study was carried out at The Royal Marsden Hospital in order to design a chart for use with chronic cancer pain and to evaluate its effectiveness (Walker *et al.*, 1987). The study indicated that the chart (Figure 28.1) was a valuable tool for pain assessment in 89% of cases. The following guidelines are written with reference to The Royal Marsden Hospital pain chart but it is recognized that nurses may modify the chart to meet the needs of their own particular branch of nursing.

References and further reading

Hunt, J.M. *et al.* (1977) Patients with protracted pain; a survey conducted at the London Hospital, *Journal of Medical Ethics*, Vol. 3, no. 2, pp. 61–73.

McCaffery, M. (1983) *Nursing the Patient in Pain*, Harper & Row, London.

Melzack, R. and Dennis, S.G. (1980) Phylogenetic evolution of pain expression in animals, in H.W. Kosterlitz and L.Y. Terenius (eds.) *Pain and Society*, Chemie, New York.

Raiman, J. (1986) Pain relief – a two way process, *Nursing Times*, Vol. 82, no. 15, pp. 24–8.

Twycross, R.G. and Fairfield, S. (1982) Pain in far advanced cancer, *Pain*, Vol. 14, pp. 303–10.

Walker, V.A. *et al.* (1987) Pain assessment charts in the management of chronic cancer pain, *Palliative Medicine*, Vol. 1, pp. 111–16.

GUIDELINES: INITIAL ASSESSMENT

Action	Rationale
1 Explain the purpose of using the chart to the patient.	To obtain the patient's consent and co-operation.
2 Where appropriate, encourage the patient to complete the pain chart himself/herself.	To encourage patient participation.
3 Where the nurse completes chart, record the patient's *own* description of his/her pain.	To reduce the risk of misrepresentation.
4 (a) Record any factors which influence the intensity of the pain, e.g. activities or interventions which reduce or increase the pain such as distractions or a heat pad. (b) Record whether or not the patient is pain free at night, at rest or on movement.	Ascertaining how and when the patient experiences pain enables the nurse to plan realistic goals. For example, relieving the patient's pain during the night and while he/she is at rest is usually easier to achieve than relief from pain on movement.

GUIDELINES: PAIN SITES

Action

Rationale

1   Encourage the patient, where appropriate, to identify pain sites himself/herself.

The body outline is ideally a vehicle for the patient to describe his/her own pain experience.

2   Index each site (A – H) in whatever way seems most appropriate, e.g. shading/ colouring of areas or arrows to indicate shooting pains.

This enables individual pain sites to be located.

GUIDELINES: MONITORING PAIN INTENSITY

Action

Rationale

1   Give each pain site a numerical value according to the key to pain intensity or to the pain scale and note time recorded.

To indicate the intensity of the pain at each site.

2   Record any analgesia given and note route and dose.

To monitor efficacy of prescribed analgesia.

3   Record any significant activities which are likely to influence the patient's pain.

Extra pharmacological or non-pharmacological interventions might be indicated.

Note: Fixed times for reviewing the pain have been intentionally omitted to allow for flexibility. It is suggested that initially the patient's pain be reviewed every 4 hours. When a patient's level of pain has stabilized, recordings may be made less frequently, e.g. 12 hourly or daily. If a patient's pain becomes totally controlled the chart should be discontinued.

29

Peritoneal Dialysis

Definition
Peritoneal dialysis is a procedure used for patients with inadequate renal function to rid the body of waste products, such as urea, using the peritoneum as a dialysing membrane.

Indications
Peritoneal dialysis is indicated for the following:
1 to aid in the removal of toxic substances and metabolic waste;
2 to assist in regulating fluid and electroyle balance;
3 to remove excessive body fluid;
4 to control blood pressure.

The use of peritoneal dialysis in chronic renal failure is now regarded as controversial (*Lancet*, 1978).

REFERENCE MATERIAL
In 1926 Rosenak, basing his work on that of Ganter, conceived the possibility of using the peritoneum of humans as a dialysing membrane. The use of peritoneal dialysis reached a peak in 1959 with the introduction of commercial dialysis solutions and tubing. With the advent of haemodialysis, however, in the 1960s, peritoneal dialysis assumed a secondary role as a form of treatment for chronic renal failure. In recent years, due to improvements in equipment and technique, peritoneal dialysis is being used to treat patients for whom haemodialysis is contraindicated.

Anatomy and physiology
The peritoneum is the largest serous membrane of the body. In adults it has a surface area of approximately $2.2m^2$. It is a closed unit consisting of two parts:
1 the parietal peritoneum that lines the inside of the abdominal wall;
2 the visceral peritoneum that is reflected over the viscera.

The space between the two parts is the peritoneal cavity. This cavity is normally a potential space containing only a small amount of serous fluid. The serous fluid lubricates the viscera and allows them to move freely upon one another and the parietal peritoneum.

The visceral peritoneum consists of five layers of fibrous and elastic connective tissue and a sixth layer called the mesothelium. Blood and lymphatic capillaries are found only in the deepest layer of tissue in adults. A substance that passes from the bloodstream into the peritoneal cavity must pass through the capillary endothelium, the mesothelium and the five layers of the visceral peritoneum. The mesothelium represents the major barrier to mass transfer for most substances.

Diffusion and osmosis are the physical processes involved in the exchange of substances across the peritoneal membrane. Diffusion is the force acting on gaseous, solid or liquid molecules to spread them from a region of high to a region of lower concentration. Osmosis is the passage of a solvent through a semipermeable membrane that separates solutions of different concentrations. The force that causes this movement of solvents is osmotic pressure and this varies directly with the concentration of the solution. As the solvent moves across the membrane, it tends to pull certain amounts of solute with it. This is known as the solvent drag effect. Solvent drag enhances the efficiency of peritoneal dialysis. Equilibration is the achievement of equalization of solute and solvent concentrations on both sides of the membrane. As equilibration is achieved, dialysis ceases and solvents and solutes can be absorbed back into the bloodstream. For peritoneal dialysis to achieve maximum effectiveness, fresh solutions must be instilled at the point of equilibration to prevent reabsorption of water and uraemic toxins.

Solution concentrations
The osmotic pressure of dextrose is utilized in peritoneal dialysis to remove water from the patient. Commercially available dialysis solutions vary in dextrose concentrations. A dextrose concentration above 1.5% will in-

crease the osmotic effect and thus increase the movement of water away from the patient. Hypertonic dextrose solutions enhance the removal of water; hypotonic solutions are used when removal of water is not the primary aim of dialysis.

Dialysis cycles
Normally a cycle consists of three stages.

STAGE I (INFLOW)
The dialysis solution is infused into the peritoneal cavity to initiate the dialysis. The fluid infuses by gravity and its rate can be controlled by lowering or raising the container in relation to the patient's abdomen or by releasing or compressing the occluding clamp on the tubing.

STAGE II (DWELL TIME)
The dwell time is the time the fluid remains in the peritoneal cavity to allow for equilibration. Different dwell times may be established to remove substances of differing molecular weights. The dwell time is relevant to the type of solute and the amount of solvent removed.

STAGE III (DRAINAGE)
The drainage stage is that of the emptying of the equilibrated solution from the peritoneal cavity to complete dialysis or to prepare for the infusion of fresh solution. Drainage is also dependent on gravity.

Types of peritoneal dialysis
INTERMITTENT
For acute peritoneal dialysis, a manual system is usually used to effect a quick and gentle dialysis. Optimal dialysis is achieved with short dialysis cycles of about 1 hour each, with a dwell time of 30 minutes. Specific numbers of exchanges are prescribed and dialysis is then discontinued temporarily, with initiation recurring as uraemia increases.

CONTINUOUS AMBULATORY PERITONEAL DIALYSIS (CAPD)
CAPD technique was first introduced in 1975. It is a closed, continuous system of peritoneal dialysis and allows the patient the independence of a life free from dialysis machines. Training in its use takes up to 3 weeks on average. Clear outlines of CAPD can be found in Ainge (1981), Sorrels (1981) and Arenz (1982).

References and further reading
Ainge, T.M. (1981) Continuous ambulatory peritoneal dialysis, *Nursing Times*, Vol. 77, pp. 1636–8.

Arenz, R. (1982) Continuous ambulatory peritoneal dialysis, *Association of Operating Room Nurses Journal*, Vol. 35, no. 5, pp. 946, 948, 950, 952, 954.

Brunner, L.S. and Suddarth D.S. (1982) *The Lippincott Manual of Medical-Surgical Nursing*, Volume 3, Harper & Row, London, pp. 253–8.

Lancet (1978) Peritoneal dialysis in chronic renal failure, *Lancet* Vol. ii, p. 303.

Nursing (US) (1982) Fear of floating to a renal unit: nurses' guide to peritoneal dialysis complications, *Nursing* (US), Vol. 12, no. 12, pp. 42–3.

Sorrels, A.J. (1981) Peritoneal dialysis: a rediscovery, *Nursing Clinics of North America*, Vol. 16, no. 3, pp. 515–29.

GUIDELINES: PERITONEAL DIALYSIS

Equipment
1 Dialysis administration set
2 Sterile peritoneal set containing forceps, blade and holder, topical swabs, towels, suturing equipment
3 Sterile gown, gloves
4 Peritoneal catheter and drainage bag
5 Local anaesthetic
6 Syringe, needle
7 Skin antiseptic
8 Supplementary drugs as ordered
9 Peritoneal dialysis fluid, as ordered, warmed to 37°C.

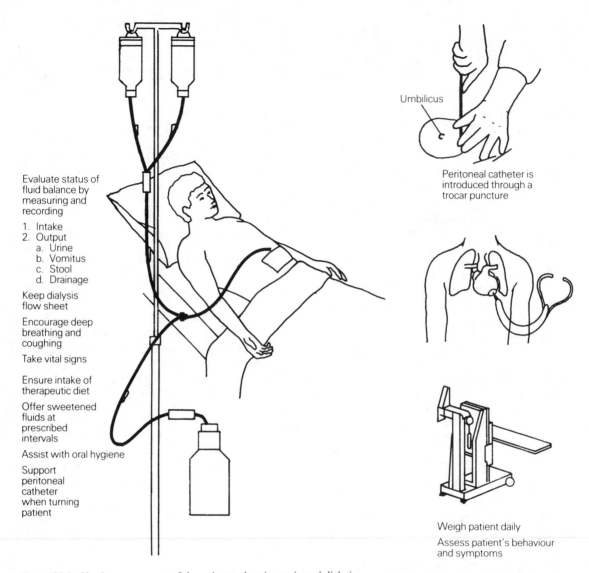

Evaluate status of
fluid balance by
measuring and
recording

1. Intake
2. Output
   a. Urine
   b. Vomitus
   c. Stool
   d. Drainage

Keep dialysis
flow sheet

Encourage deep
breathing and
coughing

Take vital signs

Ensure intake of
therapeutic diet

Offer sweetened
fluids at
prescribed
intervals

Assist with oral hygiene

Support
peritoneal
catheter
when turning
patient

Umbilicus

Peritoneal catheter is
introduced through a
trocar puncture

Weigh patient daily
Assess patient's behaviour
and symptoms

Figure 29.1   Nursing management of the patient undergoing peritoneal dialysis.

Procedure

Action

1   Explain the procedure to the patient. An acutely ill patient
may be confused and restless but every effort should be
made to inform him/her of what is about to happen.

2   Weigh the patient before the procedure begins and then
daily.

3   Record the patient's vital signs before the procedure
begins.

Rationale

To obtain the patient's consent and co-operation. Some
hospitals require a patient to sign a consent form before the
procedure can be carried out.

To obtain a baseline. Daily weighing is helpful in assessing the
state of hydration.

To obtain a baseline.

| 4 | Ask the patient to micturate and defaecate before the procedure begins. | To avoid perforation of the bladder and/or rectum when the trocar is introduced into the peritoneum. |

| 5 | Assist the patient to lie in the supine position. | To ensure that the patient is in the best position for the procedure's requirements. |

6 Continue to observe and reassure the patient throughout the procedure.

7 Assist the doctor as required.

INSERTION OF CATHETER

Action	**Rationale**
1 Using aseptic technique, the doctor prepares the abdomen surgically and injects the skin and subcutaneous tissues with a local anaesthetic.	To prevent the possibility of contamination and infection.
2 A small incision is made in the abdominal wall 3–5 cm below the umbilicus. The trocar is inserted through the incision. The patient is asked to raise his/her head from the pillow after the trocar is introduced.	This tightens the abdominal muscles and permits easier penetration of the trocar without danger of injury to the internal organs.
3 When the peritoneum is punctured, the trocar is directed to the left side of the pelvis. The stylet is removed and the catheter is inserted through the trocar and gently manoeuvred into position. Dialysis fluid is allowed to run through the catheter while it is being positioned.	To prevent the omentum from adhering to the catheter or occluding its opening.
4 Once the trocar is removed, the skin may be sutured and a sterile dressing placed around the catheter.	To prevent the loss of the catheter in the abdomen.
5 The tubing is flushed with the dialysis fluid.	To prevent air from entering the peritoneal cavity.

PREPARATION OF DIALYSIS FLUID

Action	**Rationale**
1 Wash hands. Proceed using aseptic technique.	To reduce risk of infection.
2 The dialysis fluid should have been warmed to body temperature (37 °C).	For the patient's comfort. To prevent abdominal pain. Heating causes dilation of the peritoneal vessels and increases clearance of urea.
3 Add any drugs, e.g. heparin, to the dialysis fluid if prescribed.	Heparin prevents fibrin clots from occluding the catheter.
4 Attach the dialysis fluid to the giving set.	
5 Attach the catheter connector to the giving set.	

Action

Rationale

6 Allow the dialysis fluid to flow freely into the peritoneal cavity. (This normally takes from 5 to 10 minutes.)

To ascertain whether the cathether is in the required position. The flow should be steady and brisk. If not, the tip of the catheter may be buried in the omentum or it may have been occluded by a blood clot.

7 Allow fluid to remain in the peritoneal cavity for the prescribed time. Prepare the next exchange while the first container of fluid is in the peritoneal cavity.

The fluid must remain in the peritoneal cavity for the prescribed dwell time so that potassium, urea and other waste products may be removed. The maximum concentration gradient takes place in the first 5–10 minutes. This is the most effective dwell time.

8 Unclamp the drainage tube. Drainage time will vary with each patient but, on average, should be completed in 10 minutes.

To rid the body of the required products. The abdomen is drained by a siphon effect through the closed system. Drainage is normally straw coloured.

9 Clamp off the drainage tube when outflow ceases and begin infusing the next exchange, again using aseptic technique.

To enable the next cycle to begin
To prevent local and/or systemic infection.

10 Record the following:
    (a) Time of commencement and completion of each exchange and the start and finish of the drainage stage
    (b) Amount of fluid infused and recovered
    (c) Fluid balance after each complete exchange
    (d) Any medication added to the dialysis fluid.

To detect and monitor trends and fluctuations.

11 Take and record the vital signs:
    (a) Blood pressure and pulse every 15 minutes during the first exchange and hourly thereafter, depending on the patient's condition
    (b) Temperature every 4 hours, or more frequently if condition demands.

Hypotension may be indicative of excessive fluid loss due to the glucose concentration of the dialysis fluid. Changes in pulse may indicate impending shock or overhydration.
To monitor any signs of infection. Infection is more likely to become evident after dialysis has been discontinued.

12 Record fluid balance accurately.

To prevent complications such as circulatory overload and hypertension that may occur if most of the fluid is not recovered during the drainage stage. The fluid balance should be about even or show slight fluid loss.

13 Dialysis is usually continued until blood chemistry levels are satisfactory.

The duration of dialysis is related to the severity of the condition and the size and weight of the patient. The usual time is about 12–36 hours, giving between 24–48 exchanges.

14 Ensure that the patient is comfortable during dialysis by attending to pressure area care and altering the patient's position as required. Assist the patient to sit in a chair for short periods as his/her condition allows.

The period of dialysis is lengthy and often exhausts the patient.

15 Send a specimen of peritoneal fluid for investigations daily.

To monitor any infections, etc.

NURSING CARE PLAN

Problem	Cause	Suggested action
Peritonitis, indicated by fever, persistent abdominal pain and cramping, abdominal fullness, abdominal rigidity, slow dialysis drainage, inability to obtain a predialysis ascitic fluid specimen, cloudy drainage, swelling and tenderness around the catheter, and increased white blood cell count.	Poor aseptic technique during catheter insertion or dialysis.	Aseptic technique should be used throughout the entire dialysis procedure. If peritonitis is suspected, notify the doctor immediately. Send a peritoneal fluid sample to the laboratory for fluid analysis, culture and sensitivity testing, Gram staining and cell count.
Infection at the site of entry, indicated by redness, swelling, rigidity, tenderness and purulent drainage around the catheter.	Poor aseptic technique during catheter insertion or dialysis or incomplete healing around the site of entry.	Aseptic technique should be used throughout the entire dialysis procedure. Notify a doctor. Obtain a specimen of the drainage fluid and send it to the laboratory.
Subcutaneous tunnel infection with cuffed catheter indicated by redness, rigidity and tenderness over subcutaneous tunnel.	Poor aseptic technique during catheter insertion or dialysis or incomplete healing in subcutaneous tunnel.	Aseptic technique should be used throughout the entire dialysis procedure. Notify a doctor.
Perforation of the bladder or the bowel, indicated by signs and symptoms of peritonitis, bright yellow dialysis fluid drainage (if bladder is perforated) or faeces in drainage (if bowel is perforated).	Catheter inserted when the patient had a full bladder or bowel.	Ask the patient to empty his/her bowels before the procedure begins. If perforation is suspected, notify a doctor immediately.
Bleeding through the catheter.	Minor trauma to the abdomen or minor trauma to the subcutaneous tunnel (with a cuffed catheter) or perforation of a major abdominal blood vessel during surgery.	Bleeding usually stops spontaneously. If it does not, notify the doctor, who may order blood transfusions. One-litre hourly dialysis exchanges may be ordered until the drainage fluid is clear.
Dialysis fluid leaking around the catheter.	Excessive instillation of dialysis fluid or incomplete healing.	Instill less dialysis fluid at exchanges. Drain the patient's abdomen completely during outflow.
	Incomplete healing around the cuff of the catheter. Catheter obstruction.	Bed rest may be ordered to permit healing. Use small volumes of dialysis fluid in exchanges through a new catheter. Also drain the patient's abdomen completely during outflow. Irrigate the catheter with sterile normal saline solution.
	Catheter dislodged or improperly positioned.	Inform a doctor, who will replace cathether or revise its position surgically.
Kinking of the cuffed catheter.	Subcutaneous tunnel too short or scarring in the subcutaneous tunnel.	Inform a doctor, who will remove the catheter and implant a new one.

Problem	Cause	Suggested action
Lower back pain.	Pressure and weight of dialysis fluid in the abdomen (particularly so in continuous ambulatory peritoneal dialysis (CAPD) patients)	Doctor may order analgesics. Exercises to strengthen the patient's muscles and improve his/her posture may also be ordered.
Abdominal or rectal pain (with possible referred pain in shoulder).	Improperly positioned cathether tip causing irritation. Dialysis fluid accumulating under the diaphragm. Dialysis fluid not at 37 °C. If hypertonic dialysis fluid is used, only one container should be used per cycle. With 2 litres of 6.36% solution, severe shoulder pain can occur. If air enters the peritoneal cavity, pain may occur.	Catheter position to be revised surgically. Drain the abdomen completely during outflow. Ensure that the fluid is infused at the correct temperature. Maintain a closed system.
Ileus indicated by sharp pain in abdomen, constipation, abdominal distension, nausea and vomiting, and diarrhoea.	Catheter manipulated excessively during insertion.	Notify the doctor immediately as signs and symptoms may indicate peritonitis. A nasogastric tube to suction the stomach may be ordered. Cholinergic medication, such as neostigmine, may be ordered. Administer fluids and electrolytes as ordered. Encourage the patient to walk, unless ordered otherwise by the doctor. Prepare the patient for surgery, if the doctor orders. The condition may disappear spontaneously after 12 hours.
Cramping.	Dialysis fluid warmer or cooler than 37 °C. Rapid infusion or drainage. Pressure from excess dialysis fluid in the abdomen. Chemical irritation. Air in the abdomen.	Adjust the temperature of the dialysis fluid to 37°C before infusion. Decrease the infusion or drainage rate. Infuse less dialysis fluid at exchanges. Use a dialysis fluid with a dextrose concentration lower than 7%. Clamp off the dialysis tubing before the dialysis fluid empties completely into the abdomen.
Excessive fluid loss.	Use of dialysis fluid with incorrect dextrose concentration *or* inadequate sodium intake *or* inadequate fluid intake.	Monitor the patient's weight and blood pressure. Ensure that the patient is receiving dialysis fluid with the correct dextrose concentration. The doctor may order a reduced dextrose concentration.
Fluid overload.	Use of dialysis fluid with incorrect dextrose concentration *or* excessive sodium intake *or* excessive fluid intake.	Monitor the patient's weight and blood pressure. The doctor will order a reduced fluid and sodium intake. The doctor may also order increased use of dialysis fluid with a 4.25% dextrose concentration.

Hyperglycaemia.	Use of dialysis fluid with a dextrose concentration (the dextrose is absorbed systemically).	Check plasma glucose levels after dialysis. Monitor the patient (especially if he/she has diabetes mellitus or insulin deficiency) for signs and symptoms of hyperglycaemia. The patient's insulin dose may have to be adjusted.
Respiratory difficulties.	Pressure from the fluid in the peritoneal cavity and upward displacement of the diaphragm resulting in shallow breathing.	Elevate the head of the bed. Encourage breathing exercises and coughing.

30

Pre- and Postoperative Care

Definitions

PREOPERATIVE CARE

Preoperative care is the physical and psychological preparation of a patient prior to surgery.

POSTOPERATIVE CARE

Postoperative care consists of ensuring that the patient is nursed in the greatest possible comfort, is kept free from hazards and complications during the postoperative period, and is encouraged to take an increasing responsibility for his/her care until complete recovery is effected.

Indications

PREOPERATIVE CARE

Psychological

1 To assist the patient to understand and accept the proposed surgery.
2 To assess and then control levels of anxiety.

Physical

1 To teach the patient the necessary exercises, such as deep breathing exercises, leg exercises and support of wound exercises, to reduce or prevent postoperative complications.
2 To ensure that the patient is in an optimum physical condition prior to surgery.

POSTOPERATIVE CARE

Psychological

To consolidate any psychological care offered preoperatively.

Physical

To maintain life postoperatively.

REFERENCE MATERIAL
Patient education and postoperative pain

The cause, nature and experience of pain are constantly being reviewed. Lazarus (1966) and Janis (1971) showed that the provision of information creates some anticipatory fear about a future event. It is suggested that this provides an opportunity for mental rehearsal of the stressful event that is to be experienced and results in less emotional disturbance for the subject when the event occurs. In the light of this research it has been argued that there is a need for a patient to experience and work through his/her anxiety, with support from health care professionals, preoperatively. Egbert *et al.* (1964) demonstrated how the provision of information, such as length of operation, the process of regaining consciousness, and the location and intensity of postoperative pain, could affect the recovery period. Of the two groups studied, the informed group demonstrated less postoperative pain, required less analgesia, recovered more quickly and left hospital, on average, 2.5 days earlier than the control group. This concept, referred to in psychology as locus of control, is based on the theory that if an individual feels he/she has some control over the outcome of his/her fate, he/she will function more efficiently than if he/she feels totally helpless. Zborowski (1969) has shown that cultural and racial considerations also need to be examined. Hayward (1975) suggests that nursing time spent in explanation and teaching can significantly reduce the postoperative workload.

The subjective experience of pain is extremely difficult to measure and nurses continue to underestimate its importance and severity (Seers, 1987). Bourbonnais (1981) has demonstrated the use of pain assessment scales and for further information on pain assessment see pp. 285–9. It is of interest that some centres are now placing the responsibility on patients to self-medicate or titrate their own intravenous analgesia (Hosking and Welchewe, 1985).

Skin preparation

In an effort to render the skin as clean as possible preoperatively, traditional nursing practice has placed great value on the preoperative bath. Studies have shown, however, that a single antiseptic bath has little or no effect on reducing skin flora (Clarke, 1983). Baths are reputedly difficult to clean and, in view of this, it is suggested that showering may prove a more effective means of skin cleansing preoperatively (Stokes, 1984).

Shaving is also a common preoperative procedure. Alexander *et al.* (1983) suggest that shaving produces skin damage, invisible to the naked eye, which provides entry points for micro-organisms which become focus points of infection prior to surgery. The timing of the shave is also significant; the later the shave the less incidence there is of infection postoperatively. The *Lancet* (1983) advocates the use of depilatory creams, the cost of which is phenomenally less than the cost of treating an infection.

Preoperative fasting

It has been common practice to fast patients prior to the administration of a general anaesthetic. However, Hamilton Smith (1972) has shown that the fasting rule may vary from 4 to 12 hours or more. The majority of nurses involved in the studies did not seem to grasp the essential reasons for the fast and preferred to err by prolonging the period if they were unsure. The study also revealed that in general nurses seemed unbothered by this, saw little danger to the patient and frequently operated on a routine system to withhold food and drink from 12 midnight from all patients who were scheduled for theatre the following morning. Opinions among anaesthetists and surgeons also varied in the interpretation of 'nil by mouth'. While it is commonly accepted that the contents of the stomach may be vomited or regurgitated during some period of general anaesthesia and inadvertently inhaled by the patient while the cough reflex is still absent, it is not always appreciated what factors affect gastric motility, and hence the gastric contents, at any period of time. A meal with a high fat content may take up to 20 hours to be processed in the stomach, whereas a glass of water takes little more than half an hour to pass into the duodenum. Anxiety and fear exhibit a delaying effect on peristaltic action, as do some anaesthetic agents and morphia. Furthermore, the stomach is never completely empty since gastric secretions continue to be produced at the rate of 30 ml per hour even in the absence of food, and it is not unusual for 200 ml to be present in the stomach of a fasting patient. It appeared from the study that not only were food and drink withheld from patients for significantly longer than was necessary, but often such a decision was left entirely to the whim of nurses whose level of understanding for this need varied considerably. The author concluded that there was a need for the nurse to acquire

knowledge and experience that would enable him/her to evaluate the patient's nutritional needs as part of a more holistic approach.

Anti-embolic stockings

Since the 1950s, early ambulation has been shown to reduce the incidence of postoperative deep vein thrombosis. Scurr *et al.* (1977) have demonstrated the value of anti-embolic stockings in preventing this complication, particularly among obese patients and those undergoing major abdominal or pelvic surgery. The importance of fitting the stockings correctly should be emphasized. Furthermore, their removal postoperatively from an immobile patient for as little as 3 minutes can result in a significant reduction in venous return. Stockings, therefore, should be reapplied immediately after such events as bathing.

References and further reading

Alexander, J.W. *et al.* (1983) The influence of hair removal methods on wound infections, *Archives of Surgery*, Vol. 118, pp. 347–52.

Bourbonnais, F. (1981) Pain assessment: development of a tool for the nurse and the patient, *Journal of Advanced Nursing*, Vol. 6, pp. 277–82.

Burns, R.B. (1980) *Essential Psychology*, MTP, Lancaster.

Clarke, J. (1983) The effectiveness of surgical skin preparations, *Nursing Times Theatre Nursing Supplement*, 28 Sept. pp. 8–17.

Egbert, L.D. *et al.* (1964) Reduction of postoperative pain by encouragement and instruction of patients, *New England Journal of Medicine*, Vol. 270, p. 285.

Hamilton Smith, S. (1972) *Nil by Mouth?* Royal College of Nursing, London.

Hayward, J. (1975) *Information – A Prescription Against Pain*, Royal College of Nursing, London.

Hosking, J. and Welchewe, E. (1985) *Postoperative Pain – Understanding its Nature and How To Treat It*, Faber & Faber, London.

Janis, I. (1971) *Stress and Frustration*, Harcourt Brace, New York.

Lancet (1983) Preoperative depilation, *Lancet*, Vol. i, p. 1311.

Lazarus, R.S. (1966) Some principles of psychological stress and their relations to dentistry, *Journal of Dental Research*, Vol. 45, p. 1620.

Phipps, W.J. *et al.* (1986) *Medical–Surgical Nursing: Concepts and Clinical Practice*, 3rd edn, C.V. Mosby, St. Louis.

Scurr, J. *et al.* (1977) The efficacy of graduated compression stockings in the prevention of deep vein thrombosis, *British Journal of Surgery*, Vol. 64, pp. 371–3.

Seers, K. (1987) Perceptions of pain, *Nursing Times*, Vol. 83, no. 48, pp. 37–9.

Stokes, E. (1984) Showering before surgery. Shaving before surgery, *Nursing Times*, Vol. 80, no. 20, p. 71.

Zborowski, M. (1969) *People in Pain*, Jossey Bass, San Francisco.

GUIDELINES: PREOPERATIVE CARE

Equipment

1 Theatre gown
2 Theatre hat
3 Hypo-allergenic tape for taping rings, if necessary
4 Denture container, if necessary
5 Valuables book, to record valuables the patient wishes to be kept in hospital custody during surgery
6 Any equipment and documents required by law or hospital policy if a premedication is prescribed.

Procedure

Action	Rationale
1 Ensure that the patient is wearing an identification bracelet with the correct information.	To prevent misidentification and possible harm.
2 Ascertain whether preoperative education has been assimilated by the patient.	To determine whether the patient understands the reasons for surgery and how to minimize postoperative discomfort and reduce possible postoperative complications.
3 Record the patient's vital signs. Weigh the patient. Obtain a specimen of the patient's urine for analysis.	To establish a preoperative baseline and record any preoperative abnormalities.
4 Check that the patient has undergone any preoperative examinations, e.g. X-rays, group and cross-matching of blood, and that the results are included in the patient's notes.	To ensure that all relevant material is available to the surgical team if required.
5 Perform skin preparations, if necessary.	Shaving or the removing of hairs using a depilatory cream lessens the likelihood of wound infection. Thorough skin cleansing decreases the chances of bacteria entering the skin surface at time of surgery. (For fuller information on aseptic techniques, see pp. 5–8).
6 Ensure that the patient is wearing anti-embolic stockings of the correct fit and that they are correctly applied.	To prevent venous stasis, deep venous thrombosis or pulmonary oedema.
7 Assist the patient to change into the theatre gown and theatre hat.	To minimize the risk of infection.
8 Check, by asking the patient, that: (a) Preoperative fasting has been observed. (b) Urine has been passed prior to premedication.	To prevent inhalation of undigested or semidigested food while under anaesthesia. To prevent urinary incontinence due to muscle relaxation during operation. To permit a better view of the abdominal

(c)   A good bowel motion has been achieved.

(d)   Any prostheses have been removed or noted, e.g. dental crowns or bridges. Hearing aids should be left in position until the patient has been anaesthetized.

(e)   Jewellery and cosmetics have been removed.

cavity in abdominal and pelvic surgery. To decrease the chance of inadvertent injury to the bladder in the above type of surgery.
To ensure a clear bowel before abdominal and pelvic surgery.
To prevent trauma to the patient.

Metal jewellery or hairpins may be lost accidentally, may cause damage to the patient, either directly or indirectly, and may cause diathermy burns. Cosmetics, including facial make-up and nail varnish, obscure the true colour of the patient's skin, thus camouflaging early signs of hypoxia.

9   Any valuables that the patient has not been permitted to retain during surgery should be recorded and maintained in hospital custody according to hospital policy.

To ensure their safekeeping. Wedding rings may be worn if they do not interfere with the surgery to be performed. If retained they should be taped to prevent diathermy burns.

10   Check that the form consenting to the operation has been completed and correctly signed by doctor and patient.

To comply with any legal requirements and hospital policy.

11   Conforming to legal requirements and hospital policy, check and administer any premedication prescribed.

12   Advise the patient not to get up once premedication has been administered but to use the nurse call system to attend to any of his/her needs.

To prevent trauma to the patient as premedications, generally sedatives, may make the patient drowsy and unco-ordinated.

13   Ensure that any relevant information, e.g. case notes and X-rays, accompany the patient to theatre.

To enable the surgical team to have full access to the patient's history.

GUIDELINES: POSTOPERATIVE CARE

Equipment

1   Airway
2   Oxygen supply
3   Disposable oxygen mask and tubing
4   Suction equipment
5   Selection of suction catheters
6   Disposable gloves
7   Disposable tissues
8   Receiver
9   Sphygmomanometer
10   Stethoscope
11   Intravenous infusion stand
12   Observation charts
13   Space blanket
14   Cotsides.
       Emergency cardipulmonary resuscitation equipment should also be available.

Procedure

Action	Rationale
1 Ensure that the patient is in the left lateral position if the nature of the surgery allows this. Otherwise ensure that an airway is inserted.	To ensure a clear airway.
2 Obtain full information about the nature of the surgery performed and any immediate postoperative instructions.	To ensure that the patient receives the prescribed treatment.
3 Remain with the patient until full consciousness is achieved. Orientate the patient as to time and place at frequent intervals.	To reassure the patient by informing him/her of the reality of his/her situation.
4 Record the patient's vital signs according to the anaesthetist's instructions or until the patient's condition is stable.	To establish a baseline postoperatively. To detect and monitor any fluctuations and trends in the patient's condition.
5 Note the patient's pallor.	To monitory any respiratory dysfunction.
6 Administer oxygen as prescribed.	
7 Check that intravenous fluids are infusing as prescribed and record this.	
8 Observe wound for (a) Type(s) of dressing(s) (b) Signs of oozing or oedema, which should be noted and recorded (c) Any drains, in which case record the amount of drainage if appropriate, e.g. Redivac bottles.	To establish a baseline postoperatively.
9 Suspend any drainage containers where they may be visible.	To prevent accidental trauma to the drains and to the patient. To observe whether drainage becomes excessive.
10 Record the patient's urinary output accurately.	To monitor renal function.
11 Offer the patient, if fully conscious, postoperative analgesia and/or anti-emetics if prescribed.	To alleviate any postoperative pain and/or nausea.
12 Offer mouth care.	To maintain oral cleanliness. To promote patient comfort.
13 Ensure that the patient is as comfortable as possible. If it is not too painful for the patient, carry out pressure area care.	To promote patient comfort.
14 Introduce postoperative exercises slowly, e.g. passive limb movements, if appropriate.	To prevent the postoperative complications of foot drop, muscle weakness.
15 Escort the patient back to the ward when the surgical team considers that his/her condition warrants it.	

NURSING CARE PLAN

Problem	Cause	Suggested action
Partial or total respiratory dysfunction.	Incorrect positioning. Vomitus or oral and pharyngeal secretions. Respiratory depression following prolonged general anaesthesia.	Readjust the patient's position. Remove any oral secretions using suction. Call the patient to arouse him/her. Maintain oxygen therapy as prescribed. Inform a doctor.
Primary haemorrhage and subsequent hypotension leading to cerebral anoxia and renal underperfusion. Reactionary haemorrhage.	Excessive blood and fluid loss during surgery. Slipped ligature postoperatively.	Increase the rate of intravenous infusion, if allowed. Elevate the foot of the bed. Locate the bleeding point and apply pressure. Inform a doctor.
Postoperative pain.	Tension, anxiety and disorientation. Surgical trauma.	Explain to patient where he/she is and the nature of his/her operation. Reinforce the preoperative teaching. Explain and demonstrate how the patient can support his/her wound and move with the minimum of discomfort. Give regular analgesia, providing that the patient's condition allow this, and evaluate the effects.
Nausea.	Side-effect of anaesthesia. Temporary ileus.	Maintain intravenous fluids as prescribed. Offer prescribed anti-emetics and evaluate their effect. Offer mouth care. If the patient has a nasogastric tube in position, check the position of the tube and maintain the nasogastric tube on free drainage. Aspirate the tube hourly in the presence of nausea. Give anti-emetics as prescribed and evaluate their effect. Instruct the patient not to eat or drink. Note when bowel sounds occur and flatus is passed.
Low urinary output.	If a catheter is in position check for kinking or blockage. Renal dysfunction as a result of surgery.	Readjust the position of the cathether. Irrigate the patient's bladder if appropriate. Record the patient's fluid balance and report this to a doctor.
Hypovolaemia.	Inadequate hydration following major surgery.	Increase intravenous fluids flow rate if this is allowed and inform a doctor.
Hypervolaemia and pulmonary oedema.	Overhydration via intravenous route or cardiac failure.	Assist the patient into an upright or Fowler's position, if appropriate, to facilitate breathing. Give oxygen as prescribed. Decrease intravenous fluids flow rate if this is allowed and inform a doctor.

Problem	Cause	Suggested action
Patients with a high risk of deep vein thrombosis and pulmonary embolus.	Previous history *or* position of patient during, and duration of, surgery *or* major abdominal or pelvic surgery *or* abdominal or pelvic mass *or* obesity.	Reinforce preoperative teaching about deep breathing and hourly leg exercises. On the first postoperative day, sit the patient out of bed in a comfortable chair with his/her feet supported on a stool for short periods. The amount of time which the patient remains out of bed should be increased daily, if his/her condition allows this. Check the patient's calves daily for colour, tenderness, oedema and any complaints of pain. Record the patient's temperature 4-hourly and report any abnormalities to a doctor. Anti-embolic stockings should be worn as appropriate. Administer the prescribed anti-coagulant therapy.
Wound infection.	Large open wound *or* bowel opened during surgery *or* orthopaedic surgery *or* obesity.	Maintain aseptic technique when changing the dressing. Take down the dressing only when necessary. Observe the wound for signs of infection, haematoma and pain. Report all such signs to a doctor. Record the patient's temperature and pulse 4-hourly. If signs of infection are present, take swabs for bacteriological investigation. Administer the prescribed antibiotic.
Chest infection.	Painful suture line (thoracotomy and large abdominal wounds) *or* patient is a smoker *or* chronic bronchitis or other respiratory condition *or* artificial ventilation.	Reinforce preoperative teaching about deep breathing and coughing. Alter the patient's position regularly. Observe and report the nature and amount of sputum. Send a specimen of sputum for bacteriological investigation. Record the patient's temperature, pulse and respirations 4-hourly and report any abnormalities to a doctor. Administer the prescribed antibiotics. Administer regular analgesia to ease and therefore facilitate pain.
Septicaemia.	Preoperative toxicity *or* perforated bowel *or* neutropenia *or* presence of contaminated central venous line in position.	Record the patient's temperature, pulse and blood pressure 4-hourly. Report any abnormalities to a doctor who may order blood samples for culture immediately. When administering intravenous drugs, take down the dressing each time and observe the cannula site for signs of infection. Change intravenous giving sets daily. Administer any prescribed antibiotics.

31

Pressure Sores

Definition

The term 'pressure sore' is used to describe any area of damage to the skin or underlying tissues caused by direct pressure or shearing forces. The extent of this damage can range from persistent erythema to necrotic ulceration involving muscle, tendon and bone.

REFERENCE MATERIAL
Effect of pressure on bony tissues

It is generally considered that normal capillary pressure is about 32 mmHg. Any external pressures exceeding this will cause capillary obstruction. Most healthy people experience pressures in excess of 32 mmHg over bony prominences while lying or sitting down. In a supine position the highest points of pressure are over the sacrum, the buttocks and the heels (40–60 mmHg for a healthy person with a reasonable body weight: height ratio). If external pressure is intermittent, however, capillary damage does not occur. Kosiak (1958, 1976) demonstrated that with constant pressure, even in denigrated tissues, a critical period of 1–2 hours exists before pathological changes occur.

Localized pressure does not harm living tissue directly. It is compression of the capillaries that deprives the tissue of oxygen and nutrients and allows a build-up of metabolic waste, resulting in tissue death. Death is from anoxia and not from mechanical cell disruption (Husian, 1953). Reactive hyperaemia is the normal body response to pressure ischaemia. After pressure is relieved the area shows a bright red flush as capillary dilatation occurs to return oxygen supply and remove wastes. The triggering mechanism for this is not known. After lengthy periods of unrelieved pressure, however, irreversible pathological changes occur and reactive hyperaemia becomes an insufficient compensatory system.

Relief of pressure from a body surface is the single most important factor in treating or preventing the occurrence of a pressure sore. Of prime consideration in nursing care is the positioning and regular repositioning of the patient.

Identification of patients at risk

Many predisposing factors are involved in the development of pressure sores:

1 *Continuous pressure*: see above.
2 *Shearing*: when a patient slides down a bed or a chair, unless he/she is repositioned correctly the skin often remains in contact with the supporting surface, whereas the skeleton moves over it. Superficially this friction results in epidermal damage with skin loss placing the patient at risk of infection. More serious are the effects of shearing deep in the muscle. Tissue dies due to anoxia and the result is a deep penetrating sacral sore.
3 *Immobility*: in health, numerous spontaneous readjustments are made to relieve pressure. In illness, this defence may be lost due to lethargy, brain or nerve damage, sedation, operative techniques, loss of consciousness, etc.
4 *Vascular factors*: any disruption of the flow or volume of blood will lower the skin's resistance. Shock, involving peripheral vascular failure, creates a serious danger to pressure sore formation. Venous engorgement, anteriosclerotic changes and the vascular damage caused by smoking (Barton, 1977) are all contributory factors. Anaemia impedes the effects of reactive hyperaemia.
5 *Diet*: poor nutrition increases the risk of pressure sore formation. Hypoproteinaemia, low vitamin C levels and zinc deficiences are among the most crucial factors (Tweedle, 1978).
6 *Body weight*: any deviation from ideal weight can increase risk. Thin individuals, with little subcutaneous fat, run a higher risk of sustaining relatively high local pressures over bony prominences. Obese individuals are at risk from immobility, lifting and positioning problems.

7 *Incontinence*: damp linen adds to the friction problem. Strong acids and alkalis, present in faeces or urine, damage the surface epithelium, causing a chemical burn. When skin integrity is lost, infection and further wound breakdown are likely to occur. Incontinence tends to macerate the skin, leading to tearing. Extensive washing, as occurs with incontinent patients, tends to remove most of the skin's natural lubricants, thereby causing friction between the skin and the support device. The skin becomes dry and brittle and cracks easily.

8 *Medical condition*: medical conditions, such as diabetes mellitus, that have an effect on blood vessels as well as blood sugar, render a patient more susceptible to infection.

9 *Immunosuppression*: this may occur in the malnourished, particularly the hypoproteinaemic patient, following injury or in patients with malignant disease. Immunosuppression renders the patient more likely to wound infection and delays the healing process.

10 *Age*: elderly patients are far more likely to develop pressure sores, partly because many of the above factors are involved but also due to their increased inability to repair minor tissue damage.

Patients should be assessed on admission so that appropriate precautions can be taken. Norton *et al.* (1975) developed an 'at risk' scale which is shown in Table 31.1. Patients with scores of 14 or below are considered to run the greatest risk of developing pressure sores. Patients having sores of 14–18 are not considered to be at risk but they should be reassessed immediately any deterioration in their condition is observed. Scores of 18–20 indicate patients at minimal risk.

Devices used for the relief of pressure

The most effecitve way of preventing or relieving pressure on an area is to minimize the pressure in that area. Usually it is sufficient for the patient to be nursed on alternating aspects of the body surface, provided that they are repositioned regularly. e.g. 2-hourly. Sometimes this is inappropriate or impossible due to the circumstances of individual patients, e.g. surgical intervention, body deformities, etc.

A wide variety of devices is available to help relieve pressure over susceptible areas. These devices differ in function and complexity and choice must be based on meeting the patient's individual needs (see Table 31.2).

Treatment of pressure sores

The treatment of pressure sores was shown in a national survey (David *et al.* 1983) to be the responsibility of the nurse and, despite an increasing amount of research, it remains one of the most controversial issues in nursing.

The variety of materials commercially available, together with the preferences of the individual nurse, makes the formulation of a comprehensive policy difficult. The following information should assist the nurse to make informed decisions about the individual types of wounds based on clinical judgement.

In many research studies pressure sores have been graded as shown in Table 31.3. These grades are valuable in describing the state of the sore and in determining the appropriate dressing or treatment. They should be considered in conjunction with the factors which delay healing (see p. 423).

RELIEF OF PRESSURE

A pressure sore will not heal unless the source of the pressure is removed. Correct positioning and regular repositioning of the patient are the most effective ways of relieving pressure but mechanical devices may be used as appropriate.

HYGIENE

When a pressure sore is an open wound it should be treated as such. Cleaning and dressing the wound must be carried out using an aseptic technique to minimize the risk of cross-infection.

The most commonly used cleaning solutions for noninfected wounds are normal saline and Savlodil and their advantages and disadvantages are shown in Table 31.4.

There are many commercially available products and materials suitable for dressing pressure sores. Selection should be made according to the individual needs of the patient and the nature of the sore (see Table 31.5).

Table 31.1 The Norton Scale (Norton, 1975)

Physical condition	Score	Mental condition	Score	Activity	Score	Mobility	Score	Incontinent	Score
Good	4	Alert	4	Ambulant	4	Full	4	Not	4
Fair	3	Apathetic	3	Walk/help	3	Slightly limited	3	Occasionally	3
Poor	2	Confused	2	Chairbound	2	Very limited	2	Usually/urine	2
Very bad	1	Stuporous	1	Bedfast	1	Immobile	1	Doubly	1

Table 31.2   A Selection of Mechanical Methods for Relieving Pressure

Aid	Use	Advantages	Disadvantages
Sheepskin	Low risk patients. Norton score 14 or above. Good for under heels.	Warm and comfortable. Machine washable. Decreases friction.	Does *not* relieve pressure. Hardens and matts with washing. Needs to be changed frequently. *Not recommended* for regularly incontinent patients.
Heel and elbow pads: sheepskin, foam, silicone	Norton scale 14 or less or patients on prolonged bed rest.	Reduce friction and shearing over the elbow and heel.	Often have inadequate methods of keeping them on. Become hardened by washing.
Sorbo ring	Low risk patients. Norton score 14 or above.	At first makes patient feel comfortable.	Tends to cause oedema of skin inside the hole of the ring due to pressure of the rim of the ring on surrounding tissues. Can cause venous thrombosis. *Not recommended* for patients with known vascular complications. May be a source of cross-infection.
Silicone-filled mattress pad	Norton scale 14 or less or patients on prolonged bed rest, able to move spontaneously.	Relieves pressure by distributing it over a greater area. Comfortable. Machine (industrial) washable. Acceptable in community settings as well as in hospital. Can be used for incontinent patients. Relatively cheap purchase price.	If the patient is very incontinent of urine, even if the plastic side is uppermost, there is seepage into the core material. Stitching comes undone after several launderings. Reduces self-motivated movements in very debilitated patients.
Roho air filled mattress	Norton scale 10–14, high to medium risk. To wear off pressure equalizing beds.	Interlinked air cells transfer air with movement. Patient can be nursed sitting or recumbent. Non-mechanical. Washable.	Can be punctured and is expensive to repair. Often incorrectly inflated.
Alternating pressure beds (Pegasus, ripple, Alphabed)	Medium risk, 12–14 Norton scale.	Mechanical alteration of pressure. Reduce the frequency of (but not need for) repositioning. Available on hire at short notice.	Older types prone to breakdown. Must be checked and maintained. May increase pressures in very thin patients. Punctures possible.
Mechanaid netbed	Moderate risk patients. Norton score 14 or less.	Fits any bed. Easy to assemble and dismantle. Easy to store. No servicing, maintenance or laundry difficulties. Patients can be repositioned by one nurse. Appears to encourage relaxation and sleep. Can be lowered on to the bed surface when a firm base is required.	Patients do not always like it. Wedge of pillows needed to sit patient up. Patients may lose heat. Reduces self-motivated movement. Not always easy for patients to communicate with people sitting by bed.
Water bed	Moderate risk, Norton score 12–16.	Spreads pressure. Is warm and comfortable. Available on hire at short notice.	Patient is supported on the skin of the water sac thus reducing the pressure-relieving properties. Difficult to get the patient in and out.

Table 31.2 (contd.)

Aid	Use	Advantages	Disadvantages
Water flotation bed	Moderate to high risk patients. Norton score 14 or less.	Equalizes pressure and weight. Heated.	Expensive to buy, run and maintain. Makes some patients feel 'sea-sick'. Reduces self-motivated movement. Heavy to move. If not filled correctly can create more pressure than conventional bed. Not to be confused with water trough above.
Fluidized air bed	High risk patients, Norton score 10 or less or indicated because of medical condition.	As near to levitation as possible. Warm, sterile air produces a beneficial environment for healing wounds. One nurse can manage even very heavy or debilitated patients on his/her own. Can be used for incontinent patients or those with heavy wound exudate.	Expensive to hire, run and in old buildings maintain. Need to reinforce floors before it can be installed. Minimizes self-motivation. Can be difficult for the patient to get in and out of bed even with help. Available on hire basis only.
Low air loss bed	High risk patient, Norton score 10 or less. Orientated and immobile patients.	Pressure equalizing properties equal to the fluidized air bed. Patient can be nursed in any position including prone. (Patient can control position.) Mobilization easy.	Expensive to buy but can be hired. Nurses need education in the use of the equipment.

Table 31.3 Pressure Sore Grades (David et al., 1983)

Grade	Description
1	(a) Where the skin is likely to break down (red, black and blistered areas) (b) Healed areas still covered by a scab
2	Superficial break in the skin
3	Destruction of the skin without cavity (full skin thickness)
4	Destruction of the skin with cavity (involving underlying tissues)

Table 31.4 Advantages and Disadvantages of Two Commonly Used Cleaning Solutions for Infected Wounds

Solution	Advantages	Disadvantages
Normal saline	Isotonic, non-toxic, non-irritant	Not an antiseptic
Savlodil	Antiseptic	Can be irritant; grows bacteria under certain conditions

Table 31.5   A Selection of Dressings Used in the Treatment of Pressure Sores

Dressing	Use	Advantages	Disadvantages
Topical swabs	1 Directly on to clean, dry wounds. 2 As a padding over a non-adherent type dressing.	Excellent absorbency. Sometimes air permeable. Generally good thermal insulator.	Does not provide moist interface. No barrier to infection. Can traumatize wound when removed due to exudate adherence and capillary loop instertion.
Dressing pads	As a padding over a non-adherent type dressing.	Superior absorbency. Partially air permeable. Thermal insulator.	No moist interface. No barrier to infection. Exudate often seeps through, providing a fluid pathway for infection.
Lyofoam	Non-adherent ulcer dressing.	Absorption of excess fluid without dehydration. Conformable. Non-fibrous. Also available with an activated carbon insert (Lyofoam C).	May adhere in presence of dry serum and become hard. Deodorizing dressing for infected/necrotic wounds.
Synthaderm	Non-adherent ulcer dressing.	Excellent for varicose ulcers. Air permeable. Impermeable to water. Provides moist interface. Barrier to infection. Thermal insulator. Non-adhesive. Reduces frequency of dressings.	Tends to curl away from a wound when first applied. Some adherence occurs when it is dry. Very expensive.
Melolin	Non-adherent dressing.	Absorbent. Air permeable. Thermal insulator. Minimum trauma when removed.	No moist interface. No barrier to infection. Non-adherent part of dressing tends to adhere to wound surface and separate from rest of dressing.
Release	Non-adherent dressing.	Absorbent. Air permeable. Thermal insulator. Minimum trauma at change. Moist interface.	
OpSite/Tegaderm Bioclusive	Cover for ulcerating wounds.	Air permeable. Barrier to infection. Impermeable to water. High elasticity and conformability. Moist interface. Reduces frequency of dressings. Wounds readily visible.	Needs considerable skill to apply due to its elasticity. Retention of fluid exudate causes bulging of dressing. Adhesive trauma on removal.
Granuflex Duoderm Biofilm	Cover for ulcerating wounds.	Air and water impermeable. Provide moist interface. Barrier to infection. Thermal insulator. Reduce frequency of dressings.	Adhesive trauma may occur on removal. Disliked by many nurses as they are not able to observe the wound continuously. Tend to crumble after a while.
Silastic foam	Non-adherent dressing. Can be tailor-made to wound. Best used on 'clean' wounds.	Absorbent. Moist interface. Air permeable. Thermal insulator. Barrier to infection. Minimum trauma at change. Easy to	Needs skill to mix and mould. Need to make two moulds each time (one to wear and one to clean). Not sterile.

Table 31.5   (contd.)

Dressing	Use	Advantages	Disadvantages
		clean. May be used to fill a cavity. Useful for self-caring patients.	
Scherisorb, Vigilon, Geliperm	Non-adherent ulcer and cavity dressing.	Absorbent, non-traumatic debriding of hard eschar by rehydration.	May ooze out of wound (Scherbisorb). Cold initially.
Sorbsan	Absorbent ulcer and cavity dressing.	Highly absorbent, biodegradable, easy to remove by irrigation. Non-irritant.	Expensive, may leave material in the wound, long-term effects not known.

Areas of erythema (grade 1) and the skin around the pressure sore should be treated with care and washed only as necessary for comfort and hygiene, e.g. following incontinence, sweating, etc. Frequent washing of the area is not recommended for the following reasons:

1   soap may cause excessive drying of the skin;
2   the growth of micro-organisms will be encouraged if the area is left moist;
3   friction caused by washing and drying the skin may result in tissue damage.

Preliminary trials (Willington, 1977) have indicated that the use of a non-ionic detergent is simpler and more effective than soap for cleaning the skin. The affected area should not be rubbed as this causes maceration and degeneration of the subcutaneous tissues, especially in the elderly, thus disposing of ulcer formation (Dyson, 1978).

PROMOTION OF WOUND HEALING
The treatment of pressure sores should aim at creating the ideal micro-environment for wound healing and eliminating or minimizing any factor which might delay this. Factors that tend to delay wound healing include the following:

1   *Infection*: this causes further tissue breakdown.
2   *Necrotic tissue and debris*: these predispose to infection.
3   *Dryness*: destruction of the epidermis exposes the dermis to dehydration, which in turn destroys epidermal remnants and delays epithelialization. Allowing oxygen to blow over a wound causes drying. There also appears to be more scarring in a dry wound, due perhaps to the problems of new cells having to bury beneath the scab (Winter, 1971).
4   *Excessive heat or cold.*
5   *Scab (eschar) formation*: epidermal regeneration occurs after about 18 hours. Under a suitable occlusive dressing this happens in about 6 hours (Winter, 1971).

As with dressings, many agents are commercially available for the treatment of pressure sores (see Table 31.6).

References and further reading

Barton, A.A. (1977) Prevention of pressure sores, *Nursing Times*, Vol. 73, pp. 1593–5.

David, J.A. (1983) Normal physiology from injurty to repair, *Nursing*, Vol. 2, no. 11, pp. 296–7.

David, J.A. (1986) Additions to the bed, *Nursing*, Vol. 3, no. 3, pp. 112–4.

David, J.A. (1987) Beds, *Nursing*, Vol. 3, no. 13, pp. 503–5.

David, J.A. *et al.* (1983) *An Investigation of the Current Methods Used in Nursing for the Care of Patients with Established Pressure Sores*, Nursing Practice Research Unit, Surrey University.

Dyson, R. (1978) Bed sores – the injuries hospital staff inflict on patients, *Nursing Mirror*, Vol. 146, no. 24, pp. 30–2.

Forrest, R.D. (1980) The treatment of pressure sores, *Journal of International Medical Research*, Vol. 8, pp. 430–5.

Guttman, L. (1976) The prevention and treatment of pressure sores, in R.M. Kenedi *et al.* (eds.) *Bed Sore Biomechanics*, Macmillan, London.

Husian, T. (1953) An experimental study of some pressure effects on tissues, with reference to the bed-sore problem, *Journal of Pathology and Bacteriology*, Vol. 66, pp. 347–58.

Kosiak, M. (1958) Evaluation of pressure as a factor in the production of ischial ulcers, *Archives of Physical Medicine and Rehabilitation*, Vol. 40, pp. 62–9.

Kosiak, M. (1976) A mechanical resting surface: its effect on pressure distribution, *Archives of Physical Medicine and Rehabilitation*, Vol. 57, pp. 481–3.

Norton, D. *et al.* (1975) *An Investigation of Geriatric Nursing Problems in Hospital*, Churchill Livingstone, Edinburgh.

Table 31.6   A Selection of Agents Used in the Treatment of Pressure Sores

Agent	Use	Advantages	Disadvantages
Half-strength Eusol	Infected or necrotic ulcerating wounds.	Relatively cheap to purchase. Easy to use. Some antiseptic properties.	Short shelf life (approximately 2 weeks). Relatively long healing times. Caustic to surrounding skin. 'Hospital smell'. Said to be a debriding agent but any dibridment that occurs is due to hydration of the eschar or adherence of dried-out dressing to the wound as in wet or dry dressing.
Hydrogen peroxide solution	Infected or necrotic ulcerating wounds.	Decomposes to liberate oxygen into wound. Antiseptic agent.	Caustic to surrounding skin. Considerable skill needed to judge when to discontinue its use. Any debridement which occurs is due to mechanical action of the chemical change (fizzing). Oxygen released insufficiently to have any effect on healing.
Varidase topical (streptokinase, streptodornase)	Infected or necrotic ulcerating wounds.	Excellent debriding agent. Promotes vascularization. Rapid healing times. Does not need an aseptic technique for dressings. Reduces odour from wound.	Relatively expensive to purchase. Has to be reconstituted using syringe and needle, therefore only available on prescription. Initially increases exudate. *Contraindicated* for use near blood vessels (due to potential effects of streptokinase).
Debrisan/ Iodosorb	Infected or necrotic wounds.	Good debriding agents especially on liquid slough. Bacteriostatic.	Dry preparation difficult to apply. Pastes or packaged preparations much easier. Must be kept off healthy tissue.
Povidone-iodine spray	Shallow or superficial clean wounds. Grades 1 and 2.	Quick to apply. Good antiseptic.	Potential adverse reactions.

Tweedle, D. (1978) How the metabolism reacts to injury, *Nursing Mirror*, Vol. 147, no. 21, pp. 34–6.
Willington, F.L. (1977) The use of non-ionic detergents in sanitary cleansing: a report of a preliminary trial, *Journal of Advanced Nursing*, Vol. 3, pp. 373–82.
Winter, G.D. (1971) Some factors affecting the skin and wound healing, in R.M. Kenedi *et al.* (eds.) *Bed Sore Biomechanics*, Macmillan, London.

GUIDELINES: PREVENTION OF PRESSURE SORES

Action	Rationale
1 Assess every patient on admission using a recognized scale, such as the Norton Scale.	To identify the patient at risk of developing pressure sores.
2 Reassess every patient on a regular basis.	To maintain consistency in treatment.
3 Do not rub any area at risk.	Rubbing causes maceration and degeneration of subcutaneous tissues, especially in the elderly.
4 Wash areas at risk only if the patient is incontinent or sweating profusely. Use mild soap or a liquid detergent. Ensure that all detergent or soap is rinsed off and that the area is patted dry. Use moisturizer if the skin is very dry. Ask the patient what suits his/her skin.	To maintain skin integrity and prevent the formation of sores. Excessive use of soap can be harmful to the skin. Thorough gentle drying of the skin promotes comfort and discourages the growth of micro-organisms. Dry skin cracks to allow entry of micro-organisms.
5 Use barrier creams only when indicated.	Barrier creams prevent damage to the epidermis. They are, however, occlusive and prevent correct moisture and oxygen exchange from the skin.
6 Encourage the patient to eat a nutritious diet, rich in protein and vitamin C.	Deficiencies of protein and vitamin C have been shown to render an individual more prone to pressure sores.
7 Educate the patient to shift position, to pull or push up regularly and to examine the vulnerable area.	After discharge the patient will be self-caring and possibly still vulnerable to sores. To encourage the patient to participate in his/her own care.
8 Initiate a mobility programme for the patient. Call on the physiotherapist or occupational therapist as appropriate.	Reduces further tissue damage and improves circulation.
9 Use appropriate pressure relief devices.	Use of inappropriate aids may increases pressure to that area.
10 Have the patient recumbent whenever possible. Support with bead bags or pillows in bed. reduce period spent sitting in chair if pelvic sores develop.	Avoid the use of bedrests as these increase shearing.

GUIDELINES: TREATMENT OF PRESSURE SORES

Equipment
1   Wound dressing pack
2   Solutions, dressings and tape as appropriate.

Procedure
SUPERFICIAL SORES (GRADES 2 and 3)

Action	Rationale
1 Where possible relieve the pressure on the affected area. Reposition the patient at least 2-hourly and record the position on the relevant chart.	To promote circulation and healing.

2 Clean the wound using an aseptic techniques.

To prevent infection. The wound should be disturbed as little as possible to allow healing to occur.

3 If necessary cover the wound with the dressing of choice.

To prevent leakage of exudate. To provide the optimum micro-environment for wound healing.

4 Record any changes in the appropriate documents and amend the care plan accordingly.

For accurate evaluation of the progress of wound healing.

DEEP SORES (GRADE 4)

Action	Rationale

1 Where possible relieve the pressure over the area. reposition the patient at least 2-hourly and record the position on the relevant charts. Use pressure-relieving aids.

To promote circulation and healing.
To ensure consistencyin the pattern of positions used.

2 Obtain a specimen of discharge with a wound swab or syringe, as required.

To identify any infecting organisms.

3 Clean the wound using an aseptic technique. Use gloved hand in preference to forceps.

To prevent infection.
To avoid damage to growing granulation tissue.

4 Necrotic wounds should be debrided using suitable tropical agents.

To allow epithelialization to take place.

5 Cover the wound with an appropriate dressing. Dry topical swabs are not appropriate.

To prevent leakage of exudate. To create the optimum micro-environment for healing.
Revascularization and epithelialization occur into the matrix of the topical swabs. Each time the dressing is removed the new tissue is lifted with it and bleeding occurs. Frequent dressings reduce the wound surface temperature and delay healing.

6 Cavities should be filled with an appropriate product, e.g. foam, gel or hydrocolloid. Wounds should not be tightly packed with gauze.

Tight packing increases pressure and leads to further damage.

7 Fix the dressing with hypo-allergenic tape, light bandage or Netelast.

Further damage will occur to broken skin if there is an allergic reaction or if tape cannot be removed easily.

8 Encourage the patient to eat a nutritious diet, rich in vitamin C and trace elements.

If exudate is excessive, substantial protein loss can occur. Vitamin C and trace elements promote healing.

9 Record any changes in the appropriate documents and amend the care plan accordingly.

For accurate evaluation of the progress of wound healing.

* For grade 1 sores refer to the guidelines on prevention of pressure sores, p. 312.

32

Scalp Cooling

REFERENCE MATERIAL

Doxorubicin (Adriamycin) is one of the most active cytotoxic agents currently used in cancer chemotherapy. It belongs to the anthracycline antibiotic group of drugs and has a wide spectrum of activity. Unfortunately administration of doxorubicin is associated with alopecia in approximately 90% of cases. This is often total. Hair loss is distressing for the patient and may lead to refusal to accept treatment.

Initial research into methods to prevent hair loss, using a scalp tourniquet or crushed ice, was carried out in America. Promising results led to follow-up research at The Royal Marsden Hospital. The method developed differs on a number of points from previous work and the results achieved are considerably better. The success rate in the research project was 85% and this has been maintained in everyday practice. Two factors affect the amount of hair loss experienced by the patient:

1   involvement of the liver with metastatic disease leads to elevated plasma levels of doxorubicin for a longer period. Extension of the cooling period does not seem to improve results;
2   inadequate cooling because of exceptionally thick hair may lead to partial loss. It has been demonstrated that maximum cooling occurs 20 minutes after the cap has been placed in position. The weight of the cap, as well as the temperature, is a factor, as this ensures that the contact is maintained over the complete scalp. Success does not appear to be as dose dependent as was first thought.

Scalp cooling, when doxorubicin is prescribed, is not performed routinely. The consultant's permission must be obtained as there is a risk of protecting scalp micrometastases, especially where there is the possibility of circulating cells, e.g. in cases of leukaemias and lymphomas. The patient must consent when fully informed of the nature and length of the procedure. The patient may discontinue scalp cooling at any time if he/she finds it too traumatic, physically or psychologically, or if hair loss occurs.

Patients should be selected carefully for scalp cooling and should be well motivated to undertake the procedure. Comments show that cooling can be more distressing than originally thought, and patients have reported 'ice phobias' following treatment.

The effectiveness of scalp cooling has only been demonstrated satisfactorily with doxorubicin and epirubicin. However, patients receiving other cytotoxic drugs (vincristine and vindicine), which may cause alopecia, have undergone the procedure. Unfortunately the data collected are insufficient for evaluation at the time of writing.

References and further reading

Anderson, J. et al. (1981) Prevention of doxorubicin-induced alopecia by scalp cooling in patients with advanced breast cancer, British Medical Journal, Vol. 282, pp. 423–4.

Benjamin, R.S. (1975) A practical approach to Adriamycin toxicology, Cancer Chemotherapy Reports, Vol. 6, pp. 319–27.

Benjamin, R.S. et al. (1974) Adriamycin chemotherapy – efficacy, safety and pharmacologic basis of an intermittent, single, high dosage schedule, Cancer, Vol. 33, pp. 19–27.

David, J.A. and Speechley, V. (1987) Scalp cooling to prevent alopecia, Nursing Times, Vol. 83, no. 32, pp. 36–7.

Dean, J.C. et al. (1979) Prevention of doxorubicin-induced hair loss with scalp hypothermia, New England Journal of Medicine, Vol. 301, pp. 1427–9.

Edelstyn, G.A. et al. (1977) Doxorubicin-induced hair loss and possible modification by scalp cooling, Lancet, Vol. ii, pp. 253–4.

Hayward, J.L. (1977) Assessment of response to therapy in advanced breast cancer, British Journal of Cancer, Vol. 35, pp. 292–8.

Hunt, J. *et al.* (1982) Scalp hypothermia to prevent Adriamycin-induced hair loss, *Cancer Nursing*, Vol. 5, no. 1, pp. 25–31.

Middleton, J. *et al.* (1982) Prevention of doxorubicin-induced alopecia by scalp hypothermia: relation to degree of cooling, *British Medical Journal*, Vol. 284, p. 1674.

Robinson, M.H. *et al.* (1987) Effectiveness of scalp cooling in reducing alopecia caused by epirubicin treatment of advanced breast cancer, *Cancer Treatment Reports*, Vol. 71, pp. 913–4.

Timothy, A.R. *et al.* (1980) Influence of scalp hypothermia on doxorubicin-related alopecia, *Lancet*, Vol. i, p. 663.

Tormey, D.C. (1975) Adriamycin in breast cancer. An overview of studies, *Cancer Chemotherapy Reports*, Vol. 6, pp. 319–27.

GUIDELINES: SCALP COOLING

Equipment

1   A scalp cooling cap:
    (a)   Commercial make
    (b)   Home made from eight hot/cold packs, as manufactured by 3M. These must be taped together with tape, such as Sleek, and moulded around a wig stand. When bandaged in position the cap is placed in a deep freeze (temperature approximately − 18°C) for 24 hours.
2   Ear protection – gauze, cotton wool pads
3   Two crepe bandages – 10 cm or 15 cm wide
4   Two towels
5   Comfortable chair (recliner) or bed
6   Extra pillows and blankets as required.

Procedure

Before beginning it is important to explain the procedure fully to the patient and obtain his/her consent. The patient should understand that he/she can discontinue the scalp cooling at any time and that this will not jeopardize chemotherapy. The patient may refuse the procedure.

Action	Rationale
1 Check that the cap has been in the deep freeze for 24 hours.	To ensure that the cap is cold enough to be effective.
2 Wet the patient's hair thoroughly.	To aid conduction of the cold.
3 Place the ear protection in position.	To prevent cold injury.
4 Soak one crepe bandage in cold water and use it to bandage the patient's head tightly. The bandage should be applied evenly and should provide a thin layer over the scalp.	To aid conduction of the cold. To compress the hair and prevent any trapping of air between the cap and scalp.
5 Place the cap on the patient's head, making sure it fits closely and covers the whole hairline.	To ensure cooling over the head, including all the hair roots.
6 Add supplementary packs if necessary.	
7 Bandage the cap in place.	To maintain even and close contact of the cap to the scalp and provide some insulation of the cold.

Action	Rationale
8 Add pillows, etc., as required.	To provide support for the head and neck, and reduce the weight of the cap, approximately 2–3 kg.
9 Place a dry towel around the patient's shoulders.	To catch any water if the cap defrosts.
10 Offer the patient the use of a blanket.	To prevent any chilling.
11 Leave the patient for at least 15 minutes prior to injection of the drug.	To obtain initial cooling of the scalp.
12 Administer the drug by intravenous injection.	
13 Leave the patient for a further 45 minutes.	To maintain cooling until plasma levels of drug have dropped.
14 When sufficient time has elapsed, remove the cap and bandages carefully.	To prevent damage to the scalp and hair.
15 Encourage the patient to rest, if desired.	To prevent faintness due to the weight being lifted off.
16 Towel the patient's hair dry and allow the patient to style it gently.	To prevent damage to the hair. To ensure that the patient is comfortable and has a chance to rearrange his/her hair before leaving the hospital.

NURSING CARE PLAN

Problem	Cause	Suggested action
Inadequate cooling.		Follow the procedure meticulously. Check that the cap is as cold as possible. If the patient has very thick hair, use the heaviest cap available.
Excess cooling.	Thin hair.	Use extra layers of bandage between the cap and the scalp. If it is still painful, discontinue the procedure.
Complaints of headache.	Weight and coldness of the cap.	Provide support and blankets as required.
Distressed patient.	Claustrophobia.	Support and reassure the patient. If necessary remove the cap.
Hair loss.		Offer the patient the opportunity to discontinue the scalp cooling.
		Make arrangements for the patient to see the appliance officer to obtain a wig. Discuss hair care.

'Ice phobia'.

Be aware of this possible problem; encourage the patient to discuss his/her feelings.

33

Sealed Radioactive Sources

Definition

Sealed sources are radioactive isotopes used for therapy which are permanently and completely enclosed in a metal casing.

Most radioactive isotopes used as sealed sources for brachytherapy emit both beta and gamma radiation. Beta radiation is screened out by the casting surrounding the source and it is the gamma irradiation that exerts a therapeutic effect because of its high energy and power of penetration.

Indications

Permanent or temporary insertions of small sealed sources are used to deliver very high doses of radiation into tumours or tumour-bearing tissue while giving rapidly diminishing doses to adjacent structures. This will limit the damage caused to normal tissue. A specific dose of radiation will be received by the cancer. This is delivered continuously over a period of hours or days. Small sealed sources inserted into the body may take the form of:

1 *Intracavitary applicators*: sources that are placed against tissue and usually held in place by packing.
2 *Interstitial implants*: sources that are inserted directly into the tumour-bearing tissue.

(*Note:* Surface applicators or moulds: sources are applied directly to superficial cancers.)

REFERENCE MATERIAL
Radioactive isotopes used as sealed sources
CAESIUM 137

Caesium 137 is a radioisotope that can be used in the form of implants or in applicators.

The half-life of caesium 137 is 30 years and it has largely replaced radium as a source in brachytherapy.

Oral implants

Caesium 137 may be used in a needle-like implant that can be positioned directly into the tissue surrounding the tumour. This is a fairly common treatment for early lesions of the cheek, lip and anterior two-thirds of the tongue. If bone involvement is suspected, e.g. in the mandible, alternative treatment will be given.

Gynaecological applicators

Caesium 137 may be used in applicators. The commonest malignancies treated by use of radioactive applicators are tumours of the female genital tract. Intracavity applicators are used which deliver a high dose to the region of the cervix, the paracervical tissue, the upper part of the vagina and the uterine body.

IRIDIUM 192

Iridium 192 is a radioisotope which can be used in the form of pins or wires as in interstitial therapy.

The half-life of iridium 192 is 74.2 days. It is an ideal choice because of the low energy of its gamma emission, which simplifies radiation protection, and because in the form of a platinum–iridium alloy it can be drawn into thin flexible wires. The wires consist of an active platinum–iridium alloy core encased in a sheath of platinum, 10 cm thick, which screens out the beta radiation from the iridium 192.

Modern afterloading techniques reduce the radiation exposure to the radiotherapist and other staff involved.

Iridium 192 implants are used under the following circumstances:

1 as a primary treatment for small primary lesions, especially tongue or breast lesions;
2 as a 'boost' dose after external radiotherapy for larger primary tumours or where nodes are also involved;
3 to treat recurrence.

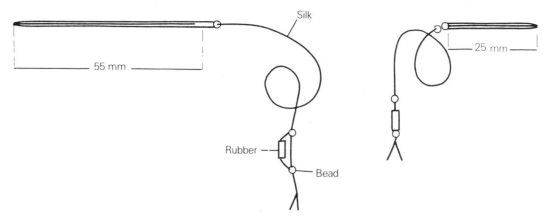

Figure 33.1   Caesium 137 needles.

GOLD 198

Gold 198 is used as an interstitial source of radiation in the form of gold grains.

The half-life of the gold 198 radioisotope is 2.76 days. Gamma and beta rays are emitted. The gamma rays are of relatively low energy and the beta rays are filtered out by the platinum casing around the gold. Gold 198 grains are used primarily in the treatment of tumours of the lung, breast, bladder neck, prostate and nodes.

When a patient is selected for interstitial or intracavitary therapy the medical staff assess the size of the tumour. The physics department is responsible for ordering the source and co-ordinating with the radiotherapists.

Intraoral implants

CAESIUM 137 NEEDLES

The sources (see Figure 33.1) are inserted in theatre under a general anaesthetic. They are inserted individually in a predetermined pattern so that the implant covers the whole growth with a safety margin of at least 1 cm. Each needle is positioned by pushers so that its eye, through which silk is threaded, is just visible beneath the mucosal surface. Each silk is then stitched to the tongue with a single suture. When all the needles have been inserted, the silks are counted and gathered together. They are threaded through a piece of rubber to prevent friction and trauma to the mouth. The silks are strapped to the cheek to prevent any needle being swallowed should it work loose. Small beads are attached to the

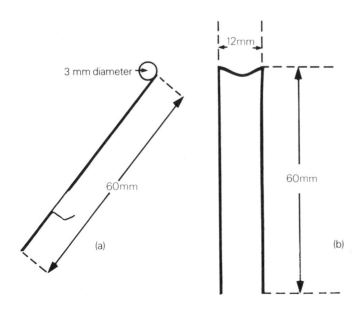

Figure 33.2   Iridium pins. *a*, Iridium single pin. *b*, Iridium 192 hair pin.

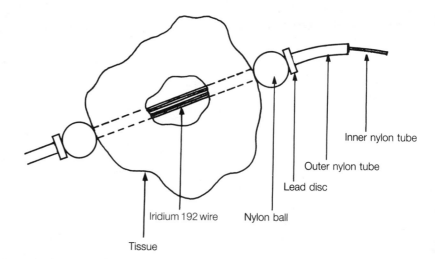

Figure 33.3   Iridium 192 wire in polythene cannula. Typical assembly in tissue.

ends of the threads to facilitate counting the needles. X-rays are always taken to check the positions of the needles and to enable estimation of the dose distribution.

IRIDIUM 192 HAIR PINS AND SINGLE PINS

These types of implants are usually used intraorally (Figure 33.2). They are slotted into tissue using steel guides to obtain accurate alignment. Radiological examination is used to check the position of the guides before the iridium is inserted. The pins are held in place by sutures.

The staff of the physics department are normally responsible for calculating how long a radioactive implant is to stay in place. This is usually about 6 days, depending on the size of the tumour. Removal is carried out in theatre by the radiotherapist.

Breast or perineal implants
IRIDIUM 192 WIRES

These are usually used for breast lesions or lesions of the vulva or perineum (Figure 33.3). Polythene cannulae are inserted under a general anaesthetic. In the case of breast lesions, both ends of each tube protrude through the skin. Correct alignment is established often with the aid of a perspex template which fits over the breast. In the case of vulval or perineal insertions only one end of the tube protrudes. For these, alignment of the sources may be achieved by using a perspex template and vaginal obtivator.

The iridium wire source is afterloaded usually on the ward and the wires are held in the cannulae with crimped lead washers.

The radiotherapist is responsible for calculating how long a radioactive implant should stay in place. This is usually for 3–6 days, depending on the size of the

tumour. Removal of the implant is usually carried out on the ward by the radiotherapist.

GOLD 198 GRAINS

Gold 198 grains are 2.5 mm long and 0.5 mm in diameter, made of gold encased in platinum. Fourteen gold 198 grains are contained in an aluminium magazine which fits into the barrel of the implantation gun (Figure 33.4). An injector needle is attached to the gun which is inserted into the tissue that is to be irradiated. The patient requires a general anaesthetic for the insertion.

Gold grains have the following advantages over more classical methods of wires and pin in the irradiation of comparatively inaccessible tumours:

1 placing gold 198 grains is easier than placing needles or pins;
2 gold 198 grains do not need any fixing sutures;
3 they are a permanent insertion, therefore the closure of any surgical wound can be immediate.

The disadvantage of this method is that higher numbers of gold 198 grains are required which means that more precautions must be taken in order to achieve a regular geometrical arrangement to ensure satisfactory distribution of the dose. This can increase the length of time the doctors, nursing staff and other personnel present are exposed to irradiation.

Intracavitary applicators

The applicators are inserted under a general anaesthetic, and the position of the applicator is checked by X-ray before the patient returns to the ward. A urinary catheter is also inserted in theatre to reduce the risk of the sources becoming dislodged by the patient when micturating.

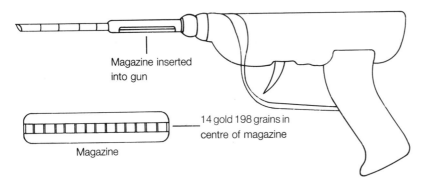

Magazine inserted
into gun

Magazine

14 gold 198 grains in
centre of magazine

Figure 33.4 Gold grain gun.

TYPES OF APPLICATOR

There are several different types of applicator available and choice is usually determined by the site of the tumour, the anatomy of the patient and the preference of the treatment centre. The most commonly used types of applicator are described below (see Figure 33.5).

Stockholm applicator

This is used for carcinoma of the body of the uterus or cervix. Usually a uterine tube and two vaginal packets are inserted. Occasionally, if the vaginal vault is small, one packet is omitted or replaced by a vaginal tube. The radioactive material is held in place with a flavine-soaked gauze pack. It is usually left in place for 22 hours. Tubes and packets have strings attached for removal and colour-coded beads indicate which should be removed first.

Modified Stockholm applicator

This is used for carcinoma of the body of the uterus and cervix. It consists of a uterine tube and a square box which connect together by a point and a hole. The vagina is then packed with gauze saturated with proflavine. They are usually left in place for 20 hours. The box should be removed first. The uterine tube is plain.

Fletcher applicator

This is used for carcinoma of the corpus or cervix, but the patient needs to have a fairly capacious vaginal vault. Hollow applicators, a uterine tube and two vaginal ovoids are inserted in theatre and loaded with the radioactive sources later, on the ward, by the radiotherapist. The apparatus is held in place with a flavine pack. Long ends project through the vulva so that afterloading can be done. These insertions are usually left in place for 60–72 hours. No strings are needed as the apparatus itself projects from the vulva.

Curietron afterloading applicator

This is used for carcinoma of the corpus or cervix, but patients need to have a fairly capacious and symmetrical vault. Hollow metal applicators, consisting of two vaginal ovoids and a uterine tube, are inserted in the theatre and are loaded with radioactive 'Curietron' sources later, on the ward, by the radiotherapist. The apparatus is held in place with approximately 90 cm of ribbon gauze flavine pack. The long ends of the applicators project through the vulva so that afterloading can be carried out. The patient may need to be nursed with a sorbo pad or pillow under the dorsal area to keep the projecting ends off the bed.

These insertions last 60–72 hours. Patients usually have two insertions but may sometimes be given a single preoperative insertion or a single insertion following external irradiation.

Heyman's capsules

These are used for carcinoma of the corpus where there is enlargement of the uterus and expanded uterine cavity. They consist of small metal capsules, each of which contains a small, radioactive source. As many capsules as possible are placed into the uterus. Usually two vaginal packets are used as well. They are held in place by a flavine gauze pack and are left in for about 12–18 hours. Each capsule has a flexible wire attached, strapped to the thigh, for removal, and a numbered tag to indicate the order of removal.

Dobbie applicator

This is used to irradiate the whole vagina. A perspex cylindrical applicator, with radioactive sources in the centre, is inserted into the vagina and sutured in place to the vulva. It is usually left in for about 18 hours. Strings are attached to the applicator for removal.

Modified Dobbie applicator

This is a polyacetal (Delrin) cylindrical applicator with a long hollow through the middle. A uterine tube is loaded and slipped into the long hollow. The applicator is inserted into the vagina and sutured in place. It is usually left in position for about 18 hours, but this will depend on the rectal dose of radiation. Strings are attached to aid removal.

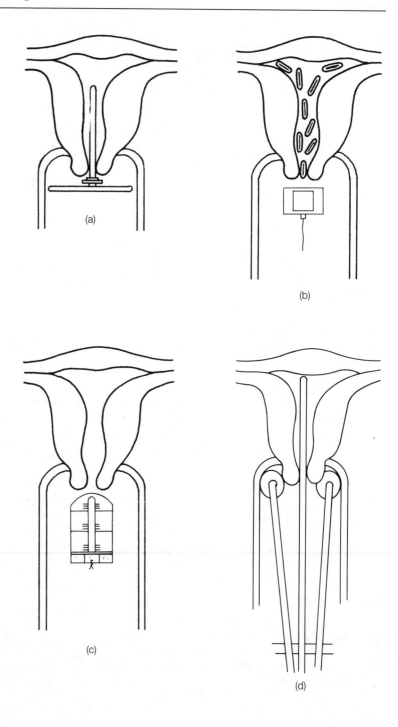

Figure 33.5   Gynaecological caesium
applicators. *a*, Modified Stockholm
applicator. *b*, Heyman's capsules and packet.
c, Dobbie applicator. *d*, Fletcher applicator.

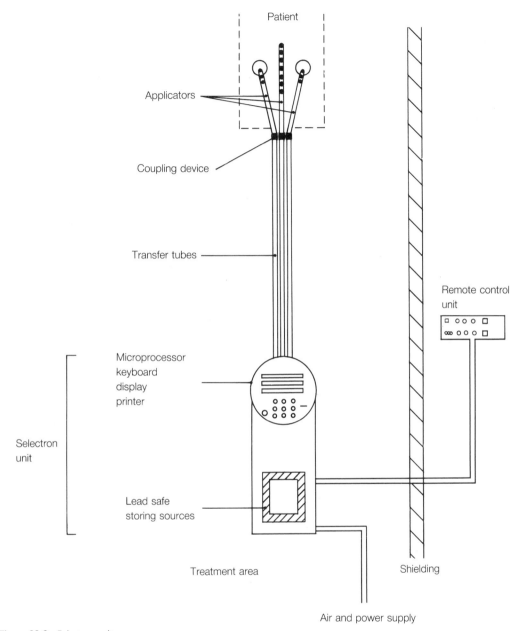

Figure 33.6 Selectron unit.

THE LOW DOSE RATE SELECTRON

Definition
The selectron is a remote-controlled afterloading system and has been designed to deliver intracavitary radiotherapy to patients without exposing hospital personnel to radiation.

Indication
It is gradually replacing conventional intracavitary radium and caesium applicators and other manual and mechanical afterloading techniques.

REFERENCE MATERIAL

The selectron unit comprises of a lead shielded safe containing caesium 137 sources in the form of small spherical pellets, a microprocessor, keyboard, display unit and printer (Figure 33.6). Leading from the selectron unit are between 3 and 6 flexible plastic transfer tubes corresponding to numbered treatment channels. Each tube ends in a fragile plastic catheter which is inserted into the appropriately numbered applicator and secured by a coupling device. The unit has a supply of compressed air and it is air pressure that the system uses to transfer the sources from the safe within the unit to the applicators along the connecting tubes. Operation of the unit is initiated from a remote-control unit situated outside the protected treatment area. Together these components form the basis of the remote-controlled afterloading system.

The selectron provides an accurate and safe method of radiotherapy treatment for cancers of the cervix, uterus and upper part of the vagina.

The advantages of the selectron system are threefold:

1   remote afterloading eliminates contact with radioactive material and protects personnel;
2   it allows highly accurate dosimetry;
3   the activity of the caesium 137 sources is such (up to 40 mCi) that treatment times for patients are considerably shorter than for conventional techniques.

While the selectron has been used predominantly for the treatment of gynaecological cancers, features of its design render it potentially useful for treating a number of other tumours such as cancers of the oesophagus, bladder or colon.

Patients have hollow lightweight stainless steel applicators positioned in the operating theatre under a general anaesthetic. These are usually modifed Fletcher-type applicators consisting of a uterine tube and two vaginal ovoids held in place with a proflavine-soaked vaginal packing. However, several other applicators are available. Accurate positioning of the applicators is confirmed by taking X-rays with dummy sources *in situ* and the optimum source configuration is selected, taking account of individual anatomical variations.

The selectron is programmed by the physicist. For each treatment channel being used, active source pellets are interspersed with inactive stainless steel space pellets to achieve the desired dose distribution. The treatment time required to reach the prescribed dose is also entered. With a six-channel selection unit it is possible to treat two patients with Fletcher-type applicators simultaneously. The radiotherapist is responsible for connecting the transfer tubes to the applicators. The transfer tubes are led over a bed bracket which supports the weight of the tubes and prevents traction being applied to the applicators in the patient. If the wrong catheter is connected to the applicator, the system will fail to operate.

Operating the selectron

Treatment is commenced by activation of the remote control unit when all staff have left the treatment area. While treatment is in progress it can be interrupted and restarted from the remote control unit by pressing the stop and start buttons. The display panel indicates which channels are being used for treatment and which are unused with red and green lights respectively. The time of the longest treatment is displayed in decimal hours and a telephone intercom system allows for communication with the patient without the need to interrupt treatment.

Interrupting the treatment by pressing the green stop button results in the sources being withdrawn into the selectron unit and stops the timer. This allows nursing staff to enter the treatment area in safety and give routine or specific care to the patient. Pressing the red start button transfers the sources back into the applicators and restarts the timer. The red lights demonstrate that the channels are operating again satisfactory.

The system has built-in safety features. In the event of a failure in the system, treatment usually stops automatically. An audible and visual alarm at the remote control unit alerts staff to a problem and indicates whether this is a fault related to the air or power supply, the pellets or the timer. There is an optional nurse station display unit with a similar alarm indicator which also emits an audible signal when treatment has been interrupted. This helps to prevent treatment being inadvertently left interrupted for long periods.

A record of any break in treatment is shown on the print-out from the unit itself, together with any programming or system fault. These appear as an error code and can be identified by reference to the selectron users' manual.

At the end of the treatment time, all sources will be automatically withdrawn from the applicators back into the selectron unit. When two patients are being treated simultaneously termination of the treatment of one patient may be some time before that of the other. This means the timer will register the longer treatment time but the channels used for the first patient will have changed from red to green.

Additional safety features include a door switch facility to retract sources immediately if the door to the treatment area is opened when treatment is in progress, and/or Geiger dose rate meters visible when entering the treatment area and approaching the patient, which indicate when there are radioactive sources either in the patient or in the connecting tubes.

Preparation of the patient

This is similar to that required prior to other gynaecological intracavitary techniques. Information given should include explanation that the patient will be connected to the selectron unit via the flexible plastic tubes and that these will restrict turning in bed. Patients should also be prepared for the various mechanical noises that the system makes, especially when the sources are being transferred in and out of the applicators. Some patients find the prospect of treatment alarming and may prefer to receive regular sedation for the duration of the treatment.

References and further reading

Amersham International Ltd (1978) *Interstitial Therapy Using Iridium-192*, Amersham International Ltd.

Amersham International Ltd (1981) *Radioisotope Sources for Brachytherapy*, Amersham International Ltd.

Baker, J. (1979) Implants and applications, In R. Tiffany (ed.) Scan-technology in nursing – radiotherapy, *Nursing Times*, Vol. 148, Suppl. pt. 10, pp. 37–40.

Hodt, H.J. *et al.* (1952) A gun for interstitial implantation of radioactive gold grains, *British Journal of Radiology*, Vol. 25, pp. 419–21.

Hussey, K. (1985) Demystifying the care of patients with radioactive implants, *American Journal of Nursing*, Vol. 85, pp. 789–92.

Nucletron Engineering (198?) *Selectron Users' Manual*, Nucleton Engineering, Chester.

Paine, C.H. (1972) Modern afterloading methods for interstitial radiotherapy, *Clinical Radiology*, Vol. 23, pp. 263–72.

Pierquin, B. *et al.* (1978) The Paris system in interstitial radiation therapy, *Acta Radiologica: Oncology, Radiation, Physics, Biology*, Vol. 17, no. 1, pp. 33–48.

Royal Marsden Hospital (1968) *Rules for the Protection of Nursing Staff Exposed to Ionising Radiation*, rev. edn, The Royal Marsden Hospital, London.

Royal Marsden Hospital (1978) *Physics Manual Protocol*, The Royal Marsden Hospital, London.

Shell, J. and Carter, J. (1987) The gynaecological implant patient, *Seminars in Oncology Nursing*, Vol. 3, no. 1, pp. 54–66.

Tiffany, R. (1979) *Cancer Nursing–Radiotherapy*, Faber & Faber, London.

Welby-Allen, M. (1982) Selectron treatment in gynaecology, *Nursing Times*, Vol. 78, no. 46, pp. 1948–50.

GUIDELINES: CARE OF PATIENTS WITH INSERTIONS OF SEALED RADIOACTIVE SOURCES

Action	Rationale
1 When transferring patients from theatre to ward, the nurse and porter should remain at the head and foot of the bed and at least 120 cm from the centre of the bed in the event of any delay in the transfer. If the source is intraoral, the nurse should stand at the foot of the bed.	To minimize the risk of exposure to radiation.
2 A yellow radiation hazard board should accompany the patient back from theatre. This must remain at the bottom of the bed or outside the cubicle until the source is removed.	To warn everybody that the patient has a radioactive source.
3 Nursing staff must calculate the time allowed with the patient in any 24-hour period. This time should be written on the yellow hazard notice on the bed or cubicle door.	To minimize exposure to radiation.
4 A Geiger counter should be available on the ward.	To monitor radioactivity if a dislodged source is suspected, e.g. in the bed linen.

Action	Rationale
5 One nurse should be delegated responsibility for the nursing care of the patient. The time spent with the patient should be shared between all of the staff on duty and time spent in nursing procedures must be kept to a minimum.	To minimize the risk of overexposure to radiation.
6 Every nurse must wear a radiation badge above the level of the lead shield.	To record the extent of exposure to radiation.
7 All bed linen and waste materials removed from the patient area should be monitored before being removed from the ward.	To prevent loss of an accidentally dislodged source.
8 If a source becomes dislodged, use the long-handled forceps to put the source into a lead pot. Care should be taken not to damage the source. It must never be handled directly with the fingers.	To minimize the dose of radiation received.
9 Visitors must remain at least 120 cm away from the patient. The visit should not last longer than the time shown on the warning notice. No children or pregnant women are allowed to visit.	To minimize the risk of overexposure to radiation.

GUIDELINES: CARE OF PATIENTS WITH INTRAORAL SOURCES

Preparation of the patient

Dental assessment of the patient is usually carried out prior to oral brachytherapy so that caries, mouth infections and dental extractions may be dealt with in case of the oral blood supply being impaired by the treatment. The patient is usually admitted 24 hours prior to the implant, during which time the nature of the procedure and the implications of having a radioactive source should be explained to the patient. Ideally, the patient should be nursed in a cubicle or in a bed away from other patients to reduce the amount of radiation exposure to other people.

Action	Rationale
1 Encourage frequent mouth care. The patient should void the solution into a bowl and not into a handbasin.	To reduce the risk of infection. To prevent the loss of a dislodged source.
2 Provide a soft, pureed or liquid diet.	To reduce the risk of the patient biting into the source or his/her tongue. Eating is often difficult when implants are present.
3 Avoid spicy and/or hot foods. Discourage the patient from smoking and/or drinking alcohol.	To prevent exacerbation of local reaction or soreness.
4 Encourage ingestion of carbonated drinks.	To alleviate dryness.
5 Provide crushed ice for the patient to suck and/or soluble aspirin as a mouthwash.	To minimize oral pain and discomfort.
6 Give steroids as prescribed.	To prevent and/or minimize swelling.

7	Provide writing equipment for the patient.	To reduce the need for oral communication. This is liable to increase soreness and alter the distribution of the sources.
8	Provide paper tissues and a bowl for saliva.	The patient may have difficulty in swallowing due to soreness and oedema.
9	The sources should be checked at regular intervals, e.g. at the beginning of a span of duty.	To make sure that the sources have not become dislodged.
10	The patient must be confined to the cubicle or the space around the bed. Washing is carried out in the bed area, but the general toilet facilities should be used, provided that the patient remains at a distance from other people.	To minimize the risk of radiation exposure to other people on the ward.

Discharge of the patient

The patient is usually discharged the day after the removal of the implant. The patient should be warned about the brisk local reaction which he/she may experience due to rapid cell breakdown induced by the radiation. In order to minimize the risk of infection or soreness the patient should be taught how to care for the treated area, e.g. frequent oral toilet.

GUIDELINES: CARE OF PATIENTS WITH GYNAECOLOGICAL SOURCES

Preparation of the patient

The patient is usually admitted 12–48 hours prior to the procedure so that any pre-anaesthetic investigations may be performed. An enema or suppositories are usually given to reduce the chance of the patient having a bowel action while the sources are in place. This could dislodge the sources. Some patients, however, have diarrhoea on admission due to previous radiotherapy and will need regular medication, such as codeine phosphate, both before and during the application of the sources. It is arguable whether the vulval area needs to be shaved. The patient should be bathed before any premedication is administered. A full explanation should be given to the patient along with information about the implications of having a radioactive source inside her.

Action	Rationale
1 The patient must remain in bed in a recumbent or semirecumbent position while the applicators or implants are in place.	To prevent the applicators becoming dislodged or changing their position with relation to the internal organs.
2 Rolling from side to side is permitted and should be encouraged if the patient is at risk of developing a pressure sore.	To promote comfort and to relieve prolonged pressure on any one area.
3 On return from theatre, the sanitary towel should be checked for discharge. Disposable pants may be worn. Check that the catheter is correctly positioned to allow drainage.	To secure the position of the sanitary towel. To ensure that urine is draining freely.
4 Observe for any blood or other discharge from the vagina. Check the temperature and pulse every 2 hours.	To monitor haemorrhage, shock and other postoperative complications.

Action	Rationale
5 Administer prescribed analgesics, anti-emetics and antidiarrhoeal agents.	For the patient's comfort.
6 Encourage fluid intake as soon as the patient is allowed to drink. If the source is to be in for longer than 24 hours:	
(a) Encourage a fluid intake of 50–100% a day over and above the patient's normal intake.	To ensure adequate hydration. To reduce the risk of urinary tract infection.
(b) A low residue diet may be taken.	To prevent the stimulation of a bowel action.

GUIDELINES: REMOVAL OF GYNAECOLOGICAL CAESIUM

The removal of applicators is usually performed by nursing staff. Only nurses holding a certificate of competence, or nurses supervised by a suitably qualified nurse, should perform this procedure.

Equipment
1   Sterile gynaecological pack containing large receiver, green towel, paper towel, long dissecting forceps, sanitary towel, cotton wool balls
2   Equipment for the administration of Entonox
3   Solutions of choice for swabbing, e.g. Savlodil, normal saline
4   Sterile gloves
5   Sterile scissors or stitch cutter
6   Clean draw sheet
7   Geiger counter.

Procedure

Action	Rationale
1 Explain the procedure to the patient.	To obtain the patient's consent and co-operation.
2 Check the date and time for removal on the form that was received from the physics department when sources were inserted.	The accurate timing of the removal is essential for the administration of the correct therapeutic dose of radiation.
3 Check that any pre-removal drugs (e.g. sedatives, analgesics) have been administered.	
4 Check, with another nurse, the exact time of removal and the number of applicators.	To reduce the risk of error.
5 Ensure that:	
(a) The lead shield is suitably positioned beside the patient.	To shield the nurse from exposure to radiation.
(b) The lead pot is also suitably positioned with the lid removed.	So that sources can be placed in the pot immediately after removal.
6 Begin the administration of Entonox at least 2 minutes before commencing the procedure.	To allow time for the effects of the gas to be felt. (For further information on Entonox administration, see pp. 145–9.)

7	Prepare a trolley, put on gloves and open the pack before going to the bedside.	This is a clinically clean, not an aseptic procedure. To reduce the time spent in close proximity to the source.
8	Working from behind the lead shield, assist the patient into the dorsal position with knees apart. Remove the sanitary towel.	To obtain access to the sources.
9	Remove any sutures, if present. Remove the vaginal packing.	
10	Remove the caesium sources in reverse order of insertion. Contact the radiotherapist immediately if difficulty is encountered in removing a source. Place the removed sources in a lead pot immediately and cover with the lid.	To contain radioactivity
11	Remove the lead pot to a designated area, e.g. an isotope sluice or safe. Ensure that the lid of the pot or the sluice door is locked.	To remove the radioactive source from the ward area. To prevent unauthorized access to the source.
12	Monitor the patient's level of radioactivity.	To ensure that no sources remain inside the patient.
13	Remove the urinary catheter.	
14	Swab the vulva and perineal area with a solution such as Savlodil or normal saline. Ensure that the patient has a clean sanitary towel in position and is made comfortable.	To promote patient hygiene and comfort.
15	Monitor the bed linen, paper bags, vaginal packing and other waste material. (Two nurses should monitor the patient independently.)	To ensure that no source has been lost or remains inside the patient.
16	The patient should remain in bed until the physics department staff are satisfied that all sources are accounted for.	To ensure that all sources have been accounted for before the patient moves around.
17	Remove the radiation warning notice.	

NURSING CARE PLAN

Problem	Cause	Suggested action
Patient has a bowel action.		Inform the radiotherapist.
Patient removes caesium source herself.	Confusion, e.g. post-anaesthetic	Using long-handled forceps place the source in the lead container or safe. Inform the radiotherapist and the physics department.

Problem	Cause	Suggested action
Pyrexia.	Pelvic cellulitis or abscess. Reaction to the proflavine pack. Urinary infection. Physiological reaction to the breakdown of the tumour. Chest infection. Peritonitis due to perforation of the uterua.	If the patient's temperature remains over 37.5 °C for two consecutive readings, inform the radiotherapist. The caesium may have to be removed if the pyrexia persists.

GUIDELINES: CARING FOR THE PATIENT WITH GOLD 198 GRAINS

Preparation of the patient

The patient is usually admitted at least 1 day before treatment: Patients should ideally be nursed in a single room but, more importantly, in a bed away from the main thoroughfare.

Gold grains are implanted permanently into the tissue and therefore the patient must agree to stay in hospital until the physics staff state that the radioactivity is at a legally permissible level for discharge.

BREAST AND LYMPH NODE IMPLANTATION

Action	Rationale
1 The dressing to be left securely in position unless special instructions are given by the radiotherapist.	Sources may become detached, dressings will prevent them from becoming lost.
2 If dressing becomes dislodged leave it at the bedside, preferably in a lead pot and inform the physics staff.	If sources have become detached and are in the dressings physics staff will take the necessary action.
3 If there is any possibility that the sources have become detached inform physics department staff immediately and do not remove anything from the room.	It is important that the source is not lost as this could result in contamination of the environment. The patient's total dose will be altered and the medical staff will need to be informed.

LUNG IMPLANTATION

Action	Rationale
1 Check all sputum and drainage from the chest with the Geiger counter. If no radioactivity is found the sputum and drainage may be disposed of in the usual way unless special instructions are given by the physics department or radiotherapy staff.	To check for radioactivity in case any gold grains are coughed up or expelled in the drainage.
2 If radioactivity is detected, inform physics department staff immediately. Save the sputum or drainage for them to deal with.	To prevent contamination of the hospital environment.

BLADDER AND PROSTATE IMPLANTATION

Action	Rationale
1 Check all urine with the Geiger counter. If no radioactivity is found the urine may be disposed of in the usual way.	To check for radioactivity in case any gold grains are expelled in the urine.
2 If radioactivity is detected inform physics staff immediately and save urine for them to deal with.	To prevent contamination of the hospital environment.
3 Leave suspect urine in a safe place at the bedside, e.g. under the bed.	To prevent accidental disposal.

GUIDELINES: CARE OF PATIENTS WITH BREAST SOURCES

Preparation of the patient

The patient will usually be admitted for local excision of the breast tumour and an axillary clearance. Redivac drains are inserted and these are usually removed before the iridium wire sources are loaded 24–48 hours after surgery. When the sources are loaded, the patient should be nursed in a bed away from other patients.

Action	Rationale
1 Any dressing is left undisturbed for the duration of treatment.	To minimize the time spent in proximity to the patient.
2 The patient is confined to the cubicle or the space around the bed. Washing is carried out at the bed area. If general toilet facilities have to be used the patient must remain at a distance from other people.	To minimize the risk of radiation to other people on the ward.
3 Administer prescribed analgesia as required throughout the treatment period and prior to removal.	For the patient's comfort.

Discharge of the patient

The patient should normally be discharged the day after the removal of the implant. The patient should be warned about the brisk local reaction which she may experience due to the rapid cell breakdown induced by the radiation. In order the minimize the risk of infection or soreness, the patient should be taught how to care for the treated area.

GUIDELINES: CARE OF PATIENTS UNDERGOING SELECTRON TREATMENT

Action	Rationale
1 Nurse the patient on a Spenco mattress or with a foam wedge under her buttocks.	To promote comfort and to relieve backache since rolling is not permitted.

Action	**Rationale**
2 Ensure the plastic transfer tubes are supported securely in the bed bracket, leaving slight slack.	To enable the patient to change position slightly without putting traction on the applicators.
3 Limit the frequency and duration of interruption to treatment. Visitors are discouraged unless the patient is markedly distressed.	To prevent unnecessary prolongation of treatment time.
4 Unless otherwise indicated by the patient's physical or mental condition, check 2-hourly:	
(a) Temperature, pulse and vaginal loss	To monitor for haemorrhage, shock or other postoperative complications.
(b) Contents of catheter drainage bag	To ensure urine is draining freely.
(c) Assist patient to adjust her position.	To promote comfort and relieve prolonged pressure on any one area.
5 Administer prescribed analgesics, anti-emetics, antidiarrhoeal and sedative agents and evaluate effect.	To promote the patient's comfort and well-being.
6 Encourage fluid intake as soon as the patient is able to drink.	To ensure adequate hydration and reduce the risk of urinary tract infection.
7 If the patient wishes to eat, a light low residue diet may be taken.	To prevent stimulation of a bowel action.

GUIDELINES: REMOVAL OF SELECTRON APPLICATORS

If two patients are being treated simultaneously, removal of the applicators may be delayed until both patients have finished treatment, depending on the individual treatment times.

Equipment
As for removal of other gynaecological applicators (items 1–7, p. 328) plus
  8 · Rubber caps for the applicators.

Procedure

Action	**Rationale**
1 Check treatment has been terminated by:	The applicators should be removed only on completion of treatment.
(a) Ensuring the appropriate channel lights are green. If the other patient's treatment is continuing, interrupt treatment.	
(b) Ensure time display on the selectron unit reads zero for the appropriate channels. Ensure the print-out indicates treatment has stopped for those channels.	
2 Record the finish time on the patient's dosimetry sheet.	This is kept as a record in the patient's notes.

3	Check the close circuit television camera is not focused on the patient.	To ensure privacy.
4	Explain the procedure to the patient.	To obtain patient's consent and co-operation.
5	Ensure any pre-removal drugs have been administered.	To allow analgesic or sedative effect to be felt.
6	Assist the patient into a comfortable position with her knees apart.	To allow access to the applicators.
7	Uncouple the plastic transfer tubes by rotating the black coupling anticlockwise in the direction of the arrow and very carefully store the tubes on the plastic supporting mantle attached to the selectron unit.	To prevent the plastic catheter becoming damaged or kinked.
8	Place rubber caps on the ends of the applicators.	To ensure no fluid or debris is allowed to enter the applicator tubes.
9	Commence administration of Entonox (see p. 145) at least 2 minutes prior to removal of the applicators.	To allow the effect of the gas to be felt.
10	Prepare the equipment and put on gloves.	The procedure is clinically clean and not aseptic.
11	Remove the vulval dressing pads, any sutures and vaginal packing.	These must be removed before the applicators can be eased out.
12	Dismantle the applicators by loosening the screws holding them together. Remove the uterine tube first ensuring it is taken out complete with its small white flange, followed by the ovoids.	To promote ease of removal. To prevent the flange being left in the patient's vagina.
13	Remove the catheter, swab the vulval area and ensure the patient has a clean sanitary pad and a fresh draw sheet.	To promote cleanliness and patient comfort.
14	The patient can then be assisted into a comfortable position and is permitted up to have a bath.	The patient is reassured that the procedure has been completed, that she is no longer radioactive and can resume normal activities.

Applicators are carefully retained for cleaning in accordance with local policies.
Remaining treatment can then be given to the second patient.

NURSING CARE PLAN

See also Nursing Care Plan for conventional gynaecological sources, p. 329.

Problem	Cause	Suggested action
Patient removes the applicators herself.	Confusion, e.g. post-anaesthetic.	Interrupt treatment. Deposit applicators and attached tubing in the lead pot. Inform radiotherapist and physicist. Restart treatment if two patients are being treated.

Problem	Cause	Suggested action
Applicator is partially dislodged.	Patient may have moved too much or too vigorously.	Interrupt treatment. Inform physicist and radiotherapist. The applicator may have to be removed as above.
Alarm sounding at nurse station.	Treatment has been interrupted and inadvertently left off.	Check patient is unattended and recommence treatment.
Sources are not transferred to the applicators.	Incorrect coupling or loose connection.	Check print-out to identify which channel is at fault. Tighten appropriate coupling device.
Alarm activated at remote control unit.	Failure in the system.	Check the error code on the print-out with the selectron users' manual. Rectify as indicated in the manual or seek technical assistance from the physics department.
Pellets stuck in the applicator or transfer tubing.	A damaged or kinked catheter.	Inform the physics department. Withdraw the plastic catheter using long-handled forceps and deposit in the protected container until technical assistance can be provided. Reassure the patient.

34

Specimen Collection

Definition

Specimen collection is the collection of a required amount of tissue or fluid for laboratory examination.

Indications

Specimen collection is required when microbiological, biochemical or other laboratory investigations are indicated. Nursing staff should be able to identify the need for microbiological investigations and, if appropriate, initiate the taking of specimens. Specimen collection is often a first crucial step in investigations that define the nature of the disease and determine diagnosis and the mode of treatment.

REFERENCE MATERIAL
General principles

Successful laboratory diagnosis depends on the collection of specimens at the appropriate time, using the correct technique and equipment and transporting them to the designated laboratory safely without delay. For this to be achieved, good liaison is essential between medical, nursing, portering and laboratory staff. The nurse's role is:

1 to identify the need and importance for microbiological investigation;
2 to initiate, if appropriate, the taking of a swab or specimen, e.g. during wound dressing it is usually the nurse who identifies signs of infection;
3 to know the appropriate investigation to be taken so as to avoid indiscriminate specimen collection which wastes time and money;
4 to collect the desired material in the correct container;
5 to arrange prompt delivery to the laboratory.

Collection of specimens

The greater the quantity of material sent for laboratory examination, the greater the chance of isolating a causative organism. Anaerobic and other fastidious micro-

organisms particularly are more likely to survive. It is, therefore, preferable to send a few millimetres of pus aspirated with a sterile syringe than to send a swab. Specimens are readily contaminated by poor technique. Cultures taken from such specimens often result in confusing or misleading results.

Specimens should always be collected in sterile containers with close-fitting lids. Swabs should never be removed from their sterile containers until everything is ready for taking the sample.

Ideally samples should be collected before beginning any treatment, e.g. antibiotics or antiseptics. If the patient is receiving such treatment at the same time the specimen is collected, the laboratory staff must be informed. Both antibiotics and antiseptics may destroy organisms that are, in fact, active in the patient and will affect the outcome of the laboratory tests.

Documentation

Requests for microbiological investigations must include the following information:

1   patient's name, ward and/or department;
2   hospital number;
3   date collected;
4   time collected;
5   diagnosis;
6   relevant signs and symptoms;
7   relevant history, e.g. recent foreign travel;
8   any antimicrobial drug being taken by the patient;
9   type of specimen;
10 consultant's name;
11 name of the doctor who ordered the investigation, as it may be necessary to telephone the result before the typed report is dispatched.

Without full information, it is impossible to examine a specimen adequately or to report it accurately.

Transportation of specimens

Guidelines are now available on the labelling, transport

and reception of specimens (Health Services Advisory Committee, 1986). The sooner a specimen arrives in the laboratory, the greater is the chance of organisms present surviving and being identified. Delays will cause changes that may radically alter the result. The laboratory count of bacteria in a delayed specimen could be out of all proportion to that of the specimen when it was collected.

If specimens cannot be sent to a laboratory immediately, they should be stored as follows:

1 blood culture samples in a 37 °C incubator;
2 all other specimens in a specimen refrigerator at a temperature of 4 °C.

In diagnostic pathology it is likely that at any given time there will be a number of specimens that present a risk of infection. Every health authority, therefore, must ensure that medical, nursing, phlebotomy, laboratory, portering and any other staff involved in handling specimens are trained to do so. Specimen containers must be sufficiently robust and must not leak when used. They must also be closed securely and any accidental spillage cleaned immediately. Ideally, all specimens should be placed in a double self-sealing bag with one compartment containing the request form and the other the specimen. Specimens should be transported to the laboratory in washable baskets or trays.

It is the responsibility of the person who requests and takes specimens that are known to be infectious to ensure that both the form and the container are labelled correctly to indicate danger of infection.

Types of investigation

BACTERIAL

A wide range of methods is available for obtaining cultures and identifying organisms from a specimen or swab. To employ all these tests would be time consuming and costly. Testing, therefore, tends to be selective. It is at this stage that the laboratory request form plays a particularly important part. A faecal specimen, for example, from a patient with diarrhoea who also has a recent history of foreign travel, would be investigated for organisms not normally looked for in faecal specimens from patients without such a history.

The majority of specimens undergo microscopic investigation. This is valuable as an early indication of the causative organisms in an infection. The specimen is often cultured for 24–48 hours longer in the case of blood cultures. This is followed by antibiotic sensitivity testing on any pathogenic organisms that are isolated. Normally this takes a further 24 hours.

VIRAL

Three types of technique are available for the diagnosis of viral infections:

1 electron microscopy;
2 culture;
3 serology.

For culture specimens the use of viral transport media and speed of delivery to the laboratory are important as viruses do not survive well outside the body. With good liaison, the nursing personnel should obtain the specimen when the laboratory staff have the transport ready to take it to the virus laboratories. If delays occur, the specimen should be refrigerated at a temperature of 4 °C.

The time at which specimens are collected for viral investigations is important. Many viral illnesses have a prodromal phase during which the multiplication and shedding of the virus are at a peak and the patient is at his/her most infectious.

SEROLOGICAL

Serological testing for the presence of antigens and antibodies is used when it is not possible to isolate the organism from the patient's tissue easily. By demonstrating serum antibodies to suspected organisms it is inferred that the patient is, or has been, infected with the organism. A single test is inadequate as if the titres are raised it is impossible to determine whether this is due to past or present infection. Two tests need to be carried out, both of which involve the collection of 10 ml of blood once at the beginning of the illness and again 10–14 days later. If a rising titre level is demonstrated it suggests the patient's infection is current.

MYCOSIS

Although many pathogenic fungi will grow on ordinary bacteriological culture media, they grow better and with less risk of bacterial overgrowth on special mycological media. Alternatively, they may be demonstrated in skin and nail scraping. The presence of fungi in clinical specimens is difficult to interpret as *Candida albicans*, for example, is commonly present in the upper respiratory, alimentary and female genital tract and on the skin of healthy people.

MYCOBACTERIOLOGICAL

For further information, please refer to the procedure on tuberculosis (pp. 37–40).

PROTOZOA

Most protozoa do not cause disease but those that do, e.g. malaria, make a formidable contribution to human illness (Akinola, 1984). Laboratory investigations depend on direct microscopy which necessitates specimens being delivered to the laboratory as quickly as possible.

BLOOD
For information on the collection of blood see the procedure on Venepuncture (pp. 404–11).

References and further reading
Akinola, J. (1984) Malaria, *Nursing Times*, Vol. 80, no. 38, pp. 40–3.
Ayton, M. (1982) Microbiological investigations, *Nursing*, Vol. 2, no. 8, pp. 26–9, 232.
Hargiss, C.O. and Larson, E. (1981) How to collect specimens and evaluate results, *American Journal of Nursing*, Vol. 81, pp. 2166–74.
Health Services Advisory Committee (1986) *Safety in Health Services Laboratories: the Labelling, Transport and Reception of Specimens*, HMSO, London.
Parker, M.J. (1982) *Microbiology for Nurses*, 6th edn, Baillière Tindall, London.
Smith, A.L. (1985) *Principles of Microbiology*, 10th edn, C.V. Mosby, St Louis.
Wilson, M.E. and Mizer, H.E. (1969) *Microbiology in Nursing Practice*, Macmillan, London.

GUIDELINES: SPECIMEN COLLECTION

Procedure

Action	Rationale
1 Explain the procedure to the patient and ensure privacy while the procedure is being carried out.	To obtain the patient's consent and co-operation.
2 Wash hands.	Hand washing greatly reduces the risk of infection transfer.
3 Place specimens and swabs in the appropriate, correctly labelled containers.	To ensure that only organisms for investigation are preserved.
4 Dispatch specimens to the laboratory with the completed request form promptly.	To ensure the best possible conditions for any laboratory examinations.

EYE SWAB

Action	Rationale
1 Using either a plastic loop or a cotton wool-covered wooden stick, hold the swab parallel to the cornea and gently rub the conjunctiva in the lower eyelid.	To ensure that a swab of the correct site is taken. To avoid contamination by touching the eyelid.
2 If possible, smear the conjunctival swab on an agar plate at the bedside.	Eye swabs are often unsatisfactory because of the action of tears, which contain the enzyme lysozyme which acts as an antiseptic. Conjunctival scrapings are preferable. This procedure is usually performed by medical staff.

NOSE SWAB

Action	Rationale
1 Moisten the swab beforehand with sterile water.	To prevent discomfort to the patient. The healthy nose is virtually dry and a dry swab may cause discomfort.

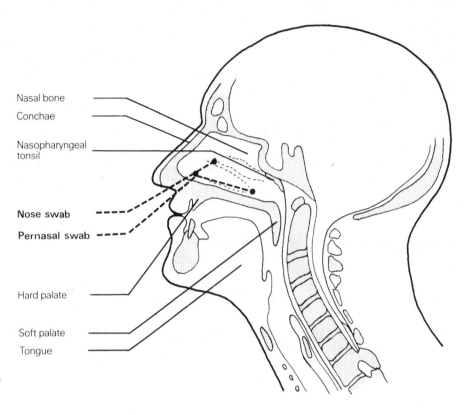

Nasal bone
Conchae
Nasopharyngeal tonsil

Nose swab

Pernasal swab

Hard palate

Soft palate
Tongue

Figure 34.1 Area to be swabbed when sampling the nose.

Action	Rationale
2 Move the swab from the anterior nares and direct it upwards into the tip of the nose (Figure 34.1).	To swab the correct site and to obtain the required sample.
3 Gently rotate the swab.	

PERNASAL SWAB (FOR WHOOPING COUGH)

Action	Rationale
1 Using a special soft-wire mounted swab, pass it along the floor of the nasal cavity to the posterior wall of the nasopharynx (see Figure 34.1).	To minimize trauma to nasal tissue. To obtain a swab from the correct site.
2 Rotate the swab gently.	

SPUTUM

Action	Rationale
1 Use a specimen container that is free from organisms of respiratory origin. This need not, therefore, be a sterile container.	Sputum is never free from organisms since material originating in the bronchi and alveoli has to pass through the pharynx and mouth, areas that have a normal commensal population of bacteria.

2 Care should be taken to ensure that the material sent for investigation is sputum, not saliva.

3 Encourage patients who have difficulty producing sputum to cough deeply first thing in the morning. Alternatively, a physiotherapist should be called to assist.

To facilitate expectoration.

4 Send any sputum specimen to the laboratory immediately.

The bacterial population alters rapidly and rapid dispatch should ensure accurate results.

THROAT SWAB

Action

1 Ask the patient to sit in such a position that he/she is facing a strong light source. Depress the patient's tongue with a spatula.

2 Quickly, but gently, rub the swab over the prescribed area, usually the onsillar fossa or any area with a lesion or visible exudate (Figure 34.2).

3 Avoid touching any other area of the mouth or tongue with the swab.

Rationale

To ensure maximum visibility of the area to be swabbed. The procedure is one that is likely to cause the patient to gag and the tongue will move to the roof of the mouth, contaminating the specimen.

To obtain the required sample.

To prevent contamination by other organisms.

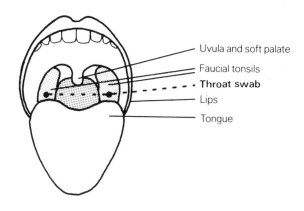

Uvula and soft palate
Faucial tonsils
Throat swab
Lips
Tongue

Figure 34.2 Area to be swabbed when sampling the throat.

EAR SWAB

Action

1 No antibiotics or other chemotherapeutic agents should have been used in the aural region 3 hours before taking the swab.

2 Place the swab into the outer ear as shown in Figure 34.3. Rotate the swab gently.

Rationale

To prevent contamination from other organisms. To prevent collection of traces of such therapeutic agents.

To avoid trauma to the ear. To collect any secretions.

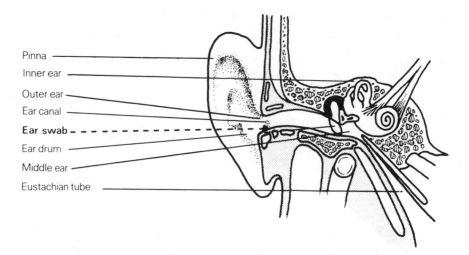

Pinna
Inner ear
Outer ear
Ear canal
Ear swab - - - - - - - -
Ear drum
Middle ear
Eustachian tube

Figure 34.3 Area to be swabbed when sampling the outer ear.

WOUND SWAB

Action	**Rationale**
1 Take any swabs required before dressing procedure begins.	To prevent collection of any therapeutic agents that may be employed in the dressing procedure.
2 Rotate the swab gently.	To collect samples. It is preferable to send samples of purulent discharge to swabs.

Note: The use of disposable gloves is recommended in the following procedures in order to prevent cross-infection.

VAGINAL SWAB

Action	**Rationale**
1 Introduce a speculum into the vagina to separate the vaginal walls. Take the swab as high as possible in the vaginal vault.	To ensure maximum visibility of the area to be swabbed. To ensure that the swab is taken from the best site. If infection by Trichomonas species is suspected, a charcoal-impregnated swab is recommended as this organism survives longer in this medium.

PENILE SWAB

Action	**Rationale**
1 Retract prepuce.	To obtain maximum visibility of area to be swabbed.
2 Rotate swab gently in the urethral meatus.	To collect any secretions.

RECTAL SWAB

Action

Rationale

1 Pass the swab, with care, through the anus into the rectum.

To avoid trauma. To ensure a rectal not an anal sample.

2 Rotate gently.

3 In patients suspected of suffering from threadworms, take the swab from the perianal region.

Threadworms lay their ova on the perianal skin.

FAECES

Action

Rationale

1 Ask the patient to defaecate into a clinically clean bedpan.

To avoid unnecessary contamination from other organisms.

2 Scoop enough material to fill a third of the specimen container using a spatula or a spoon, often incorporated in the specimen container.

To obtain a usable amount of specimen.

To prevent contamination.

3 Examine the specimen for such features as colour, consistency and odour and record your observations.

To monitor any fluctuations and trends.

4 Segments of tapeworm are easily seen in faeces and any such segments should be sent to the laboratory for identification.

Unless the head is dislodged, the tapeworm will continue to grow. Laboratory confirmation of the presence of the head is essential.

5 Patients suspected of suffering from amoebic dysentery should have any stool specimens dispatched to the laboratory immediately.

The parasite causing amoebic dysentery exists in a free-living nonmotile cyst. *Both* are characteristic in their fresh state but are difficult to identify when dead.

URINE

Action

Rationale

1 Specimens of urine should be collected as soon as possible after the patient wakens in the morning and at the same time each morning if more than one specimen is required.

The bladder will be full as urine has accumulated overnight. If specimens are taken at other times, the urine may be diluted. All specimens will be comparable if taken at the same time each morning.

2 Dispatch all specimens to the laboratory as soon after collection as possible.

Urine specimens should be examined within 2 hours of collection or 24 hours if kept refrigerated at a temperature of 4 °C. At room temperature overgrowth will occur and lead to misinterpretation. The cellular elements of urine break up quickly. Boric acid is sometimes used in specimen containers as a urine preservative.

MIDSTREAM SPECIMEN OF URINE: MALE

Action	Rationale
1 Retract the prepuce and clean the skin surrounding the urethral meatus with soap and water, saline or a solution that does not contain a disinfectant.	To prevent other organisms contaminating the specimen. Disinfectants may irritate or be painful to the urethral mucous membrane.
2 Ask the patient to direct the first and last part of his stream into a urinal or toilet but to collect the middle part of his stream into a sterile container.	To avoid contamination of the specimen with organisms normally present on the skin.

MIDSTREAM SPECIMEN OF URINE: FEMALE

Action	Rationale
1 Clean the urethral meatus with soap and water, saline or a solution that does not contain a disinfectant.	To prevent other organisms contaminating the specimen. Disinfectants may irritate or be painful to the urethral mucous membrane.
2 (a) Use a separate wool swab for each swab. (b) Swab from the front to the back.	To prevent cross-infection. To prevent perianal contamination.
3 Ask the patient to micturate into a bedpan or toilet. Place a sterile receiver or a wide-mouthed container under the stream and remove before the stream ceases.	To avoid contamination of the specimen with organisms normally present on the skin.
4 Transfer the specimen into a sterile container.	

SPECIMEN OF URINE FROM AN ILEAL CONDUIT
For further information see the relevant section in the procedure on stoma care (pp. 344–54).

CATHETER SPECIMEN OF URINE
For further information see the relevant section in the procedure on urinary catheterization (pp. 393–403).

24-HOUR URINE COLLECTION

Action	Rationale
1 Request the patient to void his/her bladder at the time appointed to begin this procedure. Discard this specimen.	To ensure the urine collected is that produced in the 24 hours stated.
2 All urine passed in the next 24 hours is collected in a large specimen bottle. The final specimen is collected at exactly the same time the bladder was voided 24 hours earlier.	Body chemistry alters constantly. A 24-hour collection will accommodate all the variables within a representative period.
3 Care must be taken to ensure the patient understands the procedure in order to eliminate the risk of an incomplete collection.	A 24-hour collection will not be obtained if one sample is lost and the results will be invalid.

SEMEN

Action	Rationale
1 Sexual intercourse should not have taken place for 3–4 days before the specimen is collected.	To ensure the sperm count will be at maximum levels. It takes between 3–4 days for the sperm count to return to normal after ejaculation.
2 A fresh masturbated specimen must be collected in a sterile container and delivered to the laboratory within 2 hours of the collection of the specimen.	Sperm will die if there is a delay in testing. Specimens must not be collected in a condom as sperm die when in contact with materials such as rubber.

CERVICAL SCRAPE

Action	Rationale
1 The ideal time for smear testing is mid-cycle.	To allow for accuracy of results as the cervix is usually free of contamination from menstrual flow at this time.
2 The menses should be avoided.	This is less uncomfortable for the patient.
3 The smear must be taken before a vaginal examination is carried out.	To ensure normal tissue samples are obtained.
4 Label the ground glass end of the slide with the patient's name.	To ensure patient identification.
5 Expose the cervix by using a dry speculum or one moistened with warm tap water.	To ensure maximum visibility. Greasy lubricants inhibit specimen collection.
6 Using the bilobed end of the cervical spatula, scrape firmly but gently around the squamocolumnar junction of the cervix. If the os is splayed open or scarred, a wider sweep with the broad end of the spatula may be necessary.	To obtain a usable amount of specimen.
7 Smear both sides of the spatula evenly on the slide with one stroke from each side of the spatula.	To ensure complete specimens.
8 Fix immediately.	To preserve the specimen and ensure accurate results.
9 Allow the fixing agents to dry for 20 minutes.	Dry specimens are less likely to be damaged.
10 Place the slides in a transport container.	To safeguard delicate glass slides.
11 Send, with a completed cervical cytology request form, to the appropriate laboratory.	

35

Stoma Care

Definition

'Stoma' is a word of Greek origin meaning 'mouth' or 'opening'. A bowel or urinary stoma is usually created on the abdominal wall as a diversionary procedure because the urinary or colonic tract beyond the position of the stoma is no longer viable.

Indications

Stoma care is required for the following purposes:
1 to achieve and maintain patient comfort and security;
2 to maintain good skin and stoma hygiene.

REFERENCE MATERIAL
Types of stoma
COLOSTOMY

In a colostomy the stoma may be formed from any section of the large bowel, e.g. 'end' or 'terminal' sigmoid colostomy (Figure 35.1).

A temporary colostomy may be raised to divert the faecal output, thus allowing healing of an anastomosis further along the colon. With a loop colostomy, a rod or bridge may be used to maintain a hold on the abdominal surface. Such a rod or bridge is removed 7–10 days after insertion (Figure 35.2).

ILEOSTOMY

In an ileostomy the ileum is brought out onto the abdominal wall (Figure 35.3), as when, for example, the large colon is affected by inflammatory disease.

ILEAL LOOP, ILEAL CONDUIT OR UROSTOMY

The performance of such operations requires the ureters to be transplanted from the bladder into a length, approximately 15 cm, of ileum which has been isolated, along with its mesentery, from the remainder of the small bowel. One end of the ileum, with the resected ureters, remains inside the abdomen, while the other is brought out on to the abdominal wall and everted to form a slightly protruding stoma (Figure 35.3).

OTHER TYPES OF URINARY DIVISION

Other types of urinary divisions include ureterostomy, a procedure that brings the ureters out onto the abdominal wall together (one stoma) or separately (two stomas).

Indications for surgery

1 Carcinoma of the bladder.
2 Carcinoma of the bowel.
3 Carcinoma of the pelvis.
4 Trauma.
5 Neurological damage.
6 Congenital disorders.
7 Ulcerative colitis.
8 Diverticular disease.
9 Familial polyposis.
10 Intractable incontinence.
11 Crohn's disease.

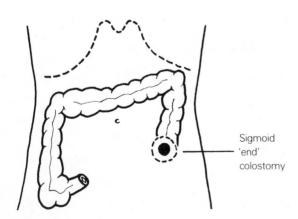

Figure 35.1 Sigmoid 'end' colostomy.

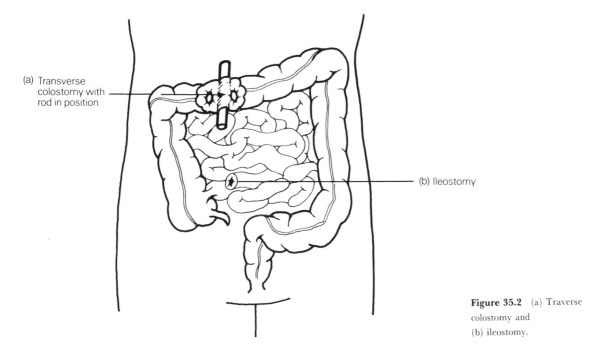

(a) Transverse colostomy with rod in position

(b) Ileostomy

Figure 35.2 (a) Traverse colostomy and (b) ileostomy.

Preoperative preparation for stoma surgery

Physical preparation of the patient will vary according to the type of operation and the policies of individual surgeons and hospitals. This will involve the usual preparation for anaesthesia, preparation of the area of the body involved and of the bowel. Other specific procedures may also be included.

Psychological preparation of the individual facing stoma surgery should begin as soon as surgery has been considered. Boore (1978) and Hayward (1978) have illustrated the importance of preoperative information

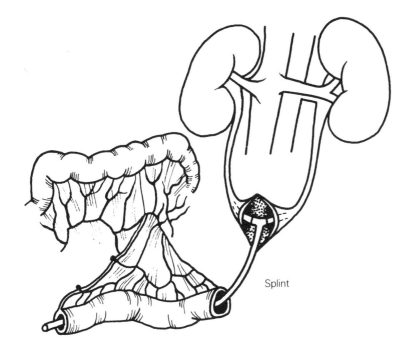

Splint

Figure 35.3 Urostomy.

and explanation in reducing postoperative physical and psychological stress. The aims of presenting such information are as follows:

1   to help the individual with a stoma to return to his/her previous place in society whenever possible;
2   to help in the process of adapting to a changed body image;
3   to reduce anxiety. The individual's perception of life with a stoma may have a positive or detrimental influence on his/her rehabilitation. There may be myths and wrong information to dispel and his/her awareness of the experiences of another ostomist to discuss;
4   to explain that the presence of a stoma need not adversely affect any previous quality of life such as hobbies, work, social life or any other interests, although the underlying disease might;
5   to prepare the individual for the appearance and likely behaviour pattern of the stoma;
6   to reassure the individual that he/she will be able to manage an appliance whatever the environment;
7   to assure the individual that he/she will be supported fully while in hospital and will not be discharged until he/she is confident about the stoma's care, and that continuing support will be available in the community.

Such preoperative education has been shown to increase co-operation and trust and to reduce anxiety, the length of time the individual remains in hospital and the amount of postoperative analgesia required. It should be borne in mind that any information given should be relevant to the patient's needs. Family and/or close friends may also be involved when appropriate, on agreement with the patient.

DIET
All patients should be encouraged to eat a wide variety of foods.

Colostomy

It should be pointed out that certain foods may cause diarrhoea or excess flatus. It is suggested that rather than eliminate these items from the diet, the foods identified should be tried again in smaller portions. No food item affects everyone in the same way and it is best for the individual to experiment. He/she may prefer to reduce the portion and prepare for the consequences. Beer may cause excess flatus. Other forms of alcohol will affect the ostomist as they do everyone else.

Ileostomy

Certain foods will cause excess flatus and pulses, cabbage, dried fruit, peanuts and coconut will be digested slowly. If eaten, therefore, they will need to be masticated well before swallowing.

Urostomy

There are no dietary restrictions. It must be stressed, however, that an adequate fluid intake must be maintained to minimize the risk of urinary infection. Approximately 1.5 litres or 12 cups per day is recommended. The slow return of both a normal appetite and bowel function is a common feature following this operation and it gives cause for much anxiety. The individual should be warned of this and advised to take small, light meals supplemented by nutritious drinks. Normal appetite may not return for 2–3 months after the operation.

FEAR OF MALODOUR
This is a common fear often based on hearsay or experience with other ostomists in hospital or the community. Appliances are usually odour free when fitted correctly. Flatus may be released via charcoal filters and deodorizers are available. The individual must be reassured, however, that any problems that occur postoperatively will be investigated, with a good possibility of them being solved by such means as the use of alternative appliances or alteration of diet.

SEX AND THE OSTOMIST
The possibility of sexual impairment for both men and women after stoma surgery depends on the nature of the operation and ensuing damage to the nerves and tissues involved. Impairment may be permanent or temporary. In the latter case, resolution of the difficulty may take anything up to 2 years. Pre- and postoperative counselling may be required for both patient and partner. In cases of male impotence, surgical intervention, such as insertion of penile implants, may be offered if impairment becomes permanent. Useful surveys of the psychosocial and sexual aspects will be found in Devlin and Plant (1979) and MacDonald (1982).

Female patients may experience narrowing or shortening of the vagina and require lubrication, for example with petroleum jelly.

Acceptance of a change in the individual's body image may take months or years, as may acceptance of the loss of bladder or bowel control.

PERSONNEL WHO MAY BE EXPECTED TO PROVIDE INFORMATION
1   Medical staff.
2   Stoma care nurse.
3   Nursing staff on the ward.
4   Primary care team.
5   Another suitable ostomist. 'Visitors' are trained by

the voluntary associations and should be, ideally, of similar age, sex and background to the patient.

USEFUL AIDS
1 Information booklets.
2 Samples of the various appliances.
3 Diagrams.

These aids are valuable to reinforce and clarify the verbal information.

Preoperative assessment
It is important to determine whether an individual will be able to manage a stoma by assessing the following:
1 eyesight;
2 manual dexterity;
3 the presence of other debilitating diseases, e.g. Parkinson's disease or arthritis;
4 mental confusion;
5 loss of limb;
6 skin conditions;
7 abdominal contours, e.g. the changes that occur with spina bifida.

Siting of the stoma is one of the most important preoperative tasks to be carried out by the doctor, stoma care nurse or experienced ward nurse (Figure 35.4). This minimizes future problems such as skin diseases or interference by the stoma with clothes. Among the priorities to be considered should be the following:
1 a flat area of the skin to facilitate safe adhesion of appliance;
2 avoidance of bony prominences such as hips or ribs;
3 avoidance of skin creases, especially in the region of the groin or the umbilicus;

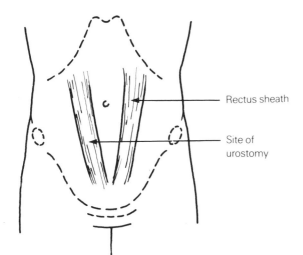

Figure 35.4 Site of urostomy.

4 avoidance of scars;
5 avoidance of waistline or belt areas;
6 maintenance of the stoma within the rectus sheath, as this reduces the risk of herniation later. The muscle may be identified by asking the patient to lie flat and then to raise his/her head. The muscle may also be palpated and easily felt when the patient coughs;
7 the individual must be able to see the stoma site.

The individual must be observed lying, sitting in a comfortable chair, with the abdominal muscles relaxed, and standing. Consideration must be given to any bending or lifting involved with his/her work and any other activities in which he/she partakes. Account must also be taken of any weight gain or loss in the postoperative period.

Postoperative period
CONTROL OF STOMA ACTION
Ileal loop
Urine will dribble from the stoma every 20–30 seconds. The output may be slightly less after periods of reduced fluid intake, e.g. at night. An appliance has to be worn at all times.

Ileostomy
The ileostomy output, normally 500–800 ml every 24 hours, is of a porridge-like consistency and contain enzymes that will excoriate the skin if contact is allowed. While the effluent cannot be controlled, the ostomist may find that the stoma is more active after main meals.

Colostomy
The transverse colostomy output may benefit from 'bulking', using one of several agents. Individuals with a sigmoid colostomy may find that wholemeal foods or synthetic agents such as Isogel and Celevac assist in producing a formed stool once or twice daily.

Medications that reduce peristaltic action, e.g. codeine phosphate, may also be used to control diarrhoea. The only means of controlling a sigmoid colostomy, however, is by regular irrigation, if used. This method must be taught under supervision to suitable ostomists.

POSTOPERATIVE STAGES
Stage I
In theatre an appropriately sized skin-protective wafer should be applied around the stoma, followed by a drainable, transparent appliance, which should be left on for approximately 5 days. For the first 48 hours postoperatively observe stoma colour (pink and healthy appearance ensures a good blood supply), size and stoma output. Appliance should always be emptied

frequently and should not be allowed to get more than half full with effluent.

If patients are unable to perform their own stoma care they will often observe those caring for them and may discuss it with them. Looking at the stoma may be very difficult for them and they may be over-aware of other people's reactions to it.

Stage II

As the individual's condition improves, he/she will be given a demonstration change of the appliance with full explanations of the principles of stoma care. This will be followed by further opportunities to discuss any problems or raise new queries. It is useful to involve the patient's partner or close friends or relatives at this stage. Their acceptance of the stoma may encourage the patient and help to restore the patient's self-esteem. In the following days patients will be encouraged to participate in and gradually assume responsibility for their own stoma care. They may now be ready to discuss appliances and choose the one that they wish to use at home. Preparation for discharge will be discussed.

Stage III

The individual should now be independent, eating a normal diet, and ready for discharge. He/she should be confident in stoma care.

The family should be closely involved during all three stages. They are also likely to require support and information so that they are in a position to help the ostomist.

SPECIFIC DISCHARGE PLANS

Follow-up support

The patient is discharged with written reminders of how to care for his/her own stoma, how to obtain supplies of appliances, and any other information that may be required. The patient should have details of non-medical stoma clinics, details about the relevant agencies and information about voluntary associations. Arrangements should also have been made for a home visit from the stoma care nurse and/or the community nurse.

Obtaining supplies

All National Health Service patients with a permanent stoma are entitled to free prescriptions for their stoma care products, and should complete the relevant exemption from payment forms. Appliances can then be obtained from the local chemist or directly from the appropriate manufacturers.

Stoma appliances and accessories

Many of the appliances available today are very similar in style, colour and efficiency and often there is very little to choose between them when the time comes for the ostomist to decide what he/she would like to wear.

The aim of good stoma care is to return the individual to his/her place in society. One of the ways in which this can be achieved is to provide him/her with a safe, reliable, appliance. This means that there must be no fear of leakage or odour and the appliance should be comfortable, unobtrusive and easy to handle. It is also necessary to ensure a problem-free skin and stoma.

APPLIANCES

Choosing the right size of appliance

Bags are labelled according to the size of the opening that fits around the stoma. To keep the skin unblemished, it must be protected from the stoma output. The size chosen, therefore, should be one that fits snugly around the stoma to within 0.5 cm of the stoma edge. This narrow edge of skin is left exposed to prevent any of the adhesives, some of which are more rigid than others, rubbing against the stoma. The appliances usually come with measuring guides to allow for correct choice of size. During the first weeks the oedematous stoma will reduce in size and the bags or flange of the two-piece type appliances will have to be changed accordingly.

Types of appliance

Although some people whose stomas were created several years ago are wearing non-disposable rubber bags, most appliances used today are made of a specially designed laminate composed of three types of plastic. This should ensure that the appliances are:

1 leak proof;
2 odourproof;
3 unobtrusive;
4 noiseless;
5 disposable.

The appliances differ slightly according to the stoma for which they are meant. All types, however, fall within one of two broad categories:

1 *One-piece*: this comprises a bag with an adhesive attached, e.g. Colodress or Coloplast. When the bag is renewed, the adhesive is removed from the skin. Its advantage is that it is easy to handle, e.g. by an ostomist suffering from rheumatism.
2 *Two-piece*: this comprises a flange, for the skin, and a bag that clips on to the flange, e.g. System 2 or Coloplast. Its advantage is that it can be used with ostomists who have a sore or sensitive skin as when bags are removed the skin is left undisturbed. Its disadvantage is that it is more difficult to handle as the bags must be clipped on securely and the flange hole needs to be cut out.

Drainable bags

1   Bowel stoma bags.
    Suitable for: ileostomy, other large bowel stomas.
    Stoma output: fluid to semiformed (volume is too great for closed bags).
    Use: emptied frequently, taking care to rinse outlet afterwards; may be left on for up to 3 days.
    Additional features: flatus filters are absent in some as the fluid would obstruct the charcoal, rendering it useless, or will leak through the small opening; the outlet may have a separate clip or fixed 'roll-up' closure.
    Colour: Clear, white, pink/beige.
2   Urinary stoma bags.
    Suitable for: urostomy.
    Stoma output: urine.
    Use: emptied frequently via a fixed tap; may be left on for up to 3 days.
    Additional features: may be used with large collecting bag and tubing for night drainage.
    Colour: clear or white.
3   Closed bags.
    Suitable for: signoid colostomy.
    Stoma output: a normal stool.
    Use: changed once or twice a day.
    Additional features: some have incorporated flatus filters that allow the release of flatus through charcoal patches that absorb the odour.
    Colour: clear, white or pink/beige.

Some may be fitted with protective adhesive especially for sensitive skin and may now have a cotton-weave backing to prevent perspiration and to prevent the plastic from sticking to the skin.

ACCESSORIES

The specific products in this section have been mentioned as examples of what aids are available and reference to them is not necessarily intended as a recommendation.

Solutions for skin and stoma cleaning

Mild soap and water, or water only, are sufficient. Detergents, disinfectants and antiseptics cause dryness and irritation and should not be used routinely. The stoma is not a wound or a lesion and should be regarded as a resited urethra or anus.

Skin barriers

1   Creams.
    Unless made specifically for use on peristomal skin, these should not be used, as the residual surface film of grease prevents adherence of the appliance.

Creams usually have a smoothing and moisturing effect.
    Use: for sensitive skin, as a preventive measure.
    Method: use sparingly; massage gently into the skin until completely absorbed, excess grease may be wiped off with a tissue.
    Example: Chiron barrier cream (aluminium chlorohydrate 2% in an emulsified base).
    Precaution: not to be used on broken or sore skin.
2   Skin gels/sealants.
    Use: Act as a film on the skin, firstly to prevent irritation, and secondly to give protection as it is removed with the adhesive of the bag, thus preventing removal of the stratum corneum of the skin.
    Method: Use sparingly; pat onto the skin gently; dries quickly.
    Example: Skin Gel, Skin Prep.
    Precaution: Should not be used on broken skin as they contain alcohol and cause stinging.
3   Lotions/sprays.
    Use: as above
    Method: applied gently.
    Example: Skin Prep spray, OpSite spray, tincture of benzoin compound lotion.
    Precaution: as above. Tincture of benzoin is a mixture of 10% benzoin and 90% alcohol. Benzoin, a balsamic resin, is ground and combined with alcohol. Sensitivities to it are common. If applied to erythematous skin it causes pain, more irritation and weeping. When applied to good skin it acts as a protective and enhances adhesion of the appliances.
4   Protective wafers.
    Use: these are hypo-allergenic and are designed to cover and protect skin, and allow healing if the skin is sore or broken. May be useful in cases of skin reaction or allergy to the adhesive of an appliance.
    Method: the wafers may be cut to the required shape and fitted on to the skin. The appliances are then attached to the wafer. The rim of the wafer should not press against the stoma but should fit to 0.5 cm around it.
    Examples: Stomahesive, Comfeel and Seel a Peel. (Stomahesive is composed of gelatin, pectin, sodium carboxymethycellulose, and polyisobutylene; it adheres painlessly to normal, erythematous, moist or broken skin; it is available in three sizes.)
    Precautions: allergy may occur, but rarely.
5   Protective rings.
    Use: protective rings are used to provide skin protection around the stoma; they will protect a smaller area than the wafers mentioned above. They are also useful to fill in 'dips' or 'gulleys' in the skin.
    Method: like the wafers, they have an adhesive side

and may be applied directly to the skin. They form an integral part of some of the appliances.

Example: Karaya rings, Seel a Peel rings and Cohesive washers (Karaya is a natural product developed from an Indian plant.)

Precautions: as for protective wafers above.

6   Pastes.

Use: useful to fill in crevices and gulleys in the skin to provide a smooth surface for an appliance.

Examples: Stomahesive paste, Karaya gum paste and Orobase paste.

Method: *Stomahesive*: either leave for 60 seconds after applying to the skin, when the surface will be dry, making the paste easier to mould into the skin contour, or apply with a spatula, or wet the finger first to prevent the paste sticking and mould the paste immediately. Will sting on raw areas as it contains alcohol. Apply a little Orahesive powder to these areas first. *Orobase*: Similar to Stomahesive in composition but with the addition of liquid paraffin. For protection of raw areas. Does not contain alcohol so will not cause local irritation.

7   Powders.

Use: for protection of sore or raw areas without impeding adhesion of the appliance.

Method: sprinkle on affected areas:

Examples: Karaya powder and Orahesive powder.

Adhesive preparations

1   Sprays.

Use: only required when appliance does not adhere well to the skin, e.g. due to leakage problems, difficult stoma site, or with abdominal fistulae.

Method: spray on appliance, not on the skin. Follow specific instructions on packaging. Removal should not be difficult.

Examples: Dow Corning Adhesive.

Precaution: the individual products differ considerably in their method of application and it is recommended that the user consults the manufacturer's instructions.

2   Lotions.

Use: as above

Method: pat gently onto skin. The individual products differ considerably in their method of application and it is recommended that the user consults the manufacturer's instructions.

Examples: Saltair solution and tincture of benzoin compound.

Deodorants

1   Aerosols.

Use: absorb odour.

Method: one or two puffs into the air before emptying or removal of appliance.

Examples: Atmacol and Oziom.

2   Drops and powders.

Use: for deodorizing bag contents.

Methods: one drop into appliance.

Examples: Dor (drops), Ostobon (powder) and Nilodor (drops).

Precaution: Beware of over enthusiastic use which may result in a strong and distinctive odour that will become associated with stoma care.

3   Other traditional methods.

Examples: Crushed aspirin, charcoal tablets and natural yoghurt.

4   Flatus filters (charcoal filled).

Use: to allow gradual release of flatus from the bag while allowing absorption of odour by the charcoal. The charcoal may only be effective for between 6 and 12 hours, depending on brand of filter. The filter will then require replacing with a fresh one.

Method: The individual products differ considerably in their method of application and it is recommended that the user consults the manufacturer's instructions.

Examples: Filtrodor and Surgicare flatus filters.

Precautions: use of flatus filters is not advised when the stoma effluent is very fluid as the charcoal may become moist and the air outlet blocked. Many bags now have built-in filters.

Useful addresses

1   Association of Spina Bifida and Hydrocephalus, Tavistock House North, Tavistock Square, London SW1V 1PS (Tel: 01–388 1382/5).

2   Colostomy Welfare Group, 38/39 Eccleston Square, London SW1V 1PB (Tel: 01–828 5175).

3   Ileostomy Association of Great Britain, Amblehurst House, Black Scotch Lane, Mansfield, Nottingham NG18 4PF.

4   Urostomy Association, Buckland, Beaumont Park, Danbury, Essex CM3 4DE.

References and further reading

Bailey, A.J. (1977) Nursing the patient with a colostomy, *Nursing Times*, Vol. 73, pp. 382–185.

Boore, J.R.P. (1978) *A Prescription for Recovery: the Effects of Preoperative Preparation of Surgical Patients on Postoperative Stress, Recovery and Infection*, Royal College of Nursing, London.

Breckman, B. (1981) *Stoma Care*, Beaconsfield Publishers, Beaconsfield.

Broadwell, D.C. and Jackson, B.S. (1982) *Principles of Ostomy Care*, C.V. Mosby, St Louis

Brooke, B.N. *et al.* (1982) *Stomas*, W.B. Saunders.

Cassel, P. (1980) Management of ulcerative colitis,

Nursing (1st series), no. 17, pp. 727–9.

Coloplast (undated) *Back on Your Feet Again*, Coloplast.

Devlin, H.B. and Plant, J. (1979) Sexual function – an aspect of stoma care, *British Journal of Sexual Medicine*, Vol. 1, pp. 33–34, 37; 2, 6, 22, 26

Gray, A. (1980) A new lease of life, *Nursing Times*, Vol. 76, pp. 1616–20.

Hayward, J. (1978) *Information – A Prescription Against Pain*, Royal College of Nursing, London.

MacDonald, L. (1982) Problems of the colostomy population, *Stoma Care News* Vol. 1, p. 45. *Nursing*

Mirror (1983) Clinical Forum 8: Stoma Care, *Nursing Mirror*, Vol. 157, no. 11, Supplement.

Squibb Surgicare (undated) *Understanding Colostomy*, Squibb Surgicare.

Squibb Surgicare (undated) *Understanding Urostomy*, Squibb Surgicare.

Turner, A.G. (1979) Urinary diversion, *Journal of Community Nursing*, Vol. 2, no. 10, pp. 20–1, 28

Whitethread, M. (1981) Ostomists: a world of difference, *Journal of Community Nursing*, Vol. 5, no. 2, pp. 4–5, 10.

GUIDELINES: STOMA CARE

These procedural guidelines contain the basic information needed for changing a stoma appliance. Modifications may be made according to the following factors:

1   the place of change, i.e. bathroom, bedside, availability of sink, etc.;
2   the person changing the appliance, i.e. nurse or patient;
3   type of appliance used, e.g. one- or two-piece, closed or drainable;
4   any accessories used, e.g. flatus filters, hypo-allergenic tape, barrier creams, etc.

Equipment

1   Clean tray holding
    (a)   tissues;
    (b)   new appliances;
    (c)   disposal bags for used appliances and tissues;
    (d)   relevant accessories, e.g. flatus filters, tape, etc.
2   Bowl of warm water
3   Soap
4   Jug for contents of appliance
5   Gloves. (It is now common practice and, in many cases, hospital policy, to wear gloves when dealing with blood and body fluids. Thus they should be worn for cleaning stomas. It is recognized that it could be difficult to attach an appliance with gloves *in situ* (due to the adhesive), but once the stoma has been cleaned of excreta and blood, the gloves may be removed to apply the bag.)

Procedure

Action	Rationale
1 Inform the patient of the proposed activity.	To obtain the patient's consent and co-operation.
2 Explain the procedure.	To familiarize the patient with the procedure.
3 Ensure that the patient is lying in a suitable and comfortable position where the patient will be able to watch the procedure, if he/she is well enough.	To allow good access to the stoma for cleaning and for secure application of the stoma bag. The patient will become familiar with the stoma and will also learn much about the care of the stoma by observation of the nurse.

Action	Rationale
4 Use a small protective pad to protect the patient's clothing from drips if the effluent is fluid and apply gloves for nurse's protection.	Prevents the necessity of renewing clothing or bedclothes and demoralization of the patient due to any soiling.
5 If the bag is of the drainable type, empty the contents into a jug before removing the bag.	For ease of handling the appliance and prevention of spillage.
6 Remove the appliance. Peel the adhesive off the skin with one hand while exerting gentle pressure on the skin with the other.	To reduce trauma to the skin. Erythema as a result of removing the appliance is normal and quickly settles.
7 Remove excess faeces or mucus from the stoma with a dry tissue.	So that the stoma and surrounding skin are clearly visible.
8 Examine the skin and stoma for soreness, ulceration or other unusual phenomena. If the skin is unblemished and the stoma is a healthy red colour, proceed.	For the prevention of complications or the treatment of existing problems.
9 Wash the skin and stoma gently until they are clean.	To promote cleanliness and prevent skin excoriation.
10 Dry the skin and stoma gently but thoroughly.	The appliance will attach more securely to dry skin.
11 Apply a clean appliance.	
12 Dispose of soiled tissues and the used bag. Rinse the bag through in the sluice with water, wrap it in a disposable bag and place it in an appropriate plastic bin. At home the bag should be emptied into the toilet; a closed bag may be cut at the lower end, then rinsed using a jug or by holding it under the flushing water. Wrap the bag in newspaper, tie it in a plastic bag and dispose of it in a rubbish bag.	Faecal material in waste bags is a potential source of infection. Excreta should be disposed of down the sluice.
13 Wash hands thoroughly.	To prevent spread of infection by contaminated hands.

GUIDELINES: COLLECTION OF A SPECIMEN OF URINE FROM AN ILEAL CONDUIT OR UROSTOMY

Equipment
1 Sterile dressing pack
2 Soft catheter – tracheal type, not larger than 12 or 14 gauge
3 Sterile gloves
4 Disposable plastic apron
5 Universal specimen container
6 Skin cleansing solution, e.g. Savlodil
7 Alcohol-based hand wash solution, e.g. Hibisol
8 Clean stoma appliance
9 Clean topical swabs.

Procedure

Action	**Rationale**
1 Explain the procedure to the patient.	To gain the patient's consent and co-operation.
2 Ensure that the patient is in a comfortable position, e.g. sitting up, supported by pillows, and that the stoma is easily accessible.	
3 Screen the bed, then wash and dry hands.	For the patient's privacy and to reduce the risk of cross-infection. Curtains are drawn at this stage so that dust and airborne organisms disturbed by the curtains do not settle on the sterile trolley.
4 Prepare the trolley and take it to the patient's bedside.	
5 Put on a disposable plastic apron.	To prevent cross-infection.
6 Remove the sterile dressing pack, catheter and receiver from their outer wrappings. Place them on the top shelf of the trolley.	
7 Remove the appliance from the stoma and cover the stoma with a clean topical swab.	To absorb spillage from the stoma.
8 Clean hands with an alcohol-based hand wash solution, such as Hibisol, and put on sterile gloves before opening the sterile field on the trolley.	To reduce the risk of introducing infection into the stoma during the procedure.
9 Remove the gauze with forceps and discard it. Arrange a sterile towel to absorb spillage from the stoma.	To keep the areas as clean as possible and to protect the patient and the bedclothes from spilled urine.
10 Clean around the stoma with a skin cleansing solution, such as Savlodil, from the centre outwards. Dry the area.	Good cleansing of the area reduces the risk of introduction of surface pathogens into the ileal loop.
11 Insert the catheter tip gently to a depth of 2.5–5 cm only and wait for urine to drain through. Collect the sample in the specimen container. The recommended volume is 3–5 ml.	Gentle handling reduces the risk of ileal perforation and is more comfortable for the patient.
12 Remove the catheter and seal in the specimen container. Remove gloves and attend to stoma care and apply a pouch as usual. Make the patient comfortable.	
13 Dispose of equipment.	
14 Wash and dry hands.	To prevent cross-infection.
15 Check that the specimen is labelled correctly and dispatch it to the laboratory with the appropriate forms.	

NURSING CARE PLAN

Problem	Cause	Suggested action
Leakage of urine or faeces.	Ill-fitting appliance.	The opening of the appliance should fit snugly around the stoma.
	Skin creases or 'gulleys' preventing correct application of adhesive.	Build up indented areas and fill in gulleys to create a smooth surface, e.g. using Stomahesive past.
	Infrequent emptying of drainable bag leading to stress on adhesion.	Drainable bags should be emptied frequently, e.g. 2–3-hourly if necessary.
Sore skin.	Leakage.	As above.
	Skin reaction to adhesive.	Change the make of appliance or apply a protective square between skin and adhesive. Anti-inflammatory agents may be required for very severe reactions.
	Poor hygiene.	Improve the technique of nurses or patient.
Odour.	Ill-fitting appliance; lack of seal between skin and adhesive.	Fit the appliance with care. Consider a change of the type of appliance.
	Poor hygiene.	Improve the technique of nurses or patient.
	Poor technique, e.g. when emptying drainable bag.	Empty the bag, then rinse the end with water to ensure that it is clean before closing.
	Ineffective flatus filters.	Use another type of filter or change the filter more frequently. (Filters should be peeled off and replaced as necessary.) Effectiveness lasts 6–12 hours.

UROSTOMY SPECIMEN

Problem	Cause	Suggested action
Stoma specimen of urine contaminated.	Contaminants introduced during specimen collection.	Take a repeat specimen, observing aseptic procedure and cleaning the stoma well.
Ileum perforated during urine specimen collection.	Catheter too hard or inserted too roughly	Report to a doctor immediately.
Difficulty passing catheter into conduit.	Small degree of retraction of ileum.	Apple gentle pressure to the area around the stoma to make it protrude.
	Unpredictable direction of ileum.	Insert your little (gloved) finger gently into the stoma to determine the direction of the conduit. Insert the catheter tip along this line.

36

Syringe Driver

Definition

The syringe driver is a portable, battery-operated device for mechanically delivering drugs at a predetermined rate, via the appropriate route.

Indications

Syringe drivers are used to deliver postoperative analgesia, heparin, insulin, cytotoxic chemotherapy, hormones, anti-emetics, milk feeds and neostigmine to patients with myasthenia gravis (Dover, 1987).

REFERENCE MATERIAL

In 1979 Dr B.M. Wright developed a portable battery-operated syringe driver, used initially to administer desferrioxamine in the management of thalassaemia (Wright and Callan, 1979).

One of the areas in which syringe drivers are used most extensively is in the management of pain in patients with advanced malignancy. Further information, therefore, will concentrate on this clinical application, though the general principles of this technique remain valid in other areas.

There are a number of syringe drivers on the market at present. The Graseby MS Series (Figure 36.1) is typical of these and will be used as an example throughout. Nurses using other types should check their user's manual for rate calculations.

The driver is lightweight (weight 175 g including 9-volt battery), compact (166 × 53 × 23 mm), and can accommodate most sizes and makes of plastic syringes. The wide variety of syringes in use means that drug delivery rates must be expressed in terms of rate of plunger travel. (MS16A model: millimetres per hour; MS26 model: millimetres per 24 hours).

Calculation of rate setting

$$\text{Set rate} = \frac{\text{fluid length in mm}}{\text{infusion time in hours}}.$$

For example: diamorphine hydrochloride 120 mg pre-scribed to be infused over 24 hours, dissolved in 8 ml of sterile water:

$$8 \text{ ml} = \frac{48 \text{ mm stroke length}}{24 \text{ hours}} = 2 \text{ mm per hour delivery rate}.$$

Indications for use

The continuous subcutaneous infusion of opioids should not be viewed merely as a convenient alternative to regular oral medication (Beswick, 1987). Strict criteria for the selection of patients who would benefit from this method of administration have been suggested by several authors (Oliver, 1985; Beswick, 1987; Dover, 1987; Latham, 1987), and are summarized in Table 36.1.

Advantages in the use of the syringe driver

1 Avoids the need for 4-hourly injections, thereby increasing patient comfort.

Table 36.1   Indications For Use of the Syringe Driver

Clinical problem	Cause
Oral route inappropriate	Dysphagia
	Diminished conscious level
Altered gastrointestinal physiology	Intractable nausea/ vomiting
	Intestinal obstruction
	Malabsorption
Rectal route inappropriate	Local disease, e.g. tumour, fistulae, haemorrhoids
	Absence of rectum
	Rectal route unacceptable to patient/family

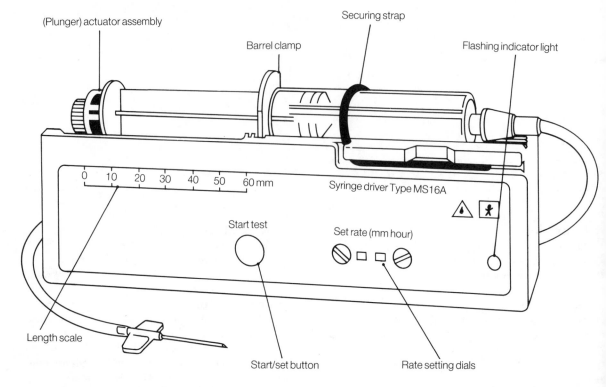

Figure 36.1   Graseby Medical MS16A syringe driver.

2   Provides stable plasma levels of analgesic without the peaks and troughs associated with intermittent parenteral therapy (Twycross and Lack, 1984).

3   This mode of administration maintains the versatility of individualized analgesic dose requirements.

4   Patients can retain mobility and independence both as inpatients and in the community.

Disadvantages in the use of the syringe driver

1   Inflammation or infection can occur at the site of cannula insertion (Oliver, 1985; Coyle *et al.*, 1986; Bruera *et al.*, 1987; Dover, 1987).

2   Rate recalculation is cumbersome if the patient's analgesic requirements are variable. This is because of the millimetre rate setting, thus making interpretation of dose titration in terms of milligramms (mgs) a complicated manoeuvre.

3   Patients may become psychologically dependent on the device, particularly if it is reserved for the control of severe exacerbations of pain. Patients will then express a reluctance to return to oral medication, fearing the return of their pain. Alternatively, some may view this mode of administration as a 'last resort', when death is imminent. Careful pa-

tient selection and preparation should minimize these misunderstandings.

4   The driver's alarm system will operate only if the pump stops for any reason, e.g. if syringe plunger has jammed or come to the end of the infusion. It does not alert the nurse in the event of skin site 'failure', cannula displacement and occlusion, or a syringe plunger out of alignment with the actuator assembly (see Figure 36.1).

5   Some problems may be experienced by ambulant patients in relation to carrying the pump. This can be overcome by the use of a shoulder holster.

Cannula selection for subcutaneous infusion

One of the most commonly used devices in the United Kingdom is the Vygon 246 100 cm Butterfly Infusion Set (21 standard wire gauge, swg; 23 swg). This is a metal cannula which appears to be reasonably well tolerated by subcutaneous tissues, although it could be argued that more inert materials, i.e. Teflon, may lengthen the lifetime of an infusion skin site (Latham, 1987). At present, no research-based information exists to either confirm or contradict this view. The 100-cm length of tubing allows the patient greatest flexibility of movement, but its 0.6-ml capacity must be taken into account when priming the system.

Skin site selection for subcutaneous infusion

The best sites to use for continuous subcutaneous infusion of drugs are the lateral aspects of the upper arms and thighs, the abdomen, the anterior chest below the clavicle and, occasionally, the back. Areas which should *not* be used for cannula placement are:

1 *Lymphoedematous limbs:* the subcutaneous tissues are 'waterlogged' with lymph fluid and the rate of absorption from a skin site would be adversely affected. A cannula breaches skin integrity thus increasing the risk of infection in a limb which is already susceptible.
2 *Site over a bony prominence*: the amount of subcutaneous tissue will be diminished, again impairing the rate of drug absorption.
3 *Previously irradiated skin area*: radiotherapy can cause sclerosis of small blood vessels, thus reducing skin perfusion (Tiffany, 1978).
4 *Site near a joint:* excessive movement may cause cannula displacement and patient discomfort.

Care of the skin site

The infusion site should be renewed when there is evidence of inflammation (erythema or reddening) or poor absorption (a hard subcutaneous swelling). The time taken for this to occur can vary from hours to over 3 weeks, dependent on the individual, and the drug(s) being infused (Regnard and Newbury, 1983; Nicholson, 1986; Coyle *et al.*, 1986; Brenneis *et al.*, 1987; Bruera *et al.*, 1987). There would appear to be a relationship between the concentration of drug(s) being infused, and the duration of a skin site (Nicholson, 1986). In one study, the average frequency of needle resiting was 5.1 days for patients receiving 7.5–30 mg of diamorphine per 24 hours, but only 2.4 days for those receiving 1,000–2,000 mg per 24 hours (Nicholson, 1986). Another study noted no statistically significant relationship between duration of skin site and sex/age of patients, type or dose of narcotic, rate of infusion, or triceps skinfold measurement (Brenneis *et al.*, 1987). Clearly, further research into the factors influencing skin site survival is required.

Drug stability and compatibility

In the context of single drug infusions, instability is not usually a clinically significant problem. The drug simply has to be:

1 available in injectable form;
2 suitable for subcutaneous administration;

3 stable in solution for the duration of the infusion (usually 24–48 hours).

For example, diamorphine hydrochloride is stable, in solution, for up to 2 weeks (Jones and Hanks, 1986).

Problems of drug instability and incompatibility arise when higher drug concentrations, and combinations of two or more drugs, are used. In addition, exposure of drug solutions to direct light and increased storage temperatures (up to 32 °C) may exacerbate the problem.

Where drug combinations (commonly an analgesic and an anti-emetic) are used, further criteria must be met:

1 the drugs must be compatible with each other;
2 the diluents must be compatible with each other;
3 each drug must be compatible with the diluent(s) of the other drug(s) in the combination.

Studies by Allwood (1984) and later work by Regnard *et al.* (1986) have examined the stability and compatibility of analgesic/anti-emetic combinations. Regnard and Davies (1986) make the following recommendations:

1 protect the syringe from direct light whenever possible;
2 visual inspection of drug solutions should be made daily, and the syringe discarded if signs of crystallization, precipitation or discoloration occur;
3 avoid high concentrations of drugs if used in combination;
4 avoid mixing more than two drugs in one syringe;
5 do not infuse anti-emetics for more than 24 hours, particularly if part of a combination of drugs.

However, it remains the responsibility of each individual practitioner to ensure that the drug(s) prescribed are suitable for continuous subcutaneous infusion, and are stable under these conditions. If in any doubt, seek advice from an appropriate professional.

References and further reading

Allwood, M.C. (1984) Diamorphine mixed with anti-emetic drugs in plastic syringes, *British Journal of Pharmaceutical Practice*, Vol. 6, pp. 88–90.

Beswick, D.T. (1987) Use of syringe driver in terminal care, *The Pharmaceutical Journal*, Vol. 239, pp. 656–8.

Brenneis, C., Michaud, M., Bruera, E. and MacDonald, R.N. (1987) Local toxicity during the subcutaneous infusion of narcotics (SCIN), *Cancer Nursing*, Vol. 10, no. 4, pp. 172–6.

Bruera, E., Brenneis, C., Michaud, M., Chadwick, S. and MacDonald, R.N. (1987) Continuous SC infusion of narcotics using a portable disposable device in patients with advanced cancer, *Cancer Treatment Reports*, Vol. 71, no. 6, pp. 635–7.

Coyle, N., Mauskop, A., Maggard, J. and Foley, K.M.

(1986) Continuous subcutaneous infusions of opiates in cancer patients with pain, *Oncology Nursing Forum*, Vol. 13, no. 4, pp. 53–7.

Dover, S.B. (1987) Syringe driver in terminal care, *British Medical Journal*, Vol. 294, pp. 553–5.

Jones, V.A. and Hanks, S.W. (1986) New portable infusion pump for prolonged administration of opioid analgesics in patients with advanced cancer, *British Medical Journal*, Vol. 292, p. 1496.

Latham, J. (1987) Syringe drivers in pain control, *The Professional Nurse*, Vol. 2, no. 7, pp. 207–9.

Nicholson, H. (1986) The success of the syringe driver, *Nursing Times*, Vol. 82, pp. 49–51.

Oliver, D.J. (1985) The use of the syringe driver in terminal care, *British Journal of Clinical Pharmacology*, Vol. 20, pp. 515–16.

Regnard, C. and Newbury, A. (1983) Pain and the portable syringe pump, *Nursing Times*, Vol. 79, pp. 25–8.

Regnard, C.F. and Davies, A. (1986) *A Guide to Symptom Relief in Advanced Cancer*, Haigh and Hochland, Manchester.

Regnard, C. *et al.* (1986) Anti-emetic/diamorphine mixture compatibility in infusion pumps, *British Journal of Pharmaceutical Practice*, Vol. 8, pp. 218–20.

Tiffany, R. (ed.) (1978) *Oncology for Nurses and Health Care Professionals*, Vol. 1, George Allen & Unwin, London.

Twycross, R.G. and Lack, S.A. (1984) *Therapeutics in Terminal Cancer*, Pitman, London.

Wright, B.M. and Callan, K. (1979) Slow drug infusions using a portable syringe driver, *British Medical Journal*, Vol. 2, p. 582.

GUIDELINES: PREPARATION OF THE SYRINGE FOR 24-HOUR DRUG ADMINISTRATION, MS16 AND MS16A

Equipment

1   Syringe driver, MS16, 16A or 26
2   9-volt battery (Duracell MN1604)
3   Syringe (Luer lock preferably)
4   100-cm butterfly infusion set
5   Mediswab
6   Transparent adhesive dressing
7   Ampoule of diluent, e.g. saline 0.9% of sterile water
8   Needle and drugs
9   Drug additive label.

Action	Rationale
1 Calculate the 24-hour dose of drug.	To ensure correct dosage.
2 Draw up the drug in a suitable syringe.	To facilitate correct administration.
3 Measure the length of the fluid in the syringe (see Figure 36.2).	This gives the stroke length necessary for calculating the rate setting.
4 If the drug can be diluted draw up sufficient diluent to give a stroke length of 24 or 48 mm.	This enables a more easily calculable and more accurate setting of the pump rate.
5 Calculate the rate setting of the pump.	To ensure the drug is given over the prescribed time period.

Note: If the set rate is a single figure, e.g. 2, this must be preceded by the figure 0 as shown, i.e. 0 2.

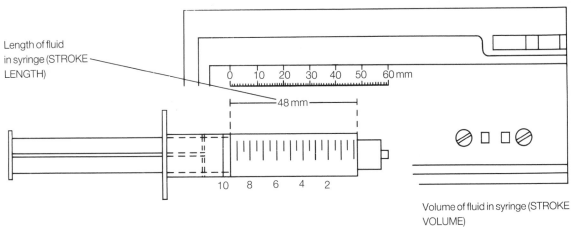

Figure 36.2 Measurement of fluid length in syringe against millimetre scale on syringe driver.

To administer drugs over time periods other than 24 hours, follow the guidelines above but substitute the alternative administration time, e.g. if the drug administration time is 6 hours, the 6-hourly drug dose should be calculated.

Similarly, in step 4, use sufficient diluent to produce a stroke length divisible by the alternative time period, e.g. for 14-hour drug administration, a stroke length of 14, 28, 42 or 56 mm could be used.

MS26 SYRINGE DRIVER

When using the MS26 syringe driver the guidelines for the MS16 and 16A models still apply. The only modification to the MS26 is a rate setting expressed in terms of mm per 24 hours and *not* mm per hour.

Calculation of the rate setting is illustrated here.

Calculation of rate setting for MS26 model

$$\text{Set rate} = \frac{\text{Fluid length in mm}}{\text{Infusion time in 24-hour periods (days)}}.$$

For example:

1   Diamorphine hydrochloride 120 mg prescribed to be infused over 24 hours, dissolved in 8 ml of sterile water.

$$8 \text{ ml} = \frac{48 \text{ mm stroke length}}{1 \times 24\text{-hour period}} = 48 \text{ mm per 24 hours}.$$

2   Diamorphine hydrochloride 360 mg prescribed to be infused over 48 hours, dissolved in 8 ml of sterile water.

$$8 \text{ mls} = \frac{48 \text{ mm stroke length}}{2 \times 24\text{-hour period}} = 24 \text{ mm per 24 hours}.$$

GUIDELINES: PRIMING THE INFUSION SET

Action	Rationale
1 Draw up a further 0.6 ml of diluent into the prepared syringe.	An extra 0.6 ml are required to prime the infusion set.
2 Connect a 100-cm winged infusion set to the syringe.	This length of tubing allows the patient greater freedom of movement.
3 Gently depress the plunger until the infusion tubing is filled up to the needle end.	This removes extraneous air from the system.
4 Recheck the stroke length.	To ensure the rate will remain as previously calculated.

GUIDELINES: INSERTING THE WINGED INFUSION SET

Action   **Rationale**

1   Explain the procedure to the patient.   To obtain the patient's consent and co-operation.

2   Assist the patient into a comfortable position.

3   Expose the chosen site for infusion (see Selection under
    Reference Material, p. 357).

4   Clean the chosen site with a swab satured with isopropyl   To reduce the number of pathogens introduced into the skin by
    alcohol and wait till alcohol evaporates.   the needle at the time of insertion.
                                                                Allowing the alcohol time to evaporate reduces pain on
                                                                insertion which may be caused by introducing alcohol.

5   Grasp the skin firmly.   To elevate the subcutaneous tissue.

6   Insert the infusion needle into the skin at an angle of 45 °C   Shallower positioning than 45 °C may shorten the life of the
    and release the grasped skin.   infusion site.

7   Tape the infusion wings firmly to the skin using   Transparent dressing allows observation of the infusion site
    transparent adhesive dressing (see Care of Skin Site   and maintains the correct position of the needle.
    under Reference Material, p. 357).

8   Connect the syringe to the syringe driver (see instructions   To ensure the syringe is correctly connected to the syringe
    below).   driver.

9   Record, in the appropriate documents, that the infusion   To comply with local drug administration policies.
    has been commenced.

Connecting the syringe to the syringe driver (see Figure 36.1)

1   Slide the actuator assembly back along the lead
    screw by pressing the actuator release button as
    shown in Figure 36.3.
2   Lay the barrel of the syringe along the grooved lines
    with a finger grip fitting in the slot above the end of
    the lead screw.
3   Secure the syringe in position using the rubber
    strap.
4   Slide the actuator assembly along the lead screw
    until it rests against the end of the plunger.
5   Press the start/test button to commence adminis-
    tration. The indicator light should flash to indicate
    a functional battery.
    Note: MS16/16A: indicator light flashes every 10.05
    seconds.
    MS26: indicator light flashes every 25.2 seconds.

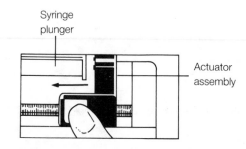

Figure 36.3   Connecting the syringe to the syringe driver.

37

Tracheostomy Care

The care of patients with a tracheostomy varies from hospital to hospital. The changing of a tracheostomy tube will usually be undertaken by a doctor or by a trained nurse who has been instructed in this procedure. It is important, however, that nurses are aware of the procedures and basic principles and know how to respond in an emergency situation.

Definition
A tracheostome is an artificial opening made into the trachea through the neck (Figure 37.1a).

Indications
Tracheostomy may be carried out:
1 to provide and maintain a patent airway;
2 to enable the removal of tracheobronchial secretions.

A tracheostomy may be performed as a temporary, permanent or emergency procedure.

REFERENCE MATERIAL
Types of tracheostomy
TEMPORARY
A temporary tracheostomy (see Figure 37.1b) is performed for patients as an elective procedure, e.g. at the time of major surgery.

PERMANENT
A permanent tracheostomy is the creation of a tracheostome following a total laryngectomy (see Figure 37.1c), The top three tracheal cartilages are brought to the surface of the skin and sutured to the skin in the form of a stoma. The 'end' tracheostome is permanent and the rigidity of the tracheal cartilage keeps the stoma open. The patient will breathe through this stoma for the remainder of his/her life. As a result, there is no connection between the nasal passages and the trachea.

EMERGENCY
A tracheostomy may be performed as an emergency procedure when a patient has an obstructed airway. Among the more common conditions causing obstruction are trauma to the airway or neck, poisoning, infections or neoplasms.

Types of tubes
The choice of tracheostomy tube depends on the type of operation performed; the patient's ability to tolerate the tube depends on various external factors. A selection of tubes is listed below.

TEMPORARY TUBES
Portex cuffed tracheostomy tube
This is a disposable plastic tracheostomy tube with introducer and inflatable cuff to give an airtight seal (Figure 37.2a). The cuff prevents blood from reaching the lungs. The seal facilitates ventilation at the time of surgery.

Portex uncuffed tracheostomy tube
This is a disposable plastic tracheostomy tube (Figure 37.2b) used, for example, during radiotherapy, when a metal tube would cause tissue reaction.

Shiley plain tracheostomy tube (Figure 37.3a)
This is a plastic tube with an introducer and two inner tubes. One inner tube has an extension at its upper aspect. This facilitates connection to other equipment, e.g. nebulizers.

Shiley cuffed tracheostomy tube (Figure 37.3b)
This is a plastic tube with an introducer and two inner tubes. One inner tube has an extension at its upper aspect to facilitate connection to other equipment. This tube has an inflatable cuff to give an airtight seal. The cuff prevents secretions from reaching the lungs. The seal facilitates ventilation.

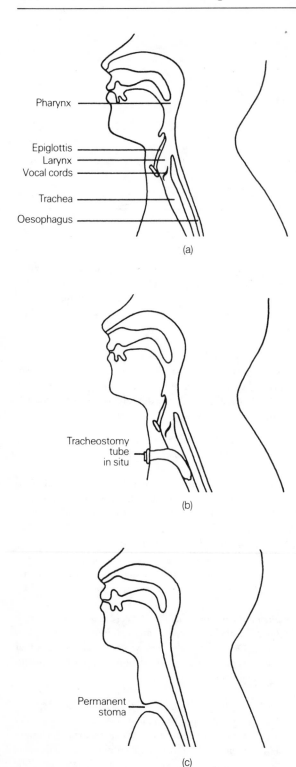

Pharynx

Epiglottis
Larynx
Vocal cords

Trachea

Oesophagus

(a)

Tracheostomy
tube
in situ

(b)

Permanent
stoma

(c)

Figure 37.1 *a*, Anatomy of the head and neck. *b*, Temporary tracheostomy. *c*, Permanent tracheostomy (total laryngectomy).

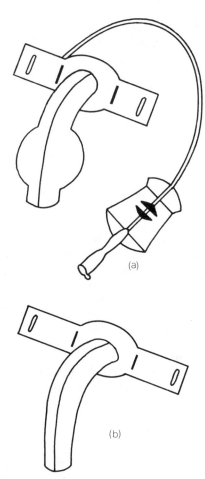

(a)

(b)

Figure 37.2 Tubes for temporary tracheostomies. *a*, Portex cuffed tube. *b*, Portex uncuffed tube.

Shiley plain fenestrated tube (Figure 37.3c)

This is a plastic tube with an introducer and two inner tubes. One inner tube has an extension at its upper end to facilitate connection to other apparatus. The outer tube has a fenestration in the middle of the cannula. This is to encourage the passage of air and secretions into the oral and nasal passage. It is useful when attempting to encourage a return to normal function following long-term use of a temporary tracheostomy.

Shiley cuffed fenestrated tube (Figure 37.3d)

This is a plastic tube with an introducer and two inner tubes. One inner tube has an extension at its upper aspect to facilitate connection to other apparatus. The outer tube has a fenestration in the middle of the cannula, again to encourage a return to normal function. The outer tube also has an inflatable cuff to give an airtight seal. The cuff prevents secretions from reaching the lungs. The seal facilitates ventilation. This tube is

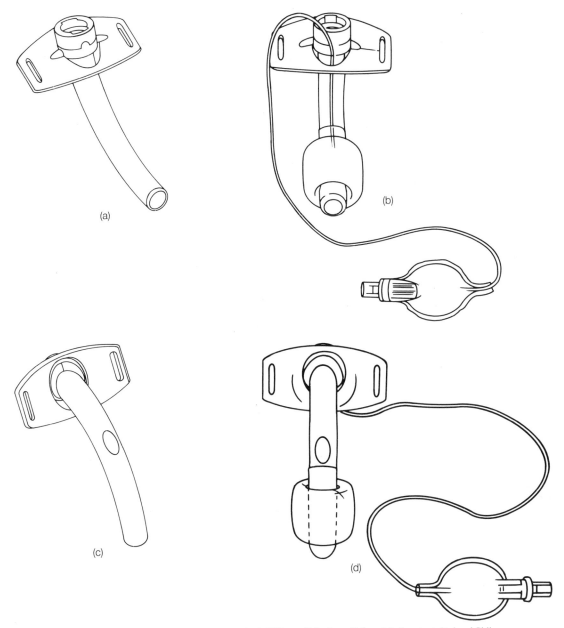

Figure 37.3 Shiley's tracheostomy tubes. *a*, Shiley plain tube. *b*, Shiley cuffed tube, *c*, Shiley plain fenestrated tube. *d*, Shiley cuffed fenestrated tube.

useful for patients with swallowing problems but who are starting to return to normal function.

Jackson's silver tracheostomy tube
This is a silver tracheostomy tube with an introducer and inner tube (Figure 37.4*a*). The inner tube is locked in position by a small catch on the outer tube and may be removed and cleaned as necessary without disturbing the outer tube.

Negus's silver tracheostomy tube
This is a silver tracheostomy tube with an introducer and a choice of inner tubes, with and without speaking valves (Figure 37.4*b*). The outer tube does not have a safety catch, consequently the inner tube may inadvertently be coughed out.

Shiley speaking valve
This is a plastic device with a two-way valve which fits

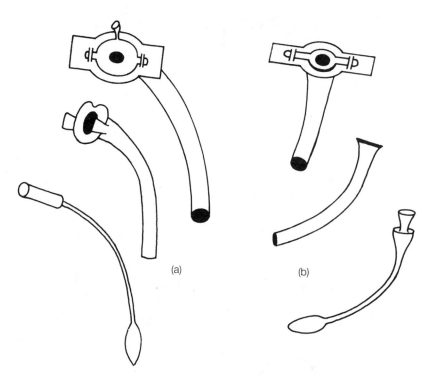

Figure 37.4   *a*, Jackson's silver tube. *b*, Negus silver tube.

(a)   (b)

onto the extended aspects of the Shiley inner tube (Figure 37.5*a*). When breathing, the valve stays open but when the patient attempts to speak the valve closes, thus redirecting air up through the normal air passages and allowing the production of voice.

Shiley decannulation plug

This is a plastic inner tube with a red blind end or a small red plastic plug (Figure 37.5*b*). It should be used when encouraging patients to breathe via normal air passages prior to removal of the tracheostomy tube.

PERMANENT TUBES
Portex cuffed tracheostomy tube

This is a disposable plastic tracheostomy tube with an introducer and inflatable cuff to give an airtight seal (Figure 37.6*a*). The cuff prevents blood from reaching the lungs. The seal facilitates ventilation at the time of surgery. This tube is used for laryngectomy patients for the first 48 hours postoperatively.

Colledge silver laryngectomy tube

This is a silver laryngectomy tube with an introducer (Figure 37.6*b*). This tube is usually fitted after drains have been removed postoperatively and bulky dressings are no longer necessary.

Shiley laryngectomy tube

This is a plastic tube with an introducer and inner tube (Figure 37.6*c*). The inner tube may be removed and cleaned frequently without disturbing the outer tube.

Shaw's silver laryngectomy tube

This is a silver laryngectomy tube with an introducer and an inner tube beyond both lower and upper aspects of the outer tube (Figure 37.6*d*). Thus pressure dressings may be secured without occluding the stoma. The lower extension of the tube ensures that crusting does not occur when the tube is changed regularly. The silver catch on the outer tube keeps the inner tube in position.

Stoma button

This is a soft Silastic 'button' (Figure 37.6*e*). It may be

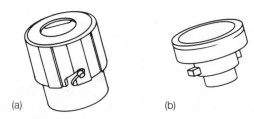

(a)   (b)

Figure 37.5   *a*, Shiley speaking valve. *b*, Shiley decannulation plug.

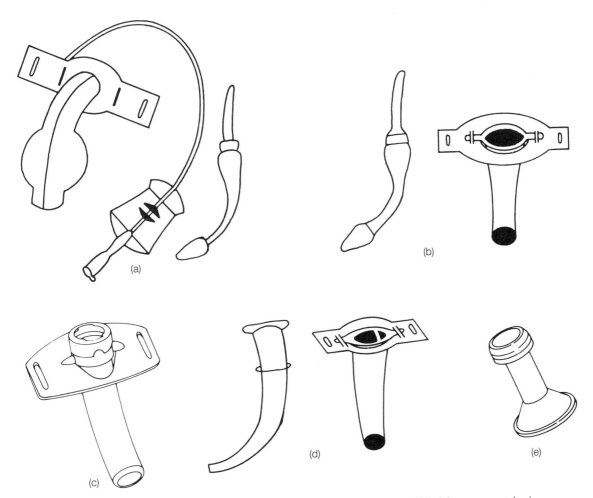

Figure 37.6 Tubes for permanent tracheostomies. *a*, Portex cuffed tube. *b*, Colledge silver tube. *c*, Shiley's laryngectomy tube. *d*, Shaw's laryngectomy tube. *e*, Stoma button.

used in place of a laryngectomy tube. It is very light and comfortable to wear.

References and further reading

Ballantyne, J.C. *et al.* (1978) *Otolaryngology*, 3rd ed, John Wright, Bristol.

Cox, S. and Jones, G. (1980) Head and neck nursing care, in R. Tiffany (ed.) *Cancer Nursing: Surgical*, Faber & Faber, London.

Davis, J. (1980) Surgical treatment – preparation of the patient, I – By the nurse, in *Laryngectomy, Rehabilitation Seminars*, Poole 1978, Abingdon 1980, National Society for Cancer Relief, pp. 67–72.

Edels, Y. (1983) *Laryngectomy – Diagnosis to Rehabilitation*, Croom Helm, London.

Freud, R.H. (1979) *Principles of Head and Neck Surgery*, Appleton Century Crofts, New York.

Harris, R.B. and Hyman, R.B. (1983) Clean vs sterile tracheostomy care and level of pulmonary infection, *Nursing Research*, Vol. 33, no. 2, pp. 80–5.

Iveson Iveson, J. (1981) Students' forum. Tracheostomy, *Nursing Mirror*, Vol. 153, no. 4, pp. 30–1.

McKelvie, P.L. (1980) Surgical aspects of laryngectomy, in *Laryngectomy Rehabilitation Seminars*, Poole 1978, Abingdon 1980, National Society for Cancer Relief, pp. 80–1.

McMinn, R.M.H. *et al.* (1981) *A Colour Atlas of Head and Neck Anatomy*, Wolfe Medical, London.

Nursing (US) (1976) Up to date survey of tracheal tubes, *Nursing* (US), Vol. 5, no. 11, pp. 66–72.

Stell, P.M. and Maran, A.G.D. (1978) *Head and Neck Surgery*, Heinemann Medical Books, London.

Tiffany, R. (1979) *Cancer Nursing: Surgical*, Faber & Faber, London.

GUIDELINES: CHANGING A TRACHEOSTOMY DRESSING

Equipment
1   Sterile dressing pack
2   Tracheostomy dressing, such as Lyofoam, or a keyhole dressing
3   Cleaning solution, such as saline
4   Alcohol-based hand wash solution, such as Hibisol.

Procedure

Action	Rationale
1 Explain the procedure to the patient.	To obtain the patient's consent and co-operation.
2 Wash hands and prepare the dressing tray or trolley.	
3 Screen the bed or cubicle.	To ensure the patient's privacy.
4 Perform the procedure using clean technique (wash hands, wear plastic gloves) (Harris and Hyman, 1983).	To prevent infection.
5 Remove the soiled dressing around the tube.	To avoid discomfort to the patient.
6 Replace with a tracheostomy dressing, such as Lyofoam, or a keyhole dressing.	To ensure the patient's comfort. To avoid pressure from the tube.

GUIDELINES: SUCTION AND TRACHEOSTOMY PATIENTS

The aim of suction is to maintain an airway and to prevent the formation of crusts. The frequency of suction varies with individual patients according to their needs.

Equipment
1   Suction machine (wall source or portable)
2   Rubber suction tube
3   Plastic connection tube
4   Y connection
5   Sterile catheters (assorted sizes; see note below)
6   Disposable gloves
7   Jug of sodium bicarbonate solution
8   Spray containing sterile normal saline
9   Disposable plastic apron
10   Alcohol-based hand wash solution, such as Hibisol.

Note: It is advisable to use the right size of catheter for the lumen of the tracheostomy tube; a 10FG catheter is appropriate for a 27–30FG tube, a 12FG catheter for a 33-36FG tube, a 14FG catheter for a 39FG tube.

Procedure

Action	Rationale
1 Instruct the patient to use his/her spray, every 2 hours, i.e. two or three sprays directly into his/her tracheostomy.	Suction will not be achieved if the secretions become too tenacious or dry. Spraying regularly minimizes this occurrence.
2 If the patient is able to perform his/her own suction, he/she should be taught this. Otherwise inform the patient precisely what to be done.	To obtain the patient's co-operation. The procedure is unpleasant and can be frightening for the patient. Reassurance is vital. Self-control of the patient's suction is preferable if the patient is able to manage it.
3 Wash hands with an ancohol-based hand wash solution, such as Hibisol, and put on a disposable plastic apron.	To reduce the risk of cross-infection. Most patients cough directly on to the nurse's clothes after spraying or suction.
4 Check that the Y connection is on the end of the suction tubing and set the suction machine to the appropriate level.	Sputum which is more tenacious requires more powerful suction.
5 Open the end of the suction catheter pack and use the pack to attach the catheter to the Y connection. Keep the rest of the catheter in the sterile packet.	To reduce the risk of transferring infection from hands to the catheter and to keep the catheter as clean as possible.
6 Put on disposable gloves and withdraw the catheter from the sleeve.	Gloves minimize the risk of infection transfer to the catheter or from the sputum to the nurse's hands.
7 Introduce the catheter to about one-third of its length and apply suction by placing the thumb over the open limb of the Y connector.	Gentleness is essential; damage to the tracheal mucosa can lead to trauma and respiratory infection. The catheter should go no further than the carina to prevent trauma. The catheter is inserted with suction off so as not to irritate mucous membrane.
8 Withdraw the catheter gently with a rotating motion. Do not suction the patient for more than 15 seconds at a time.	To remove secretions from around the mucous membranes. Prolonged suction will result in infection and the patient may experience a choking sensation.
9 Remove the catheter from the trachea having released thumb from the Y connector. Remove gloves and discard them with the catheter.	To release suction and to prevent trauma to the tracheal mucosa. Catheters are used only once to reduce the risk of introducing infection.
10 Rinse the connection tube by dipping its end in the jug of sodium bicarbonate solution with the suction turned on.	To loosen secretions which have adhered to the inside of the tube.
11 If the patient requires further suction, repeat the above actions using new gloves and a new catheter.	
12 Repeat the suction until the airway is clear.	

HUMIDIFICATION

Definition

Humidification may be defined as increasing the mois-ture content of air. In health, inspired air is filtered, warmed and moistened by the ciliated lining and mucus is produced in the upper respiratory pathways. Because the upper respiratory pathways are bypassed in patients with a tracheostomy, they need artificial humidification to ensure these pathways remain moist.

GUIDELINES: HUMIDIFICATION

Procedure

IMMEDIATE POSTOPERATIVE CARE, I.E. THE FIRST 24–48 HOURS

Action	Rationale
1 Fill a suitable nebulizer, such as an Ohio or Inspiron nebulizer, with sterile water and attach it to the oxygen supply. Set the oxygen rate at 4 litres per minute at 40%. Give a constant supply of humidified oxygen for 24–48 hours.	Constant humidification is required while new stoma adapts to the outside environment (especially for laryngectomy patients). Humidification also prevents the formation of crusts which are liable to obstruct the airway.
2 Spray saline into the trachea as necessary, using a spray or a syringe.	To loosen secretions prior to suction and to stimulate the cough reflex.
3 For patients in cubicles, a room humidifier may be placed at the bedside.	To provide a warm, humid environment.

SUBSEQUENT CARE

Action	Rationale
1 Give humidified oxygen as required. Usually patients need about 10–15 minutes of humidification every 4 hours. This may be adapted according to the patient's needs, e.g. throughout the night.	Patients begin to adapt to breathing through their tracheostomy after the first 24–48 hours. Some humidification is required according to individual needs and to prevent crust formation in the airway.
2 If the patient does not require oxygen, blow humidifiers may be used.	These provide humidified air without the need for an oxygen supply.
3 Teach the patient to keep his/her tracheostomy moist by using a spray or a syringe containing normal saline, prior to suctioning.	To loosen secretions and to prevent crust formation. To prevent contamination. Normal saline is supplied in small bottles which, if not fully used within 24 hours, should be changed. If a spray is used, this should be washed and dried each day and resterilized once the patient is discharged.
4 Provide bibs, such as Buchanan bibs, for patients.	To protect airway.

GUIDELINES: CHANGING A TRACHEOSTOMY TUBE

Equipment

1 Sterile dressing pack
2 Tracheostomy dressing, such as Lyofoam, or a keyhole dressing
3 Tracheostomy tape
4 Cleaning solution, such as Normasol
5 Barrier cream
6 Lubricating cream
7 Sterile gloves
8 Disposable plastic apron
9 Alcohol-based hand wash solution, such as Hibisol.

Procedure

Action	Rationale
1 Explain the procedure to the patient.	To obtain the patient's consent and co-operation.
2 Wash hands and prepare a dressing trolley.	
3 Screen the patient's bed.	To ensure the patient's privacy.
4 Perform the procedure using clean technique.	To prevent contamination.
5 Assist the patient to sit in an upright position, supported by pillows with his/her neck extended.	To ensure the patient's comfort and to maintain a patent airway. If the neck is not extended, skin folds may occlude the tracheostomy when the tube is removed.
6 Remove the dressing pack from its outer wrappings and open the tracheostomy dressing, such as Lyofoam.	Technique should be clean to reduce the risk of cross-infection.
7 Put on a disposable plastic apron.	
8 Clean hands with an alcohol-based hand wash solution, such as Hibisol.	
9 Put on disposable plastic gloves.	Gloves are necessary as the tube is difficult to manipulate with forceps.
10 Prepare the tracheostomy tube as outlined in steps 11–14.	So that the tube is ready for immediate insertion when required.
11 Thread one piece of tape through the silts in the flanges so that the tape passes behind the flange next to the stoma.	The tape is kept behind the flange to prevent it occluding the passage of air into the tracheostomy tube.
12 Put the tracheostomy dressing, such as Lyofoam, around the tube.	To prevent abrasion of the patient's skin by the tube.
13 Lubricate the tube sparingly with a lubricating cream, such as petroleum jelly.	

Action	**Rationale**
14 Remove the soiled tube from the patient's neck while asking the patient to breathe out.	Conscious expiration relaxes the patient and reduces the risk of coughing. Coughing can result in unwanted closure of the tracheostome.
15 Clean around the stoma with normal saline and dry gently. Apply barrier cream with topical swabs. (An aqueous cream may be used if the patient is having the site irradiated.)	To remove superficial organisms and crusts. Skin should not be left moist as this provides an ideal medium for the growth of micro-organisms.
16 Insert a clean tube with introducer in place, using an up and over action.	Introduction of the tube is less traumatic if directed along the contour of the trachea.
17 Remove the introducer immediately.	The patient cannot breathe while the introducer is in place.
18 Place the inner tube in position.	The inner tube may be changed several times when the outer tube is in position, thus minimizing the risk of trauma to trachea and stoma. The quantity of secretions present will determine the frequency with which the inner tube is changed.
19 Tie the tape securely at the side of the neck.	To secure the tube. Place the tie in an accessible place, at the same time ensuring that it will not cause discomfort to the patient.
20 Remove gloves and ask the patient to breathe out onto the palm of your hand.	Flow of air will be felt if the tube is in the correct position.
21 Ensure that the patient is comfortable.	
22 Clear away the trolley and equipment.	
23 Scrub the soiled tube with a brush under cold running water. If the tube is very soiled, then use hydrogen peroxide to remove debris. The tube must be rinsed thoroughly and stored dry at the patient's bedside.	To remove debris that may occlude the tube and/or become a source of infection.

Note: Plastic tubes should not be soaked in solutions as there is a danger that the material may absorb the solution which could then cause irritation of the trachea.

NURSING CARE PLAN

Problem	**Cause**	**Suggested action**
Profuse tracheal secretions.	Local reaction to tracheostomy tube.	Suction frequently, e.g. every 1–2 hours.
Lumen of tracheostomy tube occluded.	Tenacious mucus in tube.	Spray frequently with normal saline e.g. every 1–3 hours, and suction. Change the inner tube regularly.
	Dried blood and mucus in the tube, especially in the postoperative period.	Provide humidified air. (For further information, see the Guidelines, Humidification, p. 368).

Tracheostomy tube dislodged accidentally.	Tapes not adequately secured.	Put in a spare tube. This should be clean and ready at the bedside. *Note*: Tracheal dilators must be kept at the bedside of patients with tracheostomies.
Unable to insert clean tracheostomy tube.	Unpredicted shape or angle of stoma.	Remain calm since an outward appearance of distress may cause the patient to panic and lose confidence. Lubricate the tube well and attempt to reinsert at various angles.
	Tracheal stenosis due to patient coughing, over-reacting or because the tube has been left out too long.	Insert a smaller-size tracheostomy tube. If insertion still proves difficult, do not leave the patient but ask for a tube to be brought to the bed. Keep the tracheostomy patent with tracheal dilators if stenosis is pronounced until the tube is reinserted.
Tracheal bleeding following or during change of the tube.	Trauma due to suction or to the tube being changed. Presence of tumour.	Change the tube as planned if bleeding is minimal. For profuse bleeding, insert a cuffed tube, such as a Portex tube, and inflate. Inform the doctor. Suction the patient to remove the blood from the trachea.
Infected sputum.	Nature of surgery and condition of patient often predispose to infection.	Encourage the patient to cough up secretions and/or suction regularly. Change the tube and clean the stoma area frequently, e.g. 4-hourly. Protect permanent stomas with a bib or gauze.

38

Traction

Definition

Traction is a process whereby a force is exerted on a part or parts of the body. Countertraction is a process whereby a force is exerted that opposes the direct pull of the traction. The degree of counteraction depends on the amount of force necessary to counteract the pull of the traction.

Indications

Traction is indicated in the following circumstances:
1   to relieve pain and/or muscle spasm;
2   to ensure rest for a limb or part of the skeletal system that may be diseased or broken until healing has occurred;
3   to maintain correct anatomical alignment;
4   to restore the length of a limb where, due to disease or trauma, shortening has occurred;
5   to reduce dislocations of joints, as a preliminary measure, or in injury to the cervical vertebrae;
6   to maintain the length of a limb where a fracture is unstable;
7   as a preoperative measure prior to internal fixation;
8   as a post-operative measure to maintain the desired position.

REFERENCE MATERIAL
Types of traction
MANUAL TRACTION

Manual traction is traction applied by the hands, as when a doctor reduces a fracture or when equipment need to be reapplied.

FIXED TRACTION

Fixed traction is traction between two fixed points. Weights and pulleys are used to elevate the limb not to create the pull. The patient is attached to a device at one point and the affected part is pulled away from the point of fixation by extensions and cords which are tied to the device. The fixation point is the countertraction and the pulling extensions are the traction. This type of traction has the advantage of requiring a small degree of force only. It is frequently used to reduce or eliminate muscle spasm. An example of this type of traction would be the application of a Thomas' splint to a leg using skin extensions tied to the end of the splint.

SLIDING OR BALANCED TRACTION

This is traction exerted against a weight. Extensions and cords are applied to the affected part or parts of a patient and fixed to the foot of the bed. When the foot of the bed is elevated, an inclined plane is formed down which the patient's body will slide, away from the point of fixation. The extensions serve as counter-traction; the sliding body forms the traction. An example of this type of traction would be Pugh's traction.

WEIGHT AND PULLEY

A pulley is a wheel with a grooved edge suspended on an axle around which it rotates in a framework or block. A pulley block is a grouping of two or three pulleys on a single common axle in a frame. This type of traction may be a simple system using a single pulley to alter the direction of the force so that weights can be conveniently suspended, or a compound system using a number of pulleys in combination to increase the efficiency of the force applied as well as altering the direction. In all weighted traction, the weights must hang freely and not touch the side of the bed or the floor.

Single fixed pulley

This offers no mechanical advantage as the force (the weight) at one end of the cord is equal to the load. The advantage of this system is that traction cords can be passed in any convenient direction to reach a hanging weight, directing the force in a particular direction.

Pairs of pulley blocks

Two pulley blocks are required at each point of suspension and are used to suspend plaster beds from overhead beams. The bed can be tilted in any direction by the patient or the nurse, thus increasing mobility and convenience.

Combination of single pulleys

In Hamilton-Russell traction the arrangement of a single pulley offers the advantage of suspending the patient's legs while allowing the direction of the traction force to be altered according to the principles of the paraellelogram of forces.

Traction may be continuous, i.e. maintained without interruption, or intermittent, i.e. it may be discontinued for specified periods, such as mealtimes, or for toilet purposes.

Principal sites available for traction

SKIN TRACTION

Adhesive materials are applied to the skin and traction is achieved when a weight is added that pulls on tape, sponge rubber or plastic. The application of skin traction is contraindicated in the presence of an existing skin condition e.g. eczema or psoriasis, when the skin is thin and friable, where there are varicose veins, or where there is loss of normal skin sensation.

SKELETAL TRACTION

Traction is applied to bone using wires or pins that are placed through bone. (Tongs are attached to boney plate.) It affords a greater degree of comfort than skin traction and is the preferred method when traction is required over long periods. More weight can be applied as this is a direct pull on bone.

PULP TRACTION

A metal pin is passed through soft tissues and a stirrup is attached to the pin. Traction is applied via the stirrup.

PELVIC TRACTION

A canvas harness is fastened around the patient's pelvic region. The harness is attached to the foot of the bed by cords or straps. When the foot of the bed is elevated the patient's body slides down the inclined plane, forming the required traction. A harness may be suspended to a Balkan beam by crossed cords and weights to achieve a pull that moulds the pelvis back into the desired anatomical shape.

SKULL TRACTION

This may be applied by a harness, e.g. Glisson's sling, skull calipers or a half splint.

Application of traction

SKIN TRACTION

The application of skin traction may be painful. To minimize the patient's pain the following principles should be adhered to:

1 skill and gentleness are required in handling the affected part;
2 manual traction must be maintained;
3 the traction should be applied with speed and dexterity;
4 the length of any extension being applied is related to its purpose. If below-knee extensions (for knee tibial lesions) are applied to a hip or femoral lesion, the knee joint is strained by the traction being applied through the joint. If above-knee extensions (for femoral or hip lesions) are used, the knee joint must be supported.

ADHESIVE TYPES

Self-adhesive

A self-adhesive medium is spread in a thin layer on a supporting material. The most commonly used medium is zinc oxide. The supporting material may be non-stretch perforated cloth in the form of zinc oxide plaster, or crosswise elastic fibre that may be perforated for ventilation. A disadvantage of zinc oxide preparations is that some patients develop a reaction to them in the form of contact dermatitis.

Diachylon adhesive

This is a lead-based adhesive material spread on various supporting materials. Such materials may be of ventilated elastic cloth or Holland cloth. This form of adhesive material can be reapplied after temporary removal and is less likely to cause contact dermatitis. A disadvantage is that the lead base may impede slightly the passage of the radiation if radiological investigations are required.

Unna's paste

This is a paste composed of 15% zinc oxide in gelatin, glycerine and water stored in airtight jars. Heat reduces the paste to a fluid state; it is then painted onto prepared calico extensions before application to the affected part. Setting takes 2 hours or more.

NON-ADHESIVE TYPES

Latex foam pads or bandages

These may be improvised extensions or, more commonly, commercially supplied extension kits. They have a disadvantage in that to serve as extensions they must be firmly bandaged to the skin, with the resulting danger of constricting the part bandaged.

Gamgee tissue under a clove hitch
An anklet of gamgee padding with a calico bandage arranged as a clove hitch attaching the affected part to the foot of an elevated bed may serve as a temporary extension while permanent extensions are being replaced or Unna's paste extensions are setting.

Skeletal
Strong pins or wires are passed through the bone, often under anaesthesia, by a surgeon using full aseptic technique. Commonly used are Steinmann's pins, Kirschner wires and Denham pins. Tongs are attached to the boney plate.

Specific types of traction
Illustrated descriptions of the types of traction currently in use can be found in Hilt and Cogburn (1980) and Roaf and Hodkinson (1980).

General principles for the care of patients on traction
POSITION
Patients may be required to adopt uncomfortable or unnatural positions for long periods. This may make the management of everyday functions such as eating, drinking, personal hygiene and toileting difficult. Help and sympathy from nursing personnel will be required until the patient has adopted new ways of dealing with this situation.

STASIS
Prolonged immobilization produces many adverse reactions.

Pressure sores
Skin and underlying tissues in direct contact with the bed and equipment may break down, become infected or even become necrotic. Frequent and consistent attention to the care of pressure areas is essential.

Kidneys
Stasis of urine in the kidneys due to immobilization and position may result in renal complications. A high fluid intake is recommended to counteract any such complications.

Bowels
Patients on traction for extended periods may become constipated. A high-fibre diet should be introduced if permissible, to prevent such a complication developing.

Chest
Stasis may lead to oedema of the lungs, and respiratory distress. Physiotherapy, breathing exercises and suitable medication may be required to overcome such complications.

PSYCHOLOGICAL EFFECTS
Scant literature is available on the psychological effect of prolonged traction on patients and/or nurses. Howard and Corbo-Pelaia (1982) offer an assessment of a patient who underwent halo traction.

Daily checkup of traction equipment
1 *Balkan beams*: ensure that they are attached securely to the bed and each other.
2 *Pulleys*: ensure they are secure. The cord should pass through them and not down the side. This reduces the risk of cord fraying. Ensure knots are tied tightly.
3 *Cord*: must be without any frays.
4 *Weights*: ensure that they are of the correct amount. They must not rest on the floor or the chair. If water-type weights are used, ensure there are no leaks.

References and further reading
Brunner, L.S. and Suddarth, D.S. (1986) *The Lippincott Manual of Nursing Practice*, 4th edn, J.B. Lippincott, Philadelphia.
Cohen, S. (1979) Nursing care of a patient in traction, *American Journal of Nursing*, Vol. 79, pp. 1771–98.
Hilt, N.E. and Cogburn, S.B. (1980) *Manual of Orthopaedics*, C.V. Mosby, St Louis.
Howard, M. and Corbo-Pelaia, S.A. (1982) Psychological after effects of halo traction, *American Journal of Nursing*, Vol. 82, pp. 1839–43.
Miller, M. and Miller, J.H. (1985) *Orthopaedics and Accidents*, Hodder and Stoughton, London.
Powell, M. (1986) *Orthopaedic Nursing and Rehabilitation*, 9th edn, Churchill Livingstone, Edinburgh.
Roaf, R. and Hodkinson, L.J. (1980) *Textbook of Orthopaedic Nursing*, 3rd edn, Blackwell Scientific Publications, Oxford.

GUIDELINES: SKIN TRACTION

Equipment
Commercially prepared packs are now generally available. If this is not the case, then the section on the application of skin traction should be consulted (see p. 373).

Procedure

ADHESIVE

Action	**Rationale**
1 Explain the procedure to the patient.	To obtain the patient's consent and co-operation.
2 Ensure privacy for the patient while carrying out the procedure.	
3 Ensure that the affected part is clean.	To prevent infection from developing.
4 Shave any limb covered by thick tough hairs.	To ensure that adhesive sticks to the skin and not to the hairs. The part affected will be sore if the traction is applied to the hair follicles only.
5 If possible, leave the ankle joint free.	To allow full plantarflexion and dorsiflexion in the foot.
6 If the lower limb is for traction, apply pieces of felt or latex foam to the malleoli and other bony prominences.	To protect them from friction. To prevent the development of pressure sores.
7 Leave the patellae exposed and the knee 10–15 °C off full flexion.	To prevent limb deformity and joint stiffness.
8 The limb may be painted/sprayed with tincture of benzoin compound.	To reduce moisture through perspiration. To increase the adhesive quality of the material used. To harden the skin. To act as a barrier to the adhesive in the event of the patient developing contact dermatitis.
9 Apply the extension strapping without folds or creases.	To prevent discomfort. To prevent skin deterioration under the strapping.
10 Ensure that the part affected is in the correct anatomical position, e.g. feet and patellae pointing upwards when patient is in the supine position.	To prevent limb deformity.
11 Check the temperature and colour of the part affected as required together with the degree of sensation and movement.	To ensure that the tension of strapping is correct.

NON-ADHESIVE

As above, but omit steps 4 and 8.

SKELETAL

Action	**Rationale**
1 Use strict aseptic technique when attending to the sites of entry of pins, wires and tongs.	To prevent local and/or systemic infection.
2 Record vital signs as necessary.	To monitor development of any infection.

NURSING CARE PLAN

Problem	Cause	Suggested action
Patient is irritable, complains of pain, itching; elevated temperature; drainage through supporting material; foul odour.	Skin breakdown is occurring or has occurred.	Inform appropriate personnel. Remove supporting material if applicable.
Patient complains of paraesthesia, joint pain and/or coldness or part affected.	Supporting material bound too tightly.	Rebandage.
Increase in the distance between the sole of the foot, for example, and the spreader (a piece of wood, plastic or metal that serves to maintain the pull of the extensions along parallel lines as they are attached to the traction cord).	Skin extension material slipping.	Reapply using manual traction.
Localized sores.	Bandage or extension material causing pressure.	Reapply using manual traction.
Drop foot.	Pressure on the lateral pophliteal nerve.	Realign the limb in the correct anatomical position. Ensure correct degree of knee flexion. Attach a foot board.
Joint irritation or displacement of bone at fracture site.	Insufficient traction.	Ensure sufficient traction.
Low grade osteomyelitis.	Infection at site of entry of pin, wires or tongs.	Inform appropriate personnel. Ensure strict aseptic technique when attending to lesion.
Delayed union or non-union of fracture.	Over-distraction at fracture site.	Realign.
Necrosis of the bone adjacent to the pin, wires or tongs.	Impaired blood supply.	Inform appropriate personnel.
Pin slipping from one side to the other, carrying an area of non-sterile pin into the bone, or rotatory slipping.	Pin is loose in the bone. May be an area of necrotic or osteoporotic bone around the pin.	Report to the medical staff.
Swelling, oedema, pain, discoloration below site of insertion of pin.	May be indicative of venous thrombosis.	Report to the medical staff.

39

Transfusion of Blood and Blood Products

Definition

A transfusion consists of the administration of whole blood or any of its components to correct or treat a clinical abnormality.

Indications

The range of products currently available, those mose widely used, indications for their use and recommendations for administration are listed in Table 39.1.

REFERENCE MATERIAL

There are several problems or potential problems associated with the administration of blood or its components which can be classified as either immediate reactions or long-term complications.

Immediate reactions to blood transfusion

FEVER

There are several causes of the development of the fever:

Pyrogenic reaction

This is probably the most common cause of fever. Pyrogens are the breakdown material from bacteria in the blood before sterilization.

The normal sequence seen is a rise in the patient's temperature without the signs and symptoms of shock, followed by the pyrexia subsiding when the transfusion is slowed. It is not thought to be a serious complication.

White cell antibody and platelet antibody reaction

Just as red blood cells have genetically transmitted antigens on their surface membrane from which the blood group is determined, so too have white cells. White cell antigens are more complex and are mainly linked with the human leucocyte antigen (HLA) system.

If a patient receives a number of transfusions he/she may develop antibodies against the foreign antigens. If transfusions containing white cells with similar antigens are then administered the patient's previously manufactured antibodies will react against these.

White cell antibody reactions tend to be more severe than a pryogenic reaction, showing signs and symptoms of chill and high fever. Platelet antibody reaction is very similar to white cell antibody reactions.

Both problems are normally associated with multiple transfusions but in the case of multigravida women the same reaction may occur on their first transfusion.

Foreign protein antibody reaction

This problem is very rarely seen and is associated with the development of antibodies to proteins present in the plasma of the transfused blood.

Infection

Infection can be bacterial growth in the transfusion product or it can be inadvertently introduced during cannulation or connection of giving set and transfusion bag.

Usually there is a brief period of the patient feeling hot, often associated with chest and abdominal pain, then the patient becomes severely shocked with a fall in blood pressure and a subnormal temperature. Later a pyrexia occurs.

Allergic reactions

These are often caused by the development of anti-IgA antibodies in the patient's plasma reacting against IgA protein in the transfused blood.

The reaction may be mild where the pyrexia is minimal with a rash soon appearing, or severe with the development of oedema around the eyes and/or around the larynx with accompanying dyspnoea. A severe attack warrants urgent treatment.

It is essential to determine the exact nature and probable cause of fever as treatment, and the urgency with which it is implemented, may vary considerably.

Table 39.1   Blood and Blood Products Used for Transfusion

Type	Description	Indications	Cross-matching	Shelf life	Average infusion time	Technique	Special considerations
Whole blood	Complete unadulterated blood approx. 520 ml including anticoagulant.	To restore blood volume lost due to massive, acute haemorrhage whatever the cause.	ABO and Rh	28–35 days at 4–6°C (dependent on anticoagulant)	2–4 hours/unit	Give via a blood administration set. A Y-type set may be used to administer sodium chloride 0.9% simultaneously reducing viscosity and increasing flow.	Whole blood is rarely transfused. Volume expanders and specific components are often more appropriate and clinically effective.
*Plasma reduced blood (packed red blood cells – USA)	Whole blood minus approx. 200 ml plasma, and anticoagulant. Haematocrit 60–65%.	To correct red blood cell deficiency and improve oxygen-carrying capacity of the blood.	ABO and Rh	21 days at 4–6°C	2–4 hours/unit	As above	—
Red cells in optimal additive solutions	Red cells minus all plasma: 100 ml fluid used as replacement to give optimal red cell preservation. Haematocrit 60–65%.	As above	ABO and Rh	35 days at 4–6°C	1–2 hours/unit	As avove	An example of a replacement solution is saline/adenine/glucose/mannitol.
*Concentrated red cells	Plasma removed to produce a haematocrit of 70% plus.	To correct anaemias when expansion of blood volume will not be tolerated.	ABO and Rh	21 days at 4–6°C	1–2 hours/unit	As above	Availability varies.
*Washed red blood cells	Red cells centrifuged free of plasma and resuspended in	To increase red cell mass and prevent tissue antigen formation	ABO and Rh	Use within 12 hours or preferably immediately.	1–2 hours/unit	As above	—

Product	Description	Indication	Compatibility	Storage	Time/rate	Administration	Comments
Frozen red blood cells	1 Cells from normal healthy donor with very rare blood group. 2 Patient's own cells taken in anticipation of later illness (autologous blood transfusion).	1 immunosuppressed patients 2 patients with previous transfusion reactions. To treat transplant patients or patients with atypical antibodies which react with almost the entire population. To increase safety of tranfusion therapy.	ABO and Rh	Stored frozen cells: 3 years. Use within 12 hours of thawing.	2–3 hours/unit	As above	Available from a few centres. Freezing process and recovery are time consuming and expensive.
Leucocyte poor blood	Red cells from which accompanying leucocytes have been removed.	To prevent further reactions in patients who have had febrile attacks when receiving whole or plasma reduced blood.	ABO and Rh	4–6°C. Time stated on pack. Usually within 12 hours of preparation, preferably immediately.	2–3 hours/unit	As above	Frozen red cells may be used as an alternative.
*White blood cells (leucocyte concentrate)	Mainly granulocytes obtained by leucophoresis or by 'creaming off' the buffy layers from packs of fresh blood.	To treat patients with life-threatening granulocytopaenia, e.g. due to chemotherapy.	ABO and HLA (human leucocyte group A antigen)	24 hours after collection. Stored at 5°C.	60–90 minutes/unit	Administer via a blood administration set. Usually 1 unit only.	WBC infusion *induces* fever, may cause hypertension, rigors and confusion. Treat symptoms and reassure patient.

TABLE 39.1   (contd.)

Type	Description	Indications	Cross-matching	Shelf life	Average infusion time	Technique	Special considerations
							Preparation may be irradiated to prevent initiation of graft versus heart (GVH) disease in bone marrow transplant patients. Do not give to patients receiving amphotericin B.
*Platelets	Platelet sediment from platelet-rich plasma, resuspended in 40–60 ml plasma.	To treat thrombocyto-paenia due to 1 decreased production 2 increased destruction 3 functionally abnormal platelets 4 dilutional problems following massive transfusions	Preferred but not essential.	Up to 5 days after collection at 22°C, with continuous gentle agitation. Best within 6 hours.	20–30 minutes/unit	Administration using a component set is preferred. Flush the line with 100 ml normal saline after the infusion to ensure full dose is delivered. Do not use micro-aggregate filters.	General guide to use: 1 count less than 10 × 10⁹/litre 2 count 10–20 × 10⁹/litre with haemorrhage 3 count 20–50 × 10⁹/litre or on chemotherapy may need platelets. Prophylactic use in the absence of haemorrhage is controversial.
⁺Plasma: fresh or fresh, frozen (FFP)	Citrated plasma separated from whole blood. All coagulation factors preserved for several months.	To treat a clotting factor deficiency, when specific concentrates are unavailable or precise deficiency is unknown, e.g. DIC.	ABO compatibility. Rh preferred.	Fresh: within 6 hours after collection. FFP: 12 months at −25°C. Use immediately after thawing.	15–45 minutes/unit (approx. 200 ml)	Administer rapidly via a blood administration set.	500 mls of FFP should be transfused after 8 units of blood (when massive transfusions given) to prevent dilutional

Product	Description	Indication	Compatibility	Storage	Rate	Administration	Notes
Plasma protein fraction (PPF)	4.5% solution of selected proteins from pooled plasma in a buffered, stabilized saline diluent. Usually 400-ml bottle.	To treat hypovolaemic shock or hypoprotein-aemia due to burns, trauma, surgery or infection.	Unnecessary	3 years at 25°C. Store in the dark.	unit.	blood administration set.	for 10 hours to inactivate hepatitis virus. The solution should be crystal clear with no deposits.
Salt poor human albumin 20%	Heat treated, aqueous chemically processed fraction of pooled plasma.	To treat hypovolaemic shock or hypoprotein-aemia due to burns, trauma, surgery or infection. To maintain appropriate electrolyte balance.	Unnecessary	5 years at 2°C, 3 years at 25°C. Store in the dark.	30–60 minutes/ unit	Administer via a blood administration set undiluted or diluted with saline or 5% glucose solution. Slower administration is advised if a cardiac disorder is present to avoid gross fluid shift.	Heated at 60°C for 10 hours to inactivate hepatitis virus. The solution should be crystal clear with no deposits.
Factor VIII (cryoprecipitates, dried antihaemophilic globulin concentrates)	Cold-insoluble portion of plasma recovered from FFP – amount of factor VIII varies. Potency in freeze-dried concentrates can be assayed more reliably.	To control bleeding disorders due to lack of factor VIII or fibrinogen, e.g. haemophilia, Von Willebrand's disease.	ABO compatibility between donor plasma and recipient's RBCs.	Cryoprecipitates at –30°C for 1 year. Use immediately after thawing. Freeze-dried concentrates at +4°C. Reconstitute at room temperature and use immediately.	15–30 minutes via infusion, 10–15 minutes via intravenous push.	Administer rapidly via syringe or component set. Flush each unit with saline to obtain maximum dose.	Heat treated as above to eliminate risk of hepatitis or HIV contamination, as multiple donors and imported preparation. Limited availability.
Dried factor IX concentrate	Preparation contains factor IX, prothrombin and factor X. Some may contain factor VII.	To correct bleeding disorders due to lack of these factors, e.g. Christmas disease.	Unnecessary	Refer to individual expiry dates.	15–30 minutes	Administer via a blood administration set. Dose varies.	As above. Limited availability.

* Most commonly used blood products.

BLOOD GROUP ANTIBODIES

If a patient's blood contains blood group antibodies then haemolysis of the transfused blood can occur. This happens when blood is not cross-matched prior to transfusion or if blood is required urgently and certain antibodies are not detected in the cross-matching technique used in an emergency.

Occasionally the reaction is such that the only sign of incompatibility is no increase in the patient's haemoglobin post-transfusion.

However, the patient may experience a feeling of heat along the vein, flushing of the face, and pain in the lumbar area and chest. Shock then follows with a fall in blood pressure. Urine output falls and the patient may become anuric and renal failure may develop.

Due to the rapid destruction of transfused red cells and the thromboplastin substances released from them, intravascular coagulation occurs, clotting factors are used up and the patient may develop a haemorrhagic diathesis. Therefore if the transfusion is being performed for a bleeding episode, the condition could be worsened.

CITRATE AND POTASSIUM INTOXICATION

Due to the method used to prevent blood to be transfused from clotting, i.e. the use of ACD (acid citrate dextrose) or CPD (citrate phosphate dextrose), during storage, some potassium is passed from the red cells into the plasma. If blood is then transfused in large quantities or if the patient has hepatic or renal disease, the citrate and potassium levels in the patient's blood may become toxic and could lead to heart damage.

Long-term complications of blood transfusion

These are associated with the bacterial, parasitic and viral diseases that can be transmitted via a blood transfusion.

BACTERIAL INFECTIONS

Bacterial infections of blood are now rare due to good collection methods. The two bacterial diseases that have in the past been spread via blood transfusion are brucellosis and syphilis. Today donors with a history of brucellosis are not accepted. Since direct person-to-person transfusion was discontinued the risk of transfusion syphilis has dropped, although in very rare instances both these bacterial infections have been reported post-transfusion.

PARASITIC INFECTIONS

Of the parasitic infections transmittable by blood, malaria is the most important. Although extremely rare – 0.2 per million units in the United Kingdom – it can be a serious problem where the disease is endemic.

PLASMA-BORNE VIRUS

The two main viruses associated with transfusion are hepatitis B and human immunodeficiency virus (HIV).

Hepatitis B

The incidence of post-transfusion hepatitis varies widely throughout the world and can be very difficult to estimate as many doctors do not appreciate that a case of jaundice may be related to a previous blood tansfusion. Additionally, a vast proportion of the patients affected do not show clinical signs and symptoms and are therefore missed. It has been estimated in the United Kingdom that the incidence is about 1% but in some areas of Japan it is as high as 75%.

In the late 1960s a chance discovery by Blumberg of a particle in the serum of an Aborigine was labelled the Australian antigen. It was later found that this particle was present in the blood of multitransfused patients and that Australian antigen-positive patients were very liable to transmit hepatitis. This antigen is now called hepatitis B.

In recent years a number of tests have been devised to detect the presence of the antigen and today all blood is tested prior to transfusion so the incidence of post-transfusion hepatitis has dropped dramatically.

Human Immunodeficiency Virus (HIV)

In the United Kingdom the incidence of post-transfusion HIV transmission to the recipient is not known. Many cases have been reported regarding the use of clotting factor VIII in haemophiliacs but the major cause of this was the importation of factor VIII from the United States.

As blood cannot be effectively tested at the present time for the presence of the virus, due to the time lapse between infection and the formation of the antibodies, which then show themselves in the current test, more emphasis is placed on the confidential questionnaire which is completed by every donor. If the questionnaire shows that a donor is in the 'at-risk' category donor's unit of blood is destroyed, thus reducing the risk of the virus being transmitted via transfusions.

All blood and blood products are now heat treated as an extra precaution, so reducing the risk further.

Blood grouping and Rh factor

As noted previously, it is important that blood for transfusion is matched with the blood of the recipient to prevent a haemolytic reaction which could be life threatening. There follows a brief review of the blood group classifications.

The most commonly used blood grouping system, the ABO method, was discovered in 1901 and is based

Table 39.2 The ABO Method of Blood Grouping

Blood group	Approximate frequency % in the UK	Antigen present on cells	ISO antibodies present in serum
O	46.5	Neither A nor B	Anti-A and anti-B
A	42.0	A	Anti-B
B	8.5	B	Anti-A
AB	3.0	A and B	Neither anti-A nor anti-B

on antigens on the red cells and antibodies in the serum (Table 39.2).

In 1940 the rhesus system was discovered. It is an antigen found on the red cell and because of the ease with which the antibody against it is built up in the blood, people without the antigen, (Rh negative) need to be transfused with Rh-negative blood.

If antibodies have developed and the patient is again transfused with Rh-positive blood, then he/she will react against it.

A similar problem of antibody formation can occur during pregnancy when the mother is Rh negative and the baby is Rh positive. The mother can develop Rh antibodies due to contact with the baby's blood during delivery.

The risk of incompatibility and subsequent reaction can be minimized by following the procedures detailed in the Nursing Care Plan (p. 384).

Delivery of blood and blood products
INLINE BLOOD FILTERS
Filters are used to remove micro-aggregates present in the blood to be transfused. Micro-aggregates or micro-particles are composed mainly of red cell debris, platelets, white blood cells and fibrin strands that have clumped together.

The number and size is variable and dependent on two main factors:
1 the storage time: in general the older the blood the more micro-aggregates it contains;
2 the anticoagulant used to prevent the blood from clotting.

The size of the particles can vary between 10 and 200 microns.

There are two main problems for the patient associated with the transfusion of micro-aggregates:
1 pulmonary micro-emboli;
2 non-haemolytic fevers.

These problems are more commonly associated with large transfusions of 6 units and above, and the use of

blood stored for a long time.

The filter compartment of commonly used blood administration sets will only remove particles of 170–200 microns and above.

Three types of filter are available:
1 *Screen or surface filters*: which effectively sieve the blood. The size of the particle removed will depend on the pore size on the surface. These filters tend to become more efficient the more blood flows through them.
2 *Depth filters*: these work by absorbing the particles into the layers of fibre. They tend to be effective for the removal of smaller particles but their efficiency diminishes as the number of units used increases. They also tend to slow the rate at which blood can be adminstered.
3 *Combination filters*: which consist of a surface filter above and a depth filter below.

Filters are generally capable of removing particles of 40 microns, and some depth filters effectively remove smaller debris, down to 10 microns.

As previously stated, use of additional inline blood filters is not indicated for the majority of transfusions, and is contraindicated with certain components such as platelets.

BLOOD WARMERS
The warming of blood and blood products is not recommended as it is of limited benefit and is potentially dangerous. The use of blood warmers is indicated when:
1 massive, rapid transfusion could result in cooling of cardiac tissue, causing dysfunction;
2 frozen plasma or other components are prescribed and must be thawed prior to administration;
3 transfusion is required by patients with potent cold agglutinins;
4 exchange transfusion is indicated in the newborn.

Both waterbaths and dry heat blood warmers are available. Whatever device is chosen, the temperature should be maintained below 38 °C, as warming in excess of this can cause haemolysis of red cells and denature proteins.

The optimum effectiveness of dry heat blood warmers is reached when the rate of delivery to the patient is 150–160 ml per minute. This means that their use is restricted, and because of the greater flexibility of water baths these are more frequently used.

Wherever there is water, there is the risk of bacterial contamination of blood products, particularly with Pseudomonas. For the patient this could result in a fatal systemic infection. Therefore, certain recommendations must be adhered to:

1 waterbaths must be cleaned before and after use with disinfectant;
2 they must be stored dry and empty;
3 when needed, they should be refilled with sterile water;
4 a protective overbag should be considered for the blood product to be thawed, to prevent entry of contaminants through microscopic punctures or breaks in the seal;
5 the blood warmer should be drained after each use;
6 the blood product should be used immediately after it has been thawed.

All devices should be serviced at regular intervals.

References and further reading

Barbara, J. and Contreras, M. (1986a) Bacterial and parasitic diseases transmitted by blood transfusion, *Hospital Update*, Vol. 12, pp. 629–31.

Barbara, J. and Contreras, M. (1986b) Viral diseases transmitted by blood transfusion, *Hospital Update*, Vol. 12, pp. 697–708.

Brozovic, B. (1986) Blood and blood products: availability and indications, *Hospital Update*, Vol. 12, pp. 445–58.

Canadian Red Cross Society Blood Transfusion Service (1982) *Clinical Guide to Transfusion*, Toronto, Canada.

Department of Health and Social Security, National Blood Transfusion Service, Scottish National Blood Transfusion Service (1984) *Notes on Transfusion*, London.

Editorial (1985) Warming of blood and blood products, *Canadian Intravenous Nurses Association Journal*, Vol. 1, no. 2, p. 5.

Jenkins, N.L. and Cosentino, F. (1980) Administering whole blood and its components, *Managing I.V. Therapy Nursing Photobook Series*, Intermed Communications, Pennsylvania, USA.

Lloyd, G.M. and Marshall, L. (1986) Blood microagregates: their role in transfusion reactions, *Intensive Care World*, Vol. 3, no. 4, pp. 119–22.

Lowe, G.D. (1981) Filtration in I.V. therapy: blood filters, *British Journal of Intravenous Therapy*, Vol. 2, no. 6, pp. 24–38.

Slater, N.G.P. (1980) Blood and blood products: hazards and precautions, *Proceedings of the British Intravenous Therapy Association*, inaugural meeting, BITA, pp. 24–9.

Smith, D.S. (1987) The appropriate use of diagnostic services: a guide to blood transfusion practice, *Health Trends*, Vol. 19, pp. 12–16.

Swaffield, L. (1987) Circulating the blood, *Nursing Times*, Vol. 83, no. 11, pp. 16–17.

Webster, A. (1987) Banking your own blood, *Nursing Times*, Vol. 83, no. 31, pp. 36–7.

NURSING CARE PLAN

The problems identified in this section are those specifically associated with blood or blood product transfusion. Common problems associated with delivery of these substances are similar to those encountered in intravenous administration of any therapy and reference should be made to Chapter 17 (p. 179).

Examples of problems frequently encountered are:

1 the infusion slows or stops shortly after commencing the unit of blood. The most likely cause for this is venous spasm due to a cold solution being infused. The preventive/corrective measure would be to apply a warm compress to soothe and dilate the vein and increase blood flow;
2 the infusion slows or stops due to occlusion of the cannula. Maintenance of continuous flow is important here. If this problem is recognized early, then flushing the cannula gently with normal saline may resolve this. However, if some minutes have elapsed it may be necessary to prime a new administration set with normal saline to re-establish flow as clotting may have occurred in the tubing.

These two situations may be interrelated and are more often associated with smaller veins. Flow into these vessels may be facilitated by using a 'Y' set and decreasing the viscosity of the blood by simultaneous infusion of normal saline. Keeping the patient warm and relaxed will also increase the peripheral circulation and prevent problems.

Potential problems	Cause	Preventative measure	Suggested action
Elevated temperature after the commencement of a unit of blood with temperature falling if the blood is slowed.	Pyrogenic reaction.	Regular observation of the patient's temperature, pulse and blood pressure during the transfusion, especially at the start of each unit. If patient has had multiple transfusions or experienced this type of reaction previously, ensure 'cover' of hydrocortisone and chlorpheniramine is written up and administered prior to commencement of therapy.	Slow blood transfusion rate. Inform medical staff.
A high temperature associated with fever and rigor during a transfusion.	White cell antibody reaction.	Observation as above.	Stop transfusion. Change giving set and commence normal saline to keep vein open. Inform medical staff.
Slightly elevated temperature with associated rash, may be severe with oedema round the eyes and larynx and shortness of breath.	Allergic reaction to protein in the plasma.	Observation as above. Ensure patient is aware of symptoms to report, e.g. appearance of a rash or breathlessness. Close observation of patient for swollen eyes and signs of breathlessness.	If mild, slow the rate of transfusion. Inform medical staff. If severe, stop transfusion. Change giving set and commence normal saline to keep vein open. Lie patient flat, treat as for shock. Inform medical staff.
Patient complains of feeling hot with chest and abdominal pain. Fall in blood pressure, patient's temperature subnormal at first and later rising to a pyrexia.	Infection introduced either from bacteria in the blood or during the cannulation or connection set changes.	Adhere to strict aseptic technique when handling the blood bags and intravenous line. Use blood within 30 minutes of removal from refrigerator. Regular observations as above. Adhere to recommended delivery time for each unit of blood; discard if hanging for 8 hours.	Stop transfusion. Change giving set and commence normal saline to keep vein open. Inform medical staff and institute prescribed treatment, e.g. steroids, antibiotics. Return remaining blood for examination by the bacteriology department.

Potential problems	Cause	Preventative measure	Suggested action
Patient complaining of feeling a hot flush along the vein, facial flushing and lumbar pain. The patient may become shocked with a fall in the blood pressure and the urine output may fall.	Blood not cross-matched. Urgent cross-match completed and blood not fully compatible. Blood administered to wrong patient. Cross-matched blood sample wrongly labelled or taken from wrong patient.	Ensure blood cross-matching forms are completed correctly. If taking blood sample, check carefully that the name and number on the form matches the patient. Ensure that before a unit is checked against the cross-match form for blood group, patient's name, patient's number, ward, Rh factor, unit number of blood, when blood taken, and expiry date. Begin transfusion slowly and observe the patient carefully at the start of each unit.	Stop transfusion. Change giving set and commence normal saline to keep vein open. Lay patient flat and treat as for shock. Inform medical staff.

Note: Tranfusion risks associated with administration of massive amounts of blood include:
1   abnormal bleeding tendencies;
2   hypocalaemia;
3   increased oxygen affinity;
4   potassium intoxication;
5   elevated blood ammonia level;
6   haemosiderosis;
7   hypothermia.
Massive transfusion refers to quantities in excess of 6 units and specific texts should be consulted in these circumstances.

40

The Unconscious Patient

Definition

Plum and Posner (1978) define unconsciousness as an unrousable, unresponsive state characterized by the absence of any psychologically understandable response to external stimulus or inner need. Spielman (1981) adds that such a definition is more accurate if based on a continuum from normal consciousness to deep coma with various stages of impaired consciousness in between, e.g. confusion, lethargy and stupor. Jennett and Teasdale (1974) initiated the Glasgow Coma Scale as a means of assessing the integrity of the central nervous system on the basis of three behavioural responses that denote the patient's motor activity, verbal performance and eye-opening ability. Myco and McGilloway (1980), in the introduction to their article, have a brief survey of the ways in which 'unconsciousness' has been defined. The authors conclude that 'consciousness' and 'unconsciousness' cannot be defined simply in physiological or sociological terms, but should be approached as containing, or lacking, elements of both.

Indications

The normal reflexes that protect the conscious patient have been lost and their protective function must be taken over by the nurse until the patient can function fully in his/her environment. In order to do this it will be necessary:

1 to establish and maintain a clear airway;
2 to assess the level of consciousness;
  (a) evaluate verbal responses
  (b) evaluate motor responses;
3 to evaluate the vital signs;
4 to maintain fluid and electrolyte balance;
5 to carry out direct nursing care appropriate to the patient's condition.

REFERENCE MATERIAL
Causes of unconsciousness
POISONS AND DRUGS
1 Alcohol.
2 General anaesthetics.
3 Overdose of drugs.
4 Gases.
5 Heavy metals.

VASCULAR CAUSES
1 Ischaemia.
2 Hypertensive encephalopathy.
3 Haemorrhage – subarachnoid, cerebral haemorrhage.

INFECTIONS
1 Septicaemia.
2 Encephalitis.
3 Meningitis.
4 Protozoan (e.g. malaria).
5 Metazoan (e.g. cysticercus).
6 Fungal (e.g. torulosis).

SEIZURES
1 Epilepsy
2 Eclampsia.

OTHER CAUSES
1 Neoplastic causes.
2 Trauma, hypothermia, hyperthermia, dehydration.
3 Uraemia.
4 Hepatic coma.
5 Tetany.
6 Myxoedema.

Recording level of consciousness

There is no universally accepted method of assessing and recording a patient's level of consciousness. One of the more commonly used ones is the Glasgow coma scale. Useful descriptions of this scale may be found in Albeson (1982) and Jones (1979).

Attitudes of nurses

Leon and Smyder (1980) came to the conclusion that, in general, nurses felt acceptance for the comatose patient and were challenged by such an assignment. Calmness pervaded the respondent's attitudes when providing care for these patients. These authors also felt, however, that further research was needed to gain insight into how nurses can effectively cope with their feelings of hopelessness and despair and with the questions surrounding whether or not to prolong life.

References and further reading

Albeson, N.M. (1982) Observations of the neurosurgical patient, *Curationis*, Vol. 5, no. 3, pp. 32–7.
Jennett, B. and Teasdale, G. (1974) Assessment of coma and impaired consciousness. A practical scale, *Lancet*, Vol. ii, pp. 81–3.
Jones, C. (1979) Glasgow coma scale, *American Journal of Nursing*, Vol. 79, no. 9, pp. 1551–3.
Leon, M. and Smyder, M. (1980) Care of the long-term comatose patient: a pilot study, *Journal of Neurosurgery Nursing*, Vol. 12, no. 3, pp.134–7.
Mason, A. and Pratt, J. (1980) Touch, *Nursing Times*, Vol. 76, pp. 999–1001.
Mountjoy, P. and Wrythe, B. (1970) *Nursing Care of the Unconscious Patient*, Baillière Tindall and Cassell, London.
Myco, F. and McGilloway, F.A. (1980) Care of the unconscious patient: a complementary perspective, *Journal of Advanced Nursing*, Vol. 5, no. 3, pp. 273–83.
Plum, F. and Posner, J. (1986) *Diagnosis of Stupor and Coma*, 3rd edn, F.A. Davis, Philadelphia.
Ricci, M.M. (1979) Neurological assessment: keeping it ongoing, in *Coping with Neurological Problems Proficiently*, Intermed Communications, p. 33 ff.
Roberts, A. (1982) Systems and signs. Nervous System, Coma, *Nursing Times*, Vol. 78, Systems of Life.
Spielman, G. (1981) Coma: a clinical review, *Heart and Lung*, Vol. 10, no. 4, pp. 700–7.

GUIDELINES: CARE OF UNCONSCIOUS PATIENT

Equipment

1 Airway
2 Ambu bag with valve and mask
3 Suction equipment
4 Oxygen equipment
5 Neurological tray, thermometer, sphygmomanometer
6 Intravenous infusion equipment
7 Personal hygiene equipment
8 Eye toilet set
9 Oral toilet set
10 Catheter care set
11 Nasogastric tube feeding equipment
12 Well-lit room (observation of patient's colour important)
13 Cot sides for the bed (patient may be restless)
14 Nursing observation charts (neurological, intravenous, turning, nasogastric)
15 Intubation and tracheostomy equipment for possible emergency use.

Procedure

Action

1 The room should be well lit with an even temperature and good ventilation.

Rationale

The observation of the patient's colour is important as an indication of the patient's well-being and minimal changes will not be noticed in a dim light, e.g. early signs of skin deterioration. An even temperature aids prevention of cross-

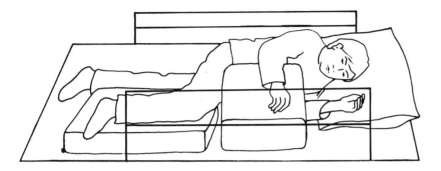

Figure 40.1 Positioning the unconscious patient.

infection and assists in the management of patients with hypothermia.

2 Nurse the patient in a bed with a firm base with a detachable head, and with padded cot sides.

To facilitate cardiac massage, if required. To prevent self-injury to a restless patient.

3 Insert a bed-cradle.

To allow for unhampered movement of limbs.

4 Place the patient in the left-lateral or semiprone position.

To prevent the tongue falling back against the pharyngeal wall, thus occluding the airway. To prevent respiratory complications by encouraging drainage of respiratory secretions and promoting oxygen and carbon dioxide exchange. To prevent contractures. Unequal strength in opposing sets of muscles fosters contractures.

5 Place the limbs as follows (Figure 40.1):
   (a) *Head*: put the patient's head on a pillow.
   (b) *Trunk*: keep the spine straight and place pillows at the patient's back for support.
   (c) *Upper Limb*: bring the uppermost arm forward in front of the patient. Bend the elbow slightly but keep the wrist extended. Support the arm on a pillow and bring the bottom arm up alongside the face with the palm facing upwards.
   (d) *Lower Limbs*: flex the uppermost leg and bring it forward. Support it on pillows.
        Keep the lower leg extended straight and in line with the spine. Make sure the patient's uppermost leg does not rest on his/her lower leg.
        Maintain the patient's feet at an angle of 90°. Use a footboard or special boots to achieve this position.

To promote comfort and maintain proper alignment of the body.

To prevent oedema by inappropriate pressure on venous flow.

To prevent internal rotation of the hip.

To avoid pressure sores.

To prevent foot-drop.

6 Remove all dental protheses.

7 Use suction to remove excess secretions and/or vomitus.

8 Clean the patient's nostrils.

9 Insert an airway.

To obtain and maintain a clear, open airway.

Note: For methods of assessing and evaluating the following, see procedures on neurological observations (pp. 252–8).

Action	Rationale
10 Evaluate the patient's verbal responses, if any.	To assess the patient's level of consciousness.
11 Evaluate the patient's motor responses.	As the patient's condition deteriorates, he/she may no longer localize pain and respond to it in a purposeful way. General restlessness may be observed.
12 Assess the patient's pupillary activity.	Any pupillary changes may indicate involvement of cranial nerve III and possible brainstem damage.
13 Assess the patient's motor function by evaluating: (a) muscle strength; (b) muscle tone; (c) posture; (d) co-ordination; (e) abnormal movements.	Damage to any part of the patient's nervous system can affect the ability to move.
14 Assess the patient's sensory function.	When disease or injury damages the sensory pathways, the sensory responses are always affected.
15 Assess the patient's vital signs: (a) respirations; (b) temperature; (c) blood pressure and pulse.	Respirations are controlled by different areas of the brain. Any injury or disease in these areas will cause respiratory changes. Damage to the hypothalamus, the temperature-regulating centre, may result in grossly abnormal body temperatures. Particularly important is unconscious patients as indicators of intracranial pressure.
16 Administer intravenous fluids as prescribed and record.	To maintain the patient's fluid and electrolyte balance.
17 Asepsis must be maintained throughout for any procedure involving the puncture site of a cannula.	To prevent local and/or systemic infection.
18 Maintain the nasogastric feeding (see the procedure on nasogastric feeding, pp. 240–51).	Feeding through a nasogastric tube ensures better nutrition than does intravenous feeding. Paralytic ileus is frequent in the unconscious patient and a nasogastric tube assists in gastric decompression.
19 Speak softly and use the patient's personal name. *Never* talk about the patient when in his/her hearing. Explain each procedure before carrying it out.	The sense of hearing frequently remains intact in the unconscious patient.
20 Touch the patient gently.	Through touch individuals establish themselves and their relationships with their environment. Being denied opportunities to touch can impair phsyiological, psychological and social development.
21 Give the patient a daily blanket bath.	To ensure that the patient's skin is kept clean, dry and supple.
22 Carry out eye toilet (see the procedure on eye care, pp. 156–64).	The blink reflex is absent during unconsciousness. This may lead to corneal drying, irritation and ulceration.

23 Carry out oral tiolet (see the procedure on mouth care, pp. 234–9).	To maintain a clean, moist mouth. To prevent the accumulation of oral secretions. To prevent the development of mouth infection.
24 Observe the patient for signs of bladder distension (see the procedure on urinary catheterization, pp. 393–403).	To prevent urinary complications. In males, an external sheath catheter may be used initially. Continuous bladder drainage may be necessary later. Catheterization may be immediately necessary for females. Regular catheter toilet will be necessary should this be the case.
25 Carry out bowel care (see the procedure on bowel care, pp. 56–70).	To prevent constipation or diarrhoea.
26 Put the patient through passive limb movements.	To prevent contractures. To aid circulation.
27 Change the patient's position regularly, e.g. every 2 hours, and record.	To relieve pressure areas. To prevent respiratory complications by allowing for postural drainage and for each side of the chest to receive a period when, free of compression by body weight, it can expand fully.

NURSING CARE PLAN

Problem	Cause	Suggested action
Restlessness and/or confusion.	A degree of restlessness may be favourable since it may indicate that the patient is regaining consciousness. When a patient is regaining consciousness there is usually a period of clouding of consciousness, with confusion and disorientation. This may present itself in the form of aggression or unco-operative behaviour. Restlessness may be a manifestation of brain injury, however. It is common in cerebral anoxia, when there is a partially obstructed airway, distended bladder, bleeding or fracture.	Be assertive. Convey confident firmness implying an expectation that the patient will follow your suggestions and requests. Ascertain that restlessness is not the result of some physical discomfort, e.g. constipation, patient too hot or cold. Carry out appropriate procedure. Summon help if the patient becomes aggressive or violent. Ensure that the patient does not harm himself, e.g. place cot-sides in position.
Seizures.	An unconscious patient is a potential candidate for seizures.	Maintain a clear, airway. Protect the patient from self-injury. Observe the patient during the seizure and record observations on a seizure chart. Administer prescribed drugs.
Cerebrospinal fluid leakage through the nose and/or ears.	May be indicative of a basilar skull fracture.	Place a sterile topical swab against the nose and/or ears to collect drainage. Inform the medical staff.

Problem	Cause	Suggested action
Vomiting.	May indicate that medulla oblongata is compromised.	Maintain a clear airway. Inform the medical staff immediately.
Distended bladder.	See the procedure on urinary catheterization (pp. 393–403) for problems associated with catheterization.	
Inability to maintain own nutritional intake.	See the procedure on nasogastric feeding (pp. 240–51) for problems associated with this type of nutrition.	

41

Urinary Catheterization

Definition

Urinary catheterization is the insertion of a special tube into the bladder, using aseptic technique, for the purpose of evacuating or instilling fluids.

Indications

MALE

In the male, urinary catheterization may be carried out for the following reasons:

1 to empty the contents of the bladder, e.g. prior to or after abdominal, pelvic or rectal surgery and prior to certain investigations;
2 to determine residual urine;
3 to allow irrigation of the bladder;
4 to bypass an obstruction;
5 to relieve retention of urine;
6 to introduce cytotoxic drugs in the treatment of papillary bladder carcinomas;
7 to enable bladder function tests to be performed;
8 to measure urinary output accurately, e.g. when a patient is in shock, undergoing bone marrow transplantation or receiving high-dose chemotherapy
9 to relieve incontinence when no other means is practicable.

FEMALE

In the female, urinary catheterization may be carried out for the nine reasons listed above and for two further reasons:

10 to empty the bladder prior to childbirth, if though necessary;
11 to avoid complications during intracavitary insertion of radioactive caesium.

REFERENCE MATERIAL
Common sites of cross-infection

The common sites of cross-infection of a catheterized patient are illustrated in Figure 41.1.

Types of material used for catheters

LATEX

Latex is a purified form of rubber and is the softest material from which catheters are made. It has a smooth surface and has a tendency to attract crust formation. Latex can also produce urethral irritation and should only be used for short-term catheterization.

TEFLON-COATED LATEX

Teflon-coated latex was produced to reduce urethral reaction. It is appropriate for short- or medium-term catheterization.

SILICONE-COATED OR ALL SILICONE

Silicone is a very soft, inert material ideal for long-term drainage. This type of catheter is more expensive than those mentioned above and must be reserved for patients who require catheterization for two or more weeks.

CATHETER SELECTION

Selection of catheter type, size and design is important if catheterization is to be effective. Careful consideration of the features required, i.e. shaft length, balloon size and materials used in manufacture, will assist the best selection. Ten millilitres fill volume balloons should be used in the majority of cases. Thirty millilitres fill volume balloons preferably should be used for patients following urological surgery.

TYPES OF CATHETERS

Types of catheters are listed in Table 41.1, together with their applications.

CATHETER SIZE

Catheter size is measured in French gauge; 1 FG indicates an external tube diameter of the catheter of 0.66 mm.

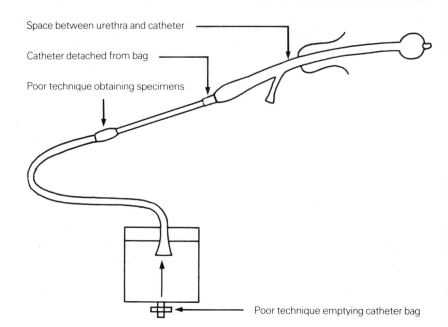

Space between urethra and catheter

Catheter detached from bag

Poor technique obtaining specimens

Poor technique emptying catheter bag

Figure 41.1 Common sites of cross-infection in a catheterized patient.

LEG DRAINAGE BAG

If an active patient has a permanent urinary catheter in position, he/she should be instructed in the use of a leg drainage bag as this will allow the resumption of a full range of normal activities. Such patient education should begin several days before his/her discharge so that any problems may be identified while the patient is still in hospital. If the patient has any physical or mental disabilities, a responsible relative or close friend should be taught the required catheter care before the patient is discharged.

Leg drainage bags have a limited capacity (350–750 ml). For nighttime drainage, connection of a larger capacity bag to the outlet portal of the leg bag allows effective drainage without interruption of the closed system.

References and further reading

Bard Ltd (1984) *Guidelines for the Management of the Catheterised Patient*, Bard Ltd.
Bard Ltd (1987) *You, Your patients, and Urinary Catheters*, Bard Ltd.

Table 41.1 Types of Catheter

Catheter type	Material	Uses
Foley two-way	Latex	The usual choice when short-term indwelling catheterization is indicated. If Teflon coated may remain in position for 1 month.
Foley three-way	Latex	For those procedures where there is a need to irrigate the bladder or instil solutions into it. Potential infection is avoided by decreasing the need to break the closed system of drainage.
Red rubber	Rubber	Non-drainage procedures, e.g. residual urine or obtaining sterile specimen from an ileal conduit. Rubber is extremely irritating to urethral mucosa.
Silastic	Silicone	Long-term indwelling catheterization with an approximate lifespan of 3 months.
Intermittent	PVC and other plastics	To empty bladder or continent urinary reservoir intermittently (cannot be used for continuous drainage) and to dilate urethral stricture.

Bielski, M. (1980) Preventing infection in the catheterised patient, *Nursing Clinics of North America*, Vol. 15, pp. 703–13.

Blannin, J.P. and Hobden, J. (1980) The catheter of choice, *Nursing Times*, Vol. 76, pp. 2092–3.

Brunner, L.S. and Suddarth, D.S. (1986) *The Lippincott Manual of Nursing Practice*, 4th edn, J.B. Lippincott, Philadelphia.

Chilman, A.M. and Thomas, M. (1987) *Understanding Nursing Care*, 3rd edn, Churchill Livingstone, Edinburgh.

Phipps, W.J. *et al.* (1986) *Medical–Surgical Nursing: Concepts and Clinical Practice*, 3rd edn, C.V. Mosby, St Louis.

GUIDELINES: URINARY CATHETERIZATION

Equipment

1 Sterile catheterization pack containing gallipots, receiver, wool balls, topical swabs, disposable towels, disposable dissecting forceps
2 Disposable pad
3 Sterile gloves
4 Selection of appropriate catheters
5 Sterile anaesthetic lubricating jelly, such as Xylocaine gel
6 Universal specimen container
7 Antiseptic solution such as Savolodil
8 Alcohol-based hand wash solution, such as Hibisol
9 Gate clip
10 Hypo-allergenic tape
11 Scissors
12 Sterile water or saline
13 Syringe and needle
14 Disposable plastic apron
15 Drainage bag and stand or holder.

Procedure

MALE

Action	**Rationale**
1 Explain the procedure to the patient.	To obtain the patient's consent and co-operation.
2 (a) Screen the bed.	To ensure the patient's privacy.
(b) Assist the patient to get into the supine position with his legs extended.	To allow dust and airborne organisms to settle before the sterile field is exposed.
(c) Do not expose the patient at this stage of the procedure.	
3 Wash hands.	
4 Put on a disposable plastic apron.	
5 Prepare the trolley, placing all equipment required on the bottom shelf.	
6 Take the trolley to the patient's bedside, disturbing screens as little as possible.	To minimize airborne contamination.

Action	Rationale
7 Remove cover that is maintaining the patient's privacy and position a disposable pad under his buttocks and thighs.	
8 Open the outer cover of the catheterization pack and slide the pack onto the top shelf of the trolley.	
9 Using an aseptic technique, open the supplementary packs.	The bladder is a sterile organ.
10 Clean hands with an alcohol-based hand wash solution, such as Hibisol.	Hands may have become contaminated by handling the outer packs.
11 Put on sterile gloves.	
12 Place sterile towels across the patient's thighs.	
13 Apply the nozzle to the tube of anaesthetic lubricating jelly.	
14 Wrap a sterile topical swab around the penis. Retract the foreskin, if necessary, and clean the glans penis with an antiseptic solution, such as Savlodil. Use forceps to manipulate the swabs.	
15 Insert the nozzle of the lubricating jelly into the urethra. Squeeze the gel into the urethra, remove the nozzle and discard the tube. Massage the gel along the urethra.	Adequate lubrication helps to prevent urethral trauma. Use of a local anaesthetic minimizes the discomfort experienced by the patient.
16 Grasp the shaft of the penis, raising it until it is almost totally extended. Maintain grasp of the penis until the procedure is finished.	This manoeuvre straightens the penile urethra and facilitates catheterization. Maintaining a grasp of the penis prevents contamination and retraction of the penis.
17 Place the receiver containing the catheter between the patient's legs. Insert the catheter for 15–25 cm until urine flows.	The male urethra is approximately 18 cm long.
18 If resistance is felt at the external sphincter, increase the traction on the penis slightly and apply steady, gentle pressure on the catheter. Ask the patient to strain gently, as if passing urine.	Some resistance may be due to spasm of the external sphincter.
19 Either remove the catheter gently when urinary flow ceases or:	
(a) When urine begins to flow, advance the catheter almost to its bifurcation.	Advancing the catheter ensures that it is correctly positioned in the bladder.
(b) Inflate the balloon according to the manufacturer's directions, having ensured that the catheter is draining properly beforehand.	Inadvertent inflation of the balloon in the urethra causes pain and urethral trauma.
(c) Withdraw the catheter slightly and attach it to the drainage system.	

(d)	Tape the catheter laterally to the thigh or on the abdomen.	This smooths out the urethral curve and eliminates pressure on the penoscrotal junction which can lead to the formation of a fistula.
(e)	Ensure that the catheter is not taut on the skin.	This allows room for movement should spontaneous erection occur.

20 Reduce or reposition the foreskin.

Retraction and constriction of the foreskin behind the glans penis (paraphimosis) may occur if this is not done.

21 Make the patient comfortable. Ensure that the area is dry.

22 Measure the amount of urine.

If the area is left wet or moist, secondary infection and skin irritation may occur.

23 Take a urine specimen for laboratory examination, if required.

For further information, see the procedure on collection of a catheter specimen of urine (p. 399).

24 Dispose of equipment in a disposable plastic bag and seal the bag before moving the trolley.

To prevent environmental contamination.

25 Draw back the curtains.

26 Record information in any relevant documents.

FEMALE

Action		**Rationale**
1	Explain the procedure to the patient.	To obtain the patient's consent and co-operation.
2	(a) Screen the bed.	To ensure the patient's privacy.
	(b) Assist the patient to get into the supine position with knees bent, hips flexed and feet resting about 60 cm apart.	
	(c) Do not expose the patient at this stage of the procedure.	To allow dust and airborne organisms to settle before the sterile field is exposed.
3	Ensure that a good light source is available.	To enable the genital area to be seen clearly.
4	Wash hands.	
5	Put on a disposable plastic apron.	
6	Prepare the trolley, placing all equipment required on the bottom shelf.	
7	Take the trolley to the patient's bedside, disturbing screens as little as possible.	To minimize airborne contamination.
8	Remove cover that is maintaining the patient's privacy and position a disposable pad under the patient's buttocks.	

Action

Rationale

9 Open the outer cover of the catheterization pack and slide the pack on the top shelf of the trolley.

10 Using an aseptic technique, open supplementary packs.

Catheterization requires the same aseptic precautions as a surgical procedure.

11 Clean hands with an alcohol-based hand wash solution, such as Hibisol.

Hands may have become contaminated by handling of outer packs, etc.

12 Put on sterile gloves.

13 Place sterile towels across the patient's thighs.

14 Separate the labia minora so that the urethral meatus is seen. Using sterile topical swabs, one hand should be used to maintain labial separation until catheterization is completed.

This manouevre helps to prevent labial contamination of the catheter and provides better access to the urethral orifice.

15 Clean around the urethral orifice with an antiseptic solution, such as Salvodil, using single downward strokes. Forceps should be used to handle the cleaning swabs.

Inadequate preparation of the urethral orifice is a major cause of infection following catheterization.

16 Dry the area well before proceeding.

17 Lubricate the catheter with sterile anaesthetic lubricating jelly, such as xylocaine gel.

Lubricating the catheter reduces friction and trauma to the urethral mucosa. Use of a local anaesthetic minimizes the patient's discomfort.

18 Place the catheter, in the receiver, between the patient's legs.

19 Introduce the tip of the catheter into the urethral orifice in an upward and backward direction. Advance the catheter until 5–6 cm have been inserted.

The direction of insertion and the length of catheter inserted should bear relation to the anatomical structure of the area.

20 *Either* remove the catheter gently when urinary flow ceases, *or*;

   (a) Advance the catheter 6–8 cm.

This prevents the balloon from becoming trapped in the urethra.

   (b) Inflate the balloon according to the manufacturer's directions, having ensured that the catheter is draining adequately.

Inadvertent inflation of the balloon within the urethra is painful and causes urethral trauma.

   (c) Withdraw the catheter slightly and connect it to the drainage system.

   (d) Tape the catheters and drainage system to the thigh.

This prevents traction and tension on the bladder and friction in the urethra.

21 Make the patient comfortable and ensure that the area is dry.

If the area is left wet or moist, secondary infection and skin irritation may occur.

22 Measure the amount of urine.

23 Take a urine specimen for laboratory examination, if required.

For further information, see the procedure on collection of a catheter specimen of urine (below).

24 Dispose of equipment in a disposable plastic bag and seal the bag before moving the trolley.

To prevent environmental contamination.

25 Draw back the curtains.

26 Record information in any relevant documents.

Note: When the bladder is very distended a gate clip should be applied to the drainage bag or catheter tubing to regulate the flow rate after 500 ml of urine have been drained. This prevents shock due to sudden reduction in intra-abdominal pressure.

An alternative way of preventing sudden emptying of the bladder on catheterization in the patient with a long history of urinary outflow obstruction would be to place the urinary collection bag at the height of the patient's bladder. This allows urine drainage to be gradual and controlled. However, once emptying has occurred, the bag should be placed below the level of the bladder to prevent pooling and potential ascending bacterial contamination.

GUIDELINES: COLLECTION OF A CATHETER SPECIMEN OF URINE

Equipment
1 Swab saturated with isopropyl alcohol 70% such as Medi Swab
2 Gate clip
3 Sterile syringe and needle
4 Universal specimen container.

Procedure

Action

Rationale

1 Explain the procedure to the patient.

To obtain the patient's consent and co-operation.

2 Screen the bed.

To ensure the patient's privacy.

3 If there is no urine in the tubing, clamp the tubing below the rubber cuff until sufficient urine collects.

To obtain an adequate urine sample.

4 Wash and dry hands.

5 Clean the rubber cuff with a swab saturated with isopropyl alcohol 70%.

To prevent cross-infection.

6 Using a sterile syringe and needle, aspirate the required amount of urine from the rubber cuff (Figure 41.2).

The rubber cuff is specially designed to occlude the puncture hole when the needle is withdrawn. If the catheter bag or tubing is punctured it causes leakage of urine and aspiration of air inwards, carrying organisms with it. Specimens collected from the catheter bag may give false results due to organisms proliferating there.

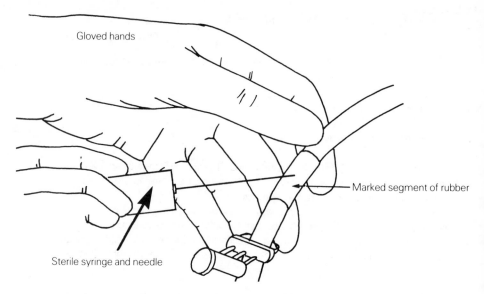

Figure 41.2   Taking a specimen.

Gloved hands

Marked segment of rubber

Sterile syringe and needle

Action	**Rationale**
7 Place the specimen in a sterile container.	
8 Wash and dry hands.	
9 Unclamp if necessary.	To allow drainage to continue.
10 Make the patient comfortable.	
11 Label the container and dispatch it to the laboratory with the completed request form.	

GUIDELINES: EMPTYING A CATHETER BAG

Equipment
1   Swabs saturated with isopropyl alcohol 70%, such as Medi Swab
2   Heat-disinfected jug or sterile jug
3   Disposable gloves.

Procedure

Action	**Rationale**
1 Explain the procedure to the patient.	To obtain the patient's consent and co-operation.
2 Wash hands and put on disposable gloves.	To prevent cross-infection.
3 Clean the outlet valve with a swab saturated with isopropyl alcohol 70%.	

4   Allow the urine to drain into the appropriate jug.

5   Close the outlet valve and clean it again with a new
alcohol-saturated swab.

To prevent cross-infection.

6   Cover the jug and dispose of contents in the sluice, having
noted the amount of urine if this is required for fluid balance
records.

To prevent environmental contamination.

7   Heat-disinfect the jug after each use or return the jub for
sterilization.

To prevent cross-infection.

8   Wash hands.

NURSING CARE PLAN
WITH THE CATHETER IN PLACE

Problem	Cause	Suggested action
Urinary tract infection introduced during catheterization.	Faulty aseptic technique. Inadequate urethral cleansing. Contamination of catheter tip.	Inform a doctor. Obtain a catheter specimen of urine.
Urinary tract infection introduced via the drainage system.	Faulty handling of equipment. Breaking the closed system. Raising the drainage bag above bladder level.	Inform a doctor. Obtain a catheter specimen of urine.
No drainage of urine.	Incorrect identification of external urinary meatus (female patients). Blockage of catheter.	Check that catheter has been correctly sited. In the female, leave the catheter in position to act as a guide, reidentify the urethra and recatheterize the patient. Remove the inappropriately-sited catheter.
	Empty bladder.	When changing the catheter, clamp the catheter 30 minutes before the procedure. On insertion of the new catheter, urine will drain.
Urethral mucosal trauma.	Incorrect size of catheter. Procedure not carried out correctly or skilfully. Movement of the catheter in the urethra. Creation of false passage as a result of too rapid insertion of catheter.	Recatheterize the patient using the correct size of catheter. Check the strapping and reapply as necessary. You may need to remove the catheter and wait for the urethral mucosa to heal.
Inability to tolerate indwelling catheter.	Urethral mucosal irritation.	You may need to remove the catheter and seek an alternative means of urine drainage.

Problem	Cause	Suggested action
	Psychological trauma.	Explain the need for and functioning of the catheter.
	Unstable bladder. Radiation cystitis.	
Inadequate drainage of urine.	Incorrect placement of a catheter. Kinked drainage tubing.	Resite the catheter. Inspect the system and straighten any kinks.
	Blocked tubing, e.g. pus, urates, phosphates, blood clots.	If a three-way catheter, such as Foley's, is in place, irrigate it. If an ordinary catheter is in use, milk the tubing in an attempt to dislodge the debris; then replace it with a three-way catheter.
Fistula formation.	Pressure on the penoscrotal angle.	Ensure that correct strapping is used.
Penile pain on erection.	Not allowing enough length of catheter to accommodate penile erection.	Ensure that an adequate length is available to accommodate penile erection.
Paraphimosis.	Failure to retract foreskin after catheterization or catheter toilet.	Always retract the foreskin.
Formation of crusts around urethral meatus.	Infection involving urea-splitting organisms that cause deposits of salts to form around the catheter.	Correct catheter toilet.
Leakage of urine around catheter.	Incorrect size of catheter.	Replace with the correct size, usually 2Ch sizes smaller.
	Incorrect balloon size.	Select catheter with 10-ml fill volume balloon.
	Bladder hyperirritability.	Use double-balloon catheter. As a last resort bladder hyperirritability can be reduced by giving diazepam or anticholinergic drugs.
Unable to deflate balloon.	Valve expansion. Valve displacement. Channel obstruction. Salt/debris deposition.	(i) Check the non-return valve on the inflation/deflation channel. If jammed, use a syringe and needle to aspirate by means of the inflation arm above the valve. (ii) Obstruction by a foreign body can sometimes be relieved by the introduction of a guidewire through the inflation channel. (iii) Inject 3.5 ml of dilute ether solution (diluted 50/50 with sterile water or normal saline) into the inflation arm.

(iv) Alternatively, the balloon can be punctured suprapubically using a needle under ultrasound visualization.

(v) Following catheter removal the balloon should be inspected to ensure it has not disintegrated leaving fragments in the bladder.

Note: Steps (ii)–(iv) should be attempted by or under the directions of a urologist. The patient may require cytoscopy following balloon deflation to remove any balloon fragments and to wash the bladder out.

AFTER REMOVAL OF THE CATHETER

Problem	Cause	Suggested action
Dysuria.	Inflammation of the urethral mucosa.	Ensure a fluid intake of 2–3 litres per day. Advise the patient that dysuria is common but will usually be resolved once micturation has occurred at least three times. Inform medical staff if the problem persists.
Retention of urine.	May be psychological.	Encourage the patient to increase his/her fluid intake. Offer the patient a warm bath. Inform medical staff if the problem persists.
Urinary tract infection.		Encourage a fluid intake of 2–3 litres a day. Collect a specimen of urine. Inform medical staff if the problem persists. Administer prescribed antibiotics.

42

Venepuncture

Definition
Venepuncture is the term used for procedure of entering a vein with a needle.

Indications
Venepuncture is carried out for two reasons:
1 to obtain a blood sample for diagnostic purposes;
2 to monitor levels of blood components.

REFERENCE MATERIAL
Venepuncture is a routine procedure that is increasingly being performed by nursing staff. In order to do this safely the nurse must have a basic knowledge of the following:
1 the relevant anatomy and physiology;
2 the criteria for choosing both the vein and device to use;
3 the potential problems which he/she may encounter.

Certain principles, such as adherence to an aseptic technique, must be applied throughout. The circulation is a closed sterile system and a venepuncture, however quickly completed, is a breach of this system providing a method of entry for bacteria.

The nurse must be aware of the physical and psychological comfort of the patient. He/she must appreciate the value of adequate explanation and simple measures to prevent haematoma formation, a complication of venepuncture, not a natural consequence of it.

Anatomy and physiology
The superficial veins of the upper limb are most commonly chosen for venepuncture. These veins are numerous and accessible, ensuring that the procedure can be performed safely and without discomfort. Occasionally the veins of a lower limb may be utilized if this is unavoidable, as blood flow in this region is diminished and the risk of ensuing complications higher.

Criteria for choosing a site for venepuncture
CONDITION AND ACCESSIBILITY OF THE PERIPHERAL VEINS
Veins may be tortuous, sclerosed, fibrosed or thrombosed, inflamed or fragile and unable to accommodate the device to be used. If the patient complains of pain or soreness over a particular site, this should be avoided, as should areas that are bruised. Veins adjacent to foci of infection must not be considered.

Preference is given to a vessel which is unused, easily detected by inspection and/or palpation, patent and healthy. These veins feel soft, bouncy and will refill when depressed.

ANATOMICAL CONSIDERATIONS
The venous anatomy of each individual differs, but care must always be taken to avoid adjacent structures, e.g. arteries and nerves. Accidental puncture of an artery may cause painful spasm and could result in prolonged bleeding. If a nerve is touched, this can result in severe pain and the attempted venepuncture at this site should be stopped.

Palpation is of value in distinguishing structures clinically, e.g. arteries and tendons, due to the presence of a pulse or resistance, and detecting deeper veins.

Use of veins which cross joints or bony prominences and those with little skin or subcutaneous cover, e.g. the inner aspect of the wrist, will subject the patient to more discomfort.

The sites of choice (Figure 42.1) are branches of:
1 the basilic vein;
2 the cephalic vein;
3 the median cubital vein in the antecubital fossa.
These are sizeable veins capable of providing copious and repeated blood specimens. The brachial artery and median nerve are in close proximity and must not be damaged.

The choice of vein, however, must be that which is

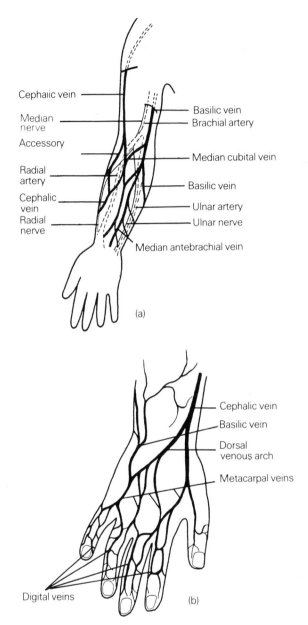

Cephalic vein

Median nerve

Accessory

Radial artery

Cephalic vein

Radial nerve

Basilic vein

Brachial artery

Median cubital vein

Basilic vein

Ulnar artery

Ulnar nerve

Median antebrachial vein

(a)

Cephalic vein

Basilic vein

Dorsal venous arch

Metacarpal veins

Digital veins

(b)

Figure 42.1 *a*, Superficial veins of the forearm, *b*, Superficial veins of the dorsal aspect of the hand.

CLINICAL STATUS OF THE PATIENT

Injury or disease may prevent the use of a limb for venepuncture. Amputation, fracture and cerebrovascular accident are good examples of conditions that affect venous access. Use of a limb may be contraindicated because of an operation on one side of the body, e.g. mastectomy. Impairment of lymphatic drainage can influence venous flow regardless of whether there is obvious lymphoedema. An oedematous limb should be avoided as there is danger of stasis predisposing to such complications as phlebitis and cellulitis. Positioning of the patient may dictate the site of venepuncture.

PHYSIOLOGICAL FACTORS

The tunica media, the middle layer of the vein wall, is composed of muscle fibres capable of constricting or dilating in response to stimuli from the vasomotor centre in the medulla via the sympathetic nerves. The nurse must be aware of the factors which can influence venous dilation. These are:

1 anxiety;
2 temperature;
3 mechanical or chemical irritation;
4 the clinical state of the patient, e.g. hypovolaemia due to dehydration.

Anxiety may be reduced by presenting a confident manner together with an adequate explanation of the procedure. Careful preparation and an unhurried approach will help to relax the patient and his/her veins.

The temperature of the environment will influence venous dilation. If the patient is cold no veins may be evident on first inspection. Application of heat, e.g. in the form of a hot compress, will increase the size and visibility of the veins, thus increasing the likelihood of a successful first attempt.

Venepuncture may cause the vein to collapse or go into a spasm. This will produce discomfort and a reduction in blood flow. Good technique will reduce the likelihood of this and stroking the vein or applying heat will help resolve it.

Good technical skill also prevents trauma to the tunica intima, the lining of the vein. Roughening of the smooth endothelium encourages the process of thrombus formation.

Choice of device

The intravenous devices commonly used to perform a venepuncture for blood sampling are a straight steel needle and a steel winged infusion device. The optimum gauge to use is 21 swg (standard wire gauge). This enables blood to be withdrawn at a reasonable speed without undue discomfort to the patient or possible damage to the blood cells.

The nurse must choose the device dependent on the

best for the individual patient. When using other sites it is advisable to avoid junctions within the venous network. Another feature in veins is the presence of valves. These are folds of the endothelium present in larger vessels to prevent a backflow of blood to the extremity. If detected, a puncture should be performed above the value in order to facilitate collection of the sample.

Table 42.1   The Choice of Intravenous Device

Device	Gauge	Advantages	Disadvantages	Use
Needle	21	Cheap. Easy to use with large veins.	Rigid. Difficult to manipulate with smaller veins in less conventional sites. May cause more discomfort.	Large, accessible veins in the antecubital fossa. When small quantities of blood are to be drawn.
Winged infusion device	21	Flexible due to small needle shaft. Easy to manipulate and insert at any site. Causes less discomfort.	More expensive than steel needles.	Veins in sites other than the antecubital fossa. When quantities of blood greater than 20 ml are required from any site.
	23	As above.	As above, plus there can be damage to cells which can cause inaccurate measurements.	Small veins in more painful sites, e.g. inner aspect of the wrist, especially if measurements are related to plasma and not cellular components.

condition and accessibility of the individual patient's veins (see Table 42.1).

Skin preparation

Asepsis is vital when performing a venepuncture as the skin is breached and an alien device introduced into a sterile circulatory system. The two major sources of microbial contamination are:

1 the hands of the practitioner;
2 the skin of the patient.

Good hand washing and drying techniques are essential on the part of the nurse. If handwashing facilities are unavailable, an alcohol-based hand wash solution is an acceptable substitute.

To remove the risk presented by the patient's skin flora, firm and prolonged rubbing with an alcohol-based solution, such as chlorhexidine 70% in spirit, is advised. This cleaning should continue for at least 30 seconds, although some authors state a minimum of 1 minute or longer. The area that has been cleaned should then be allowed to dry to facilitate coagulation of the organisms, thus ensuring disinfection. The skin must not be touched or the vein repalpated prior to puncture.

Skin cleansing is a controversial subject and it is acknowledged that a cursory wipe with an alcohol swab does more harm than no cleaning at all as it disturbs the skin flora. Good cleaning techniques in a hospital environment, where transient pathogens abound, are of value in controlling infection.

Summary

In order to perform a safe and successful venepuncture it is important that the nurse considers carefully the choice of vein and device and applies the principles of asepsis. Supervision by an experienced member of staff is essential when the nurse begins to practise.

References and further reading

Dyson, A. and Bogod, D. (1987) Minimising bruising in the antecubital fossa after venepuncture, *British Medical Journal*, Vol. 294, p. 1659.

Plumer, A.L. (1987) *Principles and Practice of Intravenous Therapy*, 4th edn, Little, Brown, Boston, USA.

Sager, D. and Bomar, S. (1980) *Intravenous Medications*, J.B. Lippincott, Philadelphia.

White, J. *et al.* (1970) Skin disinfection, *John Hopkins Medical Journal*, Vol. 126, pp. 169–70.

Yuan, R.T.W. and Cohen, M.D. (1987) Lateral antebrachial cutaneous nerve injury as a complication of phlebotomy, *Journal of Canadian Intravenous Nurses Association*, Vol. 3, no. 3, pp. 16–17.

GUIDELINES: VENEPUNCTURE

Equipment

1   Clinically clean tray or receiver
2   Tourniquet or sphygmomanometer and cuff
3   Syringe(s) of appropriate size
4   21 swg needle or 21 swg winged infusion device
5   Swab saturated with isopropyl alcohol 70%
6   Sterile cotton wool balls
7   Sterile adhesive plaster or hypo-allergenic tape
8   Labelled blood specimen bottle(s)
9   Specimen requisition forms.

Alternatively, there are a number of vacuum systems available that can be used for taking blood samples. These are simple to use and cost effective. The manufacturer's instructions should be followed carefully if one of these systems is to be used and the following items will replace syringes, needles and specimen bottles:

1   21G multiple sample needle or 21G winged infusion device and multiple sample Luer adaptor
2   Plastic shell to hold specimen tubes
3   Appropriate vacuumed specimen tubes, labelled.

Procedure

Action	Rationale
1 Approach the patient in a confident manner and explain the procedure to the patient.	To obtain the patient's consent and co-operation. To reduce anxiety.
2 Allow the patient time to ask questions and discuss any problems which have arisen previously.	A relaxed patient will have relaxed veins.
3 Assemble the equipment necessary for venepuncture.	To ensure that time is not wasted and that the procedure goes smoothly without unnecessary interruptions.
4 Carefully wash and dry hands prior to commencement.	To minimize the risk of infection.
5 Check all packaging before opening and preparing the equipment on the chosen clinically clean receptacle.	To maintain asepsis throughout and to check than no equipment is damaged.
6 Take all the requirements to the patient, exhibiting a competent manner.	To put the patient at his/her ease.
7 In both an inpatient and an outpatient situation, lighting, ventilation, privacy and positioning must be checked.	To ensure that both patient and operator are comfortable and that adequate light is available to illuminate this procedure.
8 Consult the patient as to any preferences and problems he/she may have identified at previous venepunctures.	To involve the patient in his/her treatment. To acquaint the nurse fully with the patient's previous venous history. To identify any changes in clinical status which may influence vein choice, e.g. mastectomy.
9 Support the chosen limb.	To ensure the patient's comfort.

Action	**Rationale**
10 (a) Apply a tourniquet to the upper arm on the chosen side, making sure it does not obstruct arterial flow. The position of the tourniquet may be varied, e.g. if a vein in the hand is to be used is may be placed on the forearm. A sphygomanometer cuff may be used as an alternative.	To dilate the veins by obstructing the venous return.
(b) The arm may be placed in a dependent position. The patient may assist by clenching and unclenching his/-her fist.	To increase the prominence of the veins.
(c) The veins may be tapped lightly.	
(d) If all these measures are unsuccessful, remove the tourniquet and apply moist heat, e.g. a hot compress, to the chosen limb.	To promote blood flow and therefore distend the veins.
11 Select the vein using the afore-mentioned criteria.	
12 Select the device, based on vein size, site, etc.	
13 Wash hands with soap and water or clean hands using a suitable alcohol-based solution.	To maintain asepsis.
14 Clean the patient's skin carefully for at least 30 seconds using an appropriate preparation and allow to dry. Do not repalpate the vein or touch the skin.	To maintain asepsis.
15 Inspect the device carefullly.	To detect faulty equipment, e.g. bent or barbed needles. If these are present, discard them.
16 Anchor the vein by applying manual traction on the skin a few centimetres below the proposed insertion site.	To immobilize the vein. To provide countertension, which will facilitate a smoother needle entry.
17 Insert the needle smoothly at an angle of approximately 30°. The shaft of a straight needle may be bent slightly at the hub to enable the entry to be as flush with the skin as possible.	To ensure a successful, pain-free venepuncture.
18 Level off the needle as soon as a flashback of blood is seen in the tubing of a winged infusion device or when puncture of the vein wall is felt. If you are using a needle and syringe, pull the plunger back slightly prior to venepuncture and a flashback of blood will be seen in the barrel on vein entry.	
19 Advance the needle approximately 1 mm into the vein, if possible.	To stabilize the device within the vein and prevent it becoming dislodged during venepuncture.
20 Do not exert any pressure on the needle.	To prevent a through puncture occurring.
21 Withdraw the required amount of blood.	

22	Release the tourniquet. In some instances this may be requested at the beginning of sampling as inaccurate measurements may be caused by haemostasis, e.g. blood calcium levels.	To decrease the pressure within the vein.
23	Withdraw a small amount of blood into the syringe.	To reduce the amount of static blood in the vein and therefore the likelihood of leakage.
24	Pick up a sterile wool ball and place it over the puncture point.	
25	Remove the needle.	
26	Apply digital pressure directly over the puncture point.	To stop leakage and haematoma formation.
27	Do not apply pressure until the needle has been fully removed.	To prevent pain on removal.
28	Pressure should be applied until the bleeding has ceased, approximately 1 minute. Longer may be required if current disease or treatment interferes with clotting mechanisms.	To prevent leakage and haematoma formation.
29	The patient may apply pressure with his/her finger but should be discouraged from bending his/her arm if a vein in the antecubital fossa is used.	To prevent leakage and haematoma formation.
30	Transfer the blood to appropriate specimen bottles as soon as possible, making sure that the correct quantity is placed in each container.	To prevent clotting in the syringe. To ensure that an adequate amount is available for each test.
31	Mix well if the bottle contains a chemical to prevent clotting or aid accurate measurements.	To ensure that the blood is correctly presented to the laboratory and that the patient does not have to have a repeat specimen taken.
32	Label the bottles with the relevant details.	To ensure that the specimens from the right patient are delivered to the laboratory, the requested tests are performed and the results returned to the correct patient's records.
33	Inspect the puncture point before applying a dressing.	To check that the puncture point has sealed.
34	Ascertain whether the patient is allergic to adhesive plaster.	To prevent an allergic skin reaction.
35	Apply an adhesive plaster or alternative dressing.	To cover the puncture and prevent leakage or introduction of bacteria until healing is complete.
36	Ensure that the patient is comfortable.	To ascertain whether he/she wishes to rest before leaving (if an outpatient) or whether any other measures need to be taken.
37	Discard waste, making sure it is placed in the correct containers, e.g. 'sharps' into a designed receptacle.	To ensure safe disposal and avoid laceration or other injury of staff. To prevent re-use of equipment.
38	Follow hospital procedure for collection and transportation of specimens to the laboratory.	To make sure that specimens reach their intended destination.

NURSING CARE PLAN

Problem	Cause	Suggested action
Excessive pain.	Anxiety, fear, low pain tolerance. Frequently used vein.	Confident, unhurried approach. Use all methods, including heat, to dilate veins. Avoid hesitancy and skin 'tickling'. Consider use of winged infusion device. Avoid this site, if possible, otherwise proceed as above.
	Nerve touched.	Remove the needle immediately and proceed to a different site.
Very anxious patient.	Previous trauma. Needle phobia.	Confident unhurried approach. Make sure the patient is comfortable, perhaps reclining/lying down. Use all methods, including heat, to dilate veins. Consider use of winged infusion device.
Limited venous access.	Repeated use, e.g. prolonged cytotoxic therapy. Phlebitis.	Confident, unhurried approach. Use all methods including heat to dilate veins. Use a winged infusion device of 21G or 23G. Only proceed if sure of a successful first attempt. Consider referral to a more experienced colleague.
	Bruising due to: (i) fragile veins in the elderly; (ii) anticoagulant therapy or low platelet levels.	As above plus apply tourniquet gently or do not use. Ensure adequate pressure to puncture site to prevent further damage.
	Peripheral shutdown.	Use all methods to dilate veins as listed. A sphygomomanometer and cuff may enable more effective restriction of the venous return. Work quickly if the patient is in a collapsed state. Pull blood back into the veins by massaging above the venepuncture site.
Infection.	Poor aseptic technique.	Practise good hand washing and skin cleansing and take particular care with immune-compromised patients.

PRACTICAL PROBLEMS

Problem	Cause	Suggested action
Missed vein.	Inadequate anchoring. Wrong positioning. Poor lighting. Less than 100% concentration.	Withdraw the needle almost to the bevel and manoeuvre gently to realign needle and vein. Readvance, but if it becomes painful, remove. Better preparation next time.
Spurt of blood on entry.	Bevel tip of needle entering vein before entire bevel is under the skin, due to vein being very superficial.	Ignore. Reassure the patient if a small blood blister develops.

Blood flow stops.	Overshooting vein or advancing needle while withdrawing blood.	Gently ease needle back and continue.
	Vein collapse due to contact with valve or vein wall.	Manoeuvre gently. Release and retighten tourniquet and continue.
	Poor blood flow.	As above and massage above the needle tip to pull blood into vein.
Haematoma.	Perforation of opposite wall of vein.	Insert needle at correct angle and stop when a flashback is seen in syringe or tubing of winged fashion infusion device. Do not advance needle during taking of sample.
	Forgetting to remove tourniquet before removing needle.	Remember next time.
	Inadequate pressure on puncture site.	Press. Supervise the patient doing the same.
Hardening of the veins due to scarring and thrombosis.	Prolonged use of one site.	Alternate venepuncture sites to prevent this. Do not use hard veins as this is often not successful and will cause the patient pain.
Mechanical problems.	Faulty equipment, e.g. bent needle tips, cracked syringes.	Check carefully before use and discard.
Transmittable diseases.	Viruses pose the major risk, causing hepatitis B, cytomegalovirus, acquired immune deficiency syndrome.	All blood should be handled with care and caution used when handling specimens of infection, e.g. Australia antigen-positive persons. Gloves should be worn when taking blood and handling samples. Hospital policy should be strictly observed.
Needle inoculation.	Lack of caution. Overfilling of 'sharps' containers.	Dispose of equipment safely to prevent inoculation. If it does occur, follow accident procedure and report the incident immediately. An injection of hepatitis B immunoglobulin may be required.

43

Violence: Prevention and Management

The problem of violence within public service organizations has become a matter of increasing concern to all those who work in the health service (Poyner and Warne, 1983). Incidents range from threats and abuse to permanently disabling injuries and, rarely, loss of life. This chapter is confined to the manifestation and management of violence in the hospital setting.

Definition

Stuart and Sundeen (1983) define violence as 'an act of destructive aggression which may involve injury to the self, assaulting people or objects in the environment'.

Robinson (1983) defines aggression as 'an assertive force which may be expressed through attitude or behaviour and is usually directed to external objects, though it may be turned inward, as reflected in self destructive behaviour'. She states that 'aggression is a healthy force which sometimes needs to be channelled'.

Indications

Management of violence is necessary:

1   when a patient makes a physical attack on another person;
2   when a patient becomes disturbed to the extent that his/her behaviour is considered a threat to his/her own safety or the safety of others.

REFERENCE MATERIAL
Principles

The following principles underlie the management of violent patients:

1   restraint is always therapeutic, never punitive. As far as possible the therapeutic regimen should be maintained;
2   the risk of physical injury should be minimized. Any restraint applied must be of a degree appropriate to the actual danger or resistance shown by the patient. This is particularly important with children and the elderly;

3   the agreed procedure for the nursing care of violent patients should be adhered to.

Theories of violence

Mechanisms which may combine to explain or produce a violent act are reviewed by Harrington (1972) and Gunn (1973). Generally, theories of violence may be classified as biological (Lorenz, 1966; Gray, 1971; Montague, 1979), psychological (Freud, 1955; Dollard and Miller, 1961) or sociocultural (Bandura and Walters, 1963; Wertham, 1968; Gelles, 1972). Violence may be viewed as a behaviour influenced by various factors including personality, environment and social culture. Each perspective may add to the development of a body or knowledge about the problem of violence in the hospital setting.

Physiological considerations

Under certain circumstances an individual may have little or no ability to exercise control over his/her aggression. In these instances aggression may be related to pathological physiology. Internal stressors may include endocrine imbalance as in hyperthyroidism, hypoglycaemia, convulsive disorders, dementia, and brain tumours. The effects of alcohol and drug abuse should also be considered. Preventative measures may not be appropriate and the policy for the management of violence should be adhered to.

Recently HIV involvement with the nervous system has been recognized (Royal College of Nursing, 1986), manifestations include fits, presenile dementia, personality changes and memory disturbance. Thomas (1987) suggests that the number of people with AIDS-related neuropsychiatric disorders will increase. The general principles for the management of violent patients who also happen to be HIV antibody positive or hepatitis B positive are no different to those of the management of other violent patients.

The care of violent patients

Among the guidelines recommended by the Royal College of Nursing and the National Council for Nurses of the United Kingdom (1972) for the care of violent patients, are the following:

1   prevention of violence is the goal;
2   physical confrontations should be avoided;
3   all hospital personnel within the vicinity of the violent incident are expected to render assistance;
4   staff should receive instruction and guidance in the management of violence;
5   staff should be aware of and control their own emotions;
6   the attitude of staff should be calm, non-critical and non-domineering.

There will be occasions when, for a variety of reasons, a patient will threaten violence or actually become violent. In these situations it is essential for the nurse to apply confidently the appropriate skills in order to manage the incident. Leiba (1980) isolates four aspects that need to be considered in the management of violence in the hospital setting:

1   organization of the ward, department, etc.;
2   prevention;
3   management;
4   follow-up.

ORGANIZATION

The way in which staff are deployed influences the likelihood and outcome of any violent incident. There must be adequate staff to deal with the violence. There must be a hospital policy for the management of violence. All hospital personnel should know what to do and how to do it. Teaching sessions on the management of violence should be held on a regular basis so that staff benefit from controlled practice of the required techniques for avoiding and containing violence. It is helpful if there is a team in the hospital that can be called if an emergency occurs. Teamwork is essential and the leader must be seen to be confident in making the necessary decisions.

PREVENTION

Violent incidents may be spontaneous, without apparent provocation, for example with a patient suffering from a psychotic illness or cerebral lesions which affect behaviour. However, there may be signs of warning which would alert staff to a potentially violent situation and give opportunity for prevention of violence. Megargee (1966) suggests that violent behaviour is part of a continuum of behaviour which also includes anger, frustration and aggression. Novaco (1976) attributes positive and therapeutic functions to be controlled expression of anger. Stuart and Sundeen (1983) see violence as the culmination of an escalating process, where anger and aggression are considered as precursors to violence. They suggest that preventive therapeutic interventions can be used to intercept this process, thus differing a potentially violent situation. Knowledge of the propensities of individual patients will enable a nurse to recognize many of the signs of impending violence, thus allowing steps to be taken to help patients find alternative outlets for their aggressive feelings.

MANAGEMENT

Once violence has occurred, the following may be regarded as among the important management decisions that need to be implemented:

1   all medical and nursing personnel must be involved immediately, the former because medication may be required as part of the management of the situation;
2   some nurses must be delegated to attend to the needs of the remaining patients, to telephone for help, and to prepare any required medication;
3   if immobilization is needed, the agreed policy for restricting a patient must be implemented.

FOLLOW-UP

Following the incident staff should be given an opportunity to discuss their feelings about the patient, other members of staff involved, and the way the incident was managed. This should happen as soon as possible after the incident has resolved and with as many of the staff concerned as possible. Staff injured as a result of their involvement in the incident may be entitled to industrial injuries benefits or a payment under the criminal injuries compensation scheme and will need to be informed of their rights. All documentation required by law or hospital policy should be completed and forwarded to the appropriate departments.

Summary

Violent incidents often arise from a patient feeling vulnerable. Attack may become the preferred means of defence. The manner in which a patient is approached may be crucial in determining whether the patient will feel secure enough to cease his/her behaviour or continue to feel threatened, perhaps leading him/her on to violent behaviour. The need for physical restraint should be seen as the application of the appropriate technique in a particular situation and not as a failure of other methods. Protection against any administrative or legal problems lies in following the appropriate guidelines and applying them in good faith and with due restraint.

References and further reading

Bandura, A. and Walters, R. (1963) *Social Learning and Personality Development*, Holt, Rinehart & Winston, New York.

Bethlem Royal and Maudsley Hospitals (1976) *Guidelines for the Nursing Management of Violence*, Bethlem Royal and Maudsley Hospitals.

Blackburn, R. (1970) *Personality Types Among Abnormal Homicides*, Special Hospitals Research Report No. 1, Broadmoor Hospital, Special Hospitals research Unit.

Department of Health and Social Security (1980) *Report on the Advisory Group on the Management of Potentially Violent Patients*, DHSS, London.

Dollard, J. and Miller, N.E. (1961) *Frustration and Aggression*, Yale University Press, New Haven.

Freud, S. (1955) *The Complete Psychological Works of Sigmund Freud*, Vol. 18, Hogarth Press, London.

Gelles, R.J. (1972) *The Violent Home*, Sage, Beverly Hills and London.

Gray, J.A. (1971) Sex differences in emotional behaviour in mammals including Man: endocrine basis, *Acta Psychologica*, Vol. 35, pp. 29–46.

Gunn, J. (1973) *Violence*, David & Charles, Newton Abbot.

Harrington, J.A. (1972) Violence: a clinical viewpoint, *British Medical Journal*, Vol. 1, pp. 228–31.

Leiba, P.A. (1980) Management of violent patients, *Nursing Times*, Occasional Papers, Vol. 76, no. 23, pp. 101–4.

Lorenz, K. (1966) *On Aggression*, Harcourt, Brace & World, Inc., New York.

Megargee, E.I. (1966) Under-controlled and over-controlled personality types in extreme antisocial aggression, *Psychological Monograph*, Vol. 80, pp. 1–29.

Montague, M.C. (1979) Physiology of aggressive behaviour, *Journal of Neurosurgical Nursing*, Vol. 11, pp. 10–15.

Novaco, R.W. (1976) The functions and regulation of the arousal of anger, *American Journal of Psychiatry*, Vol. 133, p. 1124.

Poyner, B. and Warne, C. (1983) *Violence to Staff: A Basis for Assessment and Prevention*, Tavistock Institute of Human Relations, Health and Safety Commission, London.

Robinson, L. (1983) *Psychiatric Nursing as a Human Experience*, W.B. Saunders Co.

Royal College of Nursing and the National Council for Nurses of the United Kingdom (1972) *The Care of the Violent Patient*, Report of the Liaison Committee, Royal College of Nursing, London.

Royal College of Nursing (1986) *Nursing Guidelines on the Management of Patients in Hospital and the Community Suffering from AIDS*, Royal College of Nursing, London.

Royal College of Psychiatrists and Royal College of Nursing (1979) *Principles of Good Medical and Nursing Practice in the Management of Acts of Violence in Hospitals*, Royal College of Psychiatrists/Royal College of Nursing, London.

Stuart, G.W. and Sundeen, S.J. (1986) *Principles and Practice of Psychiatric Nursing*, 3rd edn, C.V. Mosby, St Louis.

Surrey Area Health Authority (1979) *Guidelines to Staff on the Management of Violent or Potentially Violent Patients*, Surrey Area Health Authority.

Thomas, B.L. (1987) Medical and psychiatric nursing care in the department of sexually transmitted diseases, in L. Paine (ed.) *AIDS: Psychiatric and Psychosocial Perspectives*, Croom Helm, London.

Wertham, D.J. (1968) *A Sign For Cain*, Hale, New York.

VIDEO MATERIAL

Nursing Management of Violence (1977), produced by the South East Thames Regional Health Authority.

GUIDELINES: PREVENTION AND MANAGEMENT OF VIOLENCE

Procedure

PREVENTION OF VIOLENCE

Action	Rationale
1 (a) It is important that the nurse makes other staff aware of a potentially violent situation and does not enter it unobserved.	To maintain a safe environment.
(b) Try not to encroach upon the patient's personal space. Keep at arm's length.	

(c) Ensure that there is a clear exit from the situation.
(d) Observe the area around the patient for potential
     weapons.
(e) Try to appear confident, calm and relaxed. Do not
     fold your arms, maintain an open posture. Move
     slowly, showing that you have nothing in your hands.

2 Talk quietly and clearly to the patient. Do not argue.

The nurse may be able to gauge the patient's level of frustration
and give him/her opportunity of expressing anger verbally by
initiating conversation.

MANAGEMENT OF VIOLENCE

General principles

Action

1 Call for assistance by shouting or using any signalling
     system.

2 Ask another patient to summon help when appropriate.

3 Continue to hold on to the patient once he/she is
     immobilized.

4 Consider carefully the accessories you wear. Be aware of
     the length of your fingernails and the way long hair is
     dressed. Pens, badges and other items should be
     removed beforehand.

Rationale

It is easier to manage the situation with two or more people.

To contain the violence.

To minimize the risk of physical injury to patients.

Personal attack

Action

1 Shout to the patient: 'STOP!'

2 Call for assistance.

3 Sound any signalling alarm.

4 If the above fails, either:
     (a) Stay close to the patient.
     (b) Grasp the patient's arm at elbow level and pull
          towards you.
     (c) Change your grip quickly and encircle patient with
          your arms.
     (d) Continue pulling the patient towards you.
     (e) Quickly get behind the patient.
     (f) Push the patient towards the nearest wall.
     (g) Retain your grip and lean against the patient,
          pressing the patient to the wall (Figure 43.1).

Rationale

A sharp command may bring the patient back to the reality of
the situation.

Immobilize the patient by pressing his/her body against a wall.

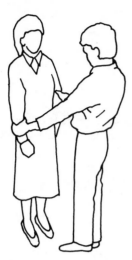
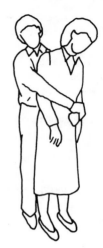

Figure 43.1   Managing the violent patient.

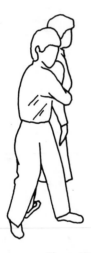
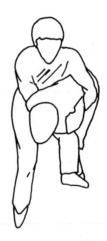

Figure 43.2   Managing the violent patient – a personal attack from behind.

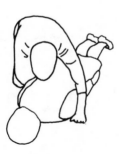
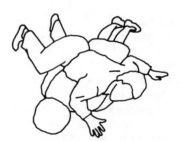

Figure 43.3   Managing the violent patient – a personal attack from behind.

Action	Rationale
5 Or (a) Move to one side. (b) Place your nearest leg behind the patient. (c) Keep your foot firmly on the ground. (d) Push the patient over your leg (Figure 43.2). (e) Lower the patient and yourself to the floor, turning the patient at the same time so that the patient's face is towards the floor. (f) Lie across the patient's trunk (Figure 43.3). (g) Wrap the patient in a blanket if possible.	Immobilize the patient by holding him/her face downwards on the floor. To restrict the use of limbs even further and to minimize the risk of physical injury to patient and staff.

Attempted choking

Action	Rationale
1 With patient in front of you (a) Bend sharply forward from the waist (Figure 43.4). (b) Cross your wrists in front of you and move back. (c) Carry out the procedure for personal attack outlined above.	To break the patient's grip. In case the patient brings his/her knee up.
2 With patient behind you (a) Grasp the little fingers on each of the patient's hands (Figure 43.5). (b) Wrench outwards to the full extent of your reach. (c) Pull the patient's arms forward, holding the patient close to your back. (d) Call for help.	To break the patient's grip.

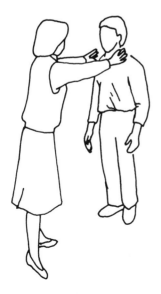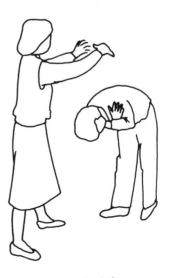

Figure 43.4   Managing the violent patient – attempted choking by a patient in front.

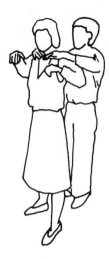

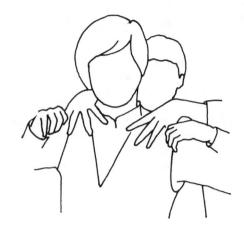

Figure 43.5   Managing the violent patient – attempted choking by a patient from behind.

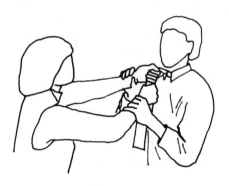

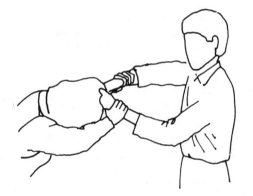

Figure 43.6   Countering hair and tie pulling.

Hair and tie pulling

Action	Rationale
1 Grasp the patient's wrists pulling his/her hands towards you (Figure 43.6).	To release the pressure on the hair or item of clothing being pulled.
2 Maintain this position.	
3 Call for help.	

Biting

Action	Rationale
1 Grasp attacker's hair and hold head still.	To minimize personal injury.

2 If possible apply firm pressure to the back of the patient's head.

To release grip of patient's jaw.

3 Call for help.

4 If blood is drawn through biting the same emergency measures should be taken as those for a needlestick injury, regardless of the patient's HIV or hepatitis B status (see Chapter 3, p. 9).

Attack with objects

Action

1 Back away from the situation.

2 Keep the patient in front of you.

3 Call for help.

4 If trapped, call for help and sound any signalling system.

5 Use a chair or similar object as a shield.

6 Keep to the middle of the room.

7 Defend yourself if attacked (Figure 43.7).

Rationale

To minimize the risk of physical injury.

To protect oneself.

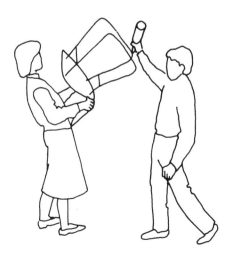

Figure 43.7   Countering an attack with a blunt object.

Blunt objects

Action

1   Close in quickly.

2   Grasp object.

3   Hold on tightly.

4   Call for help.

Sharp objects

Action

1   Pick up any piece of clothing or material, the larger and thicker the better.

2   Use the material to absorb the impact of any blow.

3   Smother the weapon if possible with the material (Figure 43.8).

4   Call for help.

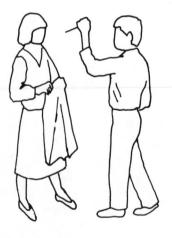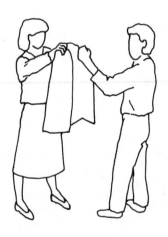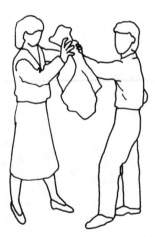

Figure 43.8   Countering an attack with a sharp object.

Threat with firearms

Action

1   Do as the patient demands.

Rationale

This is a life-threatening situation.

MANAGEMENT OF PERSONNEL INVOLVED

Action	Rationale
1 The ward manager should assess whether or not he/she has enough staff and inform the senior nurse if more are needed.	In order to contain the violence.
2 When help arrives, the staff should be organized. The manager should identify himself/herself as leader and should give a brief history of the patient and an account of the circumstances and events leading up to the incident.	Staff anxiety will need to be calmed.
3 A doctor, preferably the patient's own, should be called and must come immediately. A nurse should be allocated to draw up medication, and give injections if required.	Medication may be required in the management of the patient.
4 To restrain the patient, clear instructions should be given. The manager should indicate when the patient is to be restrained and co-ordinate staff during the procedure.	All staff must know the overall plan for restraint.
5 Specific staff should be allocated to be with the other patients, who should then be led away from the area where the patient is to be restrained.	Violent incidents are distressing and may trigger off more violence.
6 Each person should known which part of the patient's body he/she is to hold and from where to approach the patient.	To achieve full immobilization of the patient.
7 Allocate one member of staff, preferably someone the patient knows, to talk to the patient throughout the procedure.	To inform the patient about what is happening and why.
8 The first team member should help the nurse who is immobilizing the patient. They may need to disarm the patient and get them to the floor as quickly as possible in the face downwards position if this has not already been achieved. This member of staff should lie across the patient's trunk.	
9 Two other nurses should each restrain a leg.	
10 A further person should restrain the patient's head and shoulders and turn the patient's head to one side.	To ensure that the patient's airway is maintained.
11 Try to minimize discomfort. Reduce the amount of weight on the patient; use only what is necessary.	The procedure is not a punitive one.
12 As the patient calms down, the manager should indicate when restraint can be reduced. This should be done gradually, e.g. release one wrist slowly.	The patient may still be likely to strike.

Action	**Rationale**
13 The manager should withdraw staff from the patient gradually.	Restraint must be of a degree of appropriate to the actual resistance shown by the patient.
14 Some staff should stay with the patient.	To observe mood and behaviour.
15 Attend to any patients and staff injured during the incident. Inform such people of their legal rights.	To comply with legal obligations and hospital policy.
16 Record details of any violent incidents in the appropriate documents.	To comply with legal obligations and hospital policy.
17 The entire team should discuss the incident.	To ventilate feelings. Violent incidents are to be regarded as learning situations.

44

Wound Management

Definition

A wound is the superficial evidence of tissue death or damage resulting from surgical intervention or injury. The resulting wound may be classified as:

1 simple, i.e. where little or no tissue is lost and where the wound is closed by tape, stitches or clips,
2 complex, i.e. tissue has been lost or removed; these wounds may be grafted or managed an an open ulcer.

REFERENCE MATERIAL
Surgical wounds

Surgical wounds are used as the classic example for wound management and the description of the healing process.

Wound healing follows a series of interrelated and overlapping biochemical phases which commence at injury and continue for up to 1 year. The healing period is longer than is generally considered by either patient or nurse. The changes which occur are summarized in Table 44.1.

The rate and progression of healing are affected by the patient's nutritional and immunological status, age and drug therapy (Westaby, 1985; David, 1986). Contamination of the wound by bacteria also affects healing and management.

Cruse and Foord (1980) in a definitive study of the epidemiology of wound infection carried out over a 10-year peirod and embracing over 62,000 wounds, identified four types of surgical wounds:

1 clean wounds;
2 clean contaminated wounds;
3 contaminated wounds;
4 dirty wounds.

CLEAN WOUNDS

In clean wounds, no infection is encountered; there is no break in the aseptic technique during surgery, and no hollow muscular organ has been opened. Three opera-tions, namely cholecystectomy, appendicectomy in passing and hysterectomy are included in this category, provided that no acute inflammation is present.

CLEAN CONTAMINATED WOUNDS

In these wounds a hollow muscular organ has been opened but minimal spillage of contents has occurred.

CONTAMINATED WOUNDS

In contaminated wounds a hollow muscular organ has been opened accompanied by gross spillage of contents or acute inflammation, without pus, is en-countered. Also included in this category are fresh (within 4 hours) traumatic wounds, wounds that result from opening of the colon or wounds resulting from surgery where there has been a major break in aseptic technique.

DIRTY WOUNDS

Dirty wounds include those where pus or a perforated viscus is encountered at surgery, and traumatic wounds of longer than 4 hours duration.

Suture removal

Where wounds are closed by sutures, clips or tape these are removed when the tensile strength of the wound is adequate. This time ranges from 4 days for clean super-ficial wounds to 14 or more days when the patient has poor healing potential, e.g. in old age, obesity, neoplasm or infection. Dehiscence is fortunately not a common problem. In a study quoted by Westaby (1985) of 1,129 laparotomy wounds the rate for burst abdomen was 1.68%, for incisional hernia 6.73% and for wound sinus 6.73%.

Surgical wound drains

A drain may be used to carry fluid from the wound bed, preventing accumulation which would delay healing.

Table 44.1   Phases of Wound Healing

Phase	Time	Activity
Inflammatory	Days 1–3	The wound is red, swollen and hot. Blood vessels bleed and platelets and fibrin cause clotting. Histamine is released, causing dilation of capillary blood vessels and thus allowing serum and white blood cells to enter the injured area, which results in oedema, increased colour and heat. In closed surgical wounds epithelial cells proliferate to close and seal the surface skin.
Destructive	Days 1–6	Polymorphonuclear leucocytes and macrophages clear the wound of dead tissue. Wounds cannot heal in the absence of macrophages, which not only remove bacteria but are responsible for the formation and replication of fibroblasts, whithout which collagen cannot be produced.
Reconstructive	Days 3–24	Macrophages continue to clear the wound of debris. Fibroblasts continue to produce collagen, the main constituent of many body tissues. Vitamin C is essential for normal fibroblast activity. Adequate nutrition is, therefore, essential. The interaction of the various tissues during this period helps produce non-specific granulation tissue to fill gaps in tissue continuity. Excessive inflammation may lead to overgranulation with increased scar tissue (keloid and hypertrophic scars). Budding capilaries develop within the granulation tissue to carry oxygen and nutrients. In this phase the wound is very fragile and care must be exercised during dressings and mobilization. Epithelial cells proliferate and 'roll' across the surface of the granulation tissue to close the wound.
Maturation	Days 24 onwards	The scar changes colour from pink to white due to decrease in the activities of the healing process already mentioned. Collagen continues to be produced for some months to strengthen the wound. The scar tissue remains non-specific and is generally weaker than the surrounding tissue. The superficial skin develops a normal texture.

TYPES OF DRAIN

1 *Vacuum*: closed vacuum drainage via a stab wound into the wound bed (e.g. Redivac).
2 *Wick*: soft latex tube with a gauze wick (Penrose).
3 *Paul's tubing*: soft rubber tubing.
4 *Corrugated*: flat corrugated rubber, plastic or latex strip.
5 *Naunton Morgan* (Penrose): Paul's tubing with a corrugated drain inserted.
6 *Suction*: rubber or latex catheter attached to a suction pump.

INDICATIONS FOR USE

The use of surgical wound drains is indicated under the following conditions:

1 to drain intra-abdominal collections of pus, empyema or purulent pericarditis;
2 whenever collections of fluid are likely to occur postoperatively, when an anastomosis or closure of a large organ produces a discharge or when haemostasis has not been achieved at surgery;
3 to redirect body fluids to allow a new suture line time to heal.

Open wounds

In wounds where tissue has been lost such as burns, leg ulcers and trauma, the speed of healing will depend on the size and depth of the wound, the degree of infection or trauma and the patient's general potential to heal.

Local measures to treat the wound may be ineffective if the patient is not capable, due to illness, poor circulation or malnutrition, of delivering the necessary materials for wound healing to the site. With longstanding wounds such as venous ulcers compliance with measures to improve circulation is essential.

Tissue grafting

Grafts of skin, muscle, tendon or bone may be used to replace tissue lost.

TYPES OF GRAFT
Free graft
This is where tissue is transferred from a healthy site to the wound. The transferred tissue must develop links with the local circulation or be connected by microsurgery.

Flap graft
This is where the grafted tissue is lifted and remains connected to the site of removal until local circulation has developed.

The process of linkage between the graft and the wound bed is similar to wound healing in both process and duration.

Care of all wounds should be aimed at providing the ideal micro-environment in which wound healing can take place. Management must be relevant and the nurse should be able to support nursing interventions by written evidence or nursing research findings.

There are numerous wound agents and dressings available at present. New products constantly appear on the market with varying claims about their efficacy. Nurses must not accept such claims at face value until they themselves have evaluated the product or dressing in the clinical situation.

References and further reading
Bernhard, L.A. (1982) Wound healing, *Association of Operating Room Nurses Journal*, Vol. 35, p. 1067.

Brubacher, L.L. (1982) To heal a draining wound, *Registered Nurse*, Vol. 45, no. 3, pp. 30–5.

Brunner, L.S. and Suddarth, D.K. (1982) *Lippincott Manual of Medical Surgical Nursing*, Vol. 1, Harper & Row, London.

Cruse, P.J.E. and Foord, R. (1980) The epidemiology of wound infection, *Surgical Clinics of North America*, Vol. 60, no. 1, pp. 27–40.

David, J.A. (1986) *Wound Management*, Martin Dunitz, London.

Hunt, T.K. and Dunphy, J.E. (1979) *Fundamentals of Wound Management*, Appleton-Century-Crofts, New York.

Knight, B. (1981) The history of wound treatment, Wound care no. 2, *Nursing Times*, Vol. 77, pp. 5–8.

Westaby, S. (ed.) (1985) *Wound Care*, Heinemann, London.

GUIDELINES: CLOSED WOUND OR EPIDERMAL INJURY

Equipment
1 As for aseptic technique (see p. 7)
2 Wound swab or sterile syringe.

Procedure

Action	Rationale
1 Explain the procedure to the patient.	To obtain the patient's consent and co-operation.
2 Perform dressing using an aseptic technique.	To prevent infection. (For further information on asepsis, see the procedure on aseptic technique, pp. 5–8).
3 Moisten the dressing with an appropriate sterile solution, such as normal saline.	To facilitate removal of the dressing without destruction of granulation tissue.
4 Obtain a specimen of any discharge with a wound swab or syringe.	To ascertain whether infection is present.

Action	Rationale
5 Clean the wound with an appropriate sterile solution, such as normal saline.	To prevent cross-infection, and remove debris.
6 If exudate is excessive, cover the wound with a sterile dressing pad.	To prevent escape of, and to absorb, the exudate.
7 Assess the condition of the surround skin.	To preclude deterioration of skin leading to excoriation.
8 Attach dressing with hypo-allergenic tape.	To prevent damage to surrounding skin.
9 Describe the wound and the exudate in appropriate documentation and amend the care plan accordingly.	For accurate evaluation of progress in healing of the wound.

GUIDELINES: DEHISCENT WOUND OR ULCER

Equipment
1   As for Aseptic Technique (see p. 7)
2   Wound swab
3   Appropriate dressing materials (see Table 31.5, p. 309)
4   Cleansing fluid for irrigation such as saline
5   Sterile syringe for irrigation
6   Adhesive sutures such as Steristrips if required.

Procedure

Action	Rationale
1 Explain the procedure to the patient.	To obtain the patient's co-operation.
2 Perform dressing using an aseptic technique.	To prevent infection. (For further information on aseptic technique see pp. 5–8).
3 Moisten the dressing with appropriate sterile solution, such as normal saline.	To facilitate removal of the dressing without destruction of granulation tissue.
4 Clean the sound with an appropriate sterile solution, such as normal saline.	To prevent cross-infection.
5 Warm irrigation solution.	To prevent wound cooling and discomfort.
6 Irrigate the wound using syringe or infusion set with gentle pressure.	To remove debris from the wound.
7 For continuous or intermittent irrigation use a device such as the Squib wound irrigator.	A well-fitted device prevents exudate washing surrounding tissue leading to excoriation. Irrigation can be performed as required and wound can be observed through device.
8 Copious drainage can be managed using a closed wound drainage bag such as Convatec wound manager.	Surrounding skin is protected and odour reduced.

	Action	Rationale
9	Assess the condition of the surrounding skin.	To preclude deterioration of skin leading to excoriation.
10	For dehiscent wound, where possible close with adhesive sutures, such as Steristrips.	To maintain apposition of wound edges, thus promoting healing.
11	Encourage the patient to take a nutritious diet, ensuring sufficient intake of vitamin C and trace elements.	Where exudate output is excessive there may be severe protein depletion. Vitamin C and trace elements help to promote healing.
12	Describe the wound and type of dressing used in the appropriate documentation.	For accurate evaluation of progress in healing of the wound.

GUIDELINES: REMOVAL OF SUTURES OR CLIPS

Equipment

1   As for Aseptic Technique (see p. 7).
2   Sterile scissors or stitch cutter or Michel clip-removing forceps.
3   Sterile adhesive sutures (such as Steristrips).

Procedure

Action

Rationale

	Action	Rationale
1	Explain the procedure to the patient.	To obtain the patient's consent and co-operation.
2	Perform dressing using an aseptic technique.	To prevent infection. (For further information see procedure on aseptic technique, pp. 5–8).
3	Moisten the dressing with an appropriate sterile solution, such as normal saline.	To facilitate removal of the dressing without destruction of granulation tissue.
4	Clean the wound with an appropriate sterile solution such as normal saline.	To prevent infection.

FOR REMOVAL OF SUTURES

	Action	Rationale
5	Lift knot of suture in forceps and snip stitch close to the skin. Pull suture out gently (see Figure 44.1).	To prevent infection by drawing exposed suture through the wound.

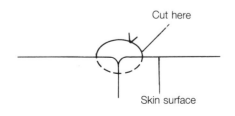

Cut here

Skin surface

Figure 44.1   Suture removal.

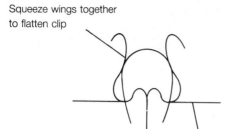

Figure 44.2   Kifa clip removal.

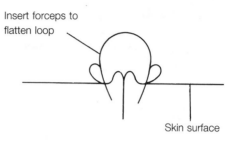

Figure 44.3   Michel clip removal.

FOR REMOVAL OF CLIPS

	Action	Rationale
6	Squeeze wings of Kifa clips together with forceps to release from skin (see Figure 44.2). For Michel clips use special forceps under the clips to flatten the loop (see Figure 44.3).	To release clips atraumatically from the wound.
7	If the wound gapes use adhesive sutures to oppose the wound edges.	To prevent wound breakdown and improve the cosmetic effect.
8	When necessary cover the wound with a non-adherent dressing.	To provide the best possible environment for wound healing to take place. To reduce the risk of infection. To prevent a suture line rubbing against clothing.
9	Describe the wound carefully in the appropriate documentation.	For accurate evaluation of progress in wound healing.

GUIDELINES: DRAIN DRESSING (REDIVAC AND CLOSED DRAINAGE SYSTEMS)

Equipment
1   As for Aseptic Technique (p. 7)
2   Keyhole dressing
3   Sterile padded dressing.

Procedure

Action

Rationale

	Action	Rationale
1	Explain the procedure to the patient.	To obtain the patient's consent and co-operation.
2	Perform dressing using an aseptic technique.	To prevent infection. (For further information on asepsis, see the procedure on aseptic technique, pp. 5–8).
3	Clean the surrounding skin with an appropriate sterile solution, such as normal saline.	To prevent infection.
4	Ensure that the skin suture holding the drain site in position is intact.	To prevent the drain from leaving the wound.

5 Cover the drain site with a keyhole dressing.	To protect the drain site and to prevent infection entering the site.
6 Tape securely.	To ensure continuity of drainage.
7 Ensure that the drain is primed or that the suction pump is in working order.	

GUIDELINES: CHANGE OF VACUUM BOTTLE (REDIVAC AND CLOSED DRAINAGE SYSTEMS)

Equipment
1 Sterile topical swabs
2 Artery forceps – tip to be covered with rubber
3 Sterile drainage bottle.

Procedure

Action	**Rationale**
1 Explain the procedure to the patient.	To obtain the patient's consent and co-operation.
2 Wash hands.	To minimize the risk of infection.
3 Clean the nozzle of wall suction apparatus with an appropriate antiseptic solution and prime a sterile vacuum bottle.	To ensure sterility and to prepare the bottle for attachment to the drainage tube.
4 Measure the contents of the bottle to be changed and record this in the appropriate documents.	To maintain an accurate record of drainage from the wound.
5 Clamp the tube with artery forceps and remove the bottle.	To prevent air and contamination entering the wound via the drain.
6 Clean the end of the tube and attach it to the sterile bottle.	To maintain sterility.
7 Remove the artery forceps.	To re-establish the drainage system.
8 Ensure that the bottle is primed.	To ensure that drainage continues.
9 If the vacuum is constantly lost, take down the dressing and examine the entry site of the drain.	To ensure that the drain has not become dislodged.
10 Re-dress as for a closed drainage system.	

GUIDELINES: REMOVAL OF DRAIN (REDIVAC AND CLOSED DRAINAGE SYSTEMS)

Equipment
1   As for aseptic technique (see p. 7)
2   Sterile scissors or suture cutter.

Procedure

Action	Rationale
1 Check the patient's operation notes.	To establish the number and site(s) of sutures.
2 Explain the procedure to the patient.	To obtain the patient's consent and co-operation.
3 Perform the procedure using an aseptic technique.	To prevent infection. (For further information on asepsis, see the procedures on aseptic technique, pp. 5–8.)
4 Where the wound is covered with an occlusive dressing (e.g. OpSite) lift and snip the dressing. Do not remove it from the entire wound.	To prevent disturbing the incision or contaminating the wound.
5 Only clean the wound if necessary, using an appropriate sterile solution, such as normal saline.	To prevent micro-organisms invading the suture pathway at removal.
6 Hold the knot of the suture with forceps and gently lift it upwards.	To allow space for the scissors or suture cutter to be placed underneath.
7 Cut the shortest end of the suture as close to the skin as possible.	To allow the suture to be liberated from the drain without any part of the exposed suture travelling through subcutaneous tissue.
8 Release vacuum and remove drain gently.	To prevent pulling at the wound tissue.
9 Cover the drain site with a sterile dressing and tape securely.	To prevent infection entering the drain site.
10 Measure and record the contents of the drainage bottle in the appropriate documents.	To maintain an accurate record of drainage from the wound.

GUIDELINES: DRAINAGE DRESSING (PENROSE, PAUL'S TUBING, CORRUGATED AND NAUNTON MORGAN DRAINAGE SYSTEMS)

Equipment
1   As for aseptic technique (see p. 7)
2   Sterile padded dressings
3   Stomahesive wafers
4   Keyhole dressing
5   Drainage stoma bag.

Procedure

MINIMUM DRAINAGE

Action	**Rationale**
1 Explain the procedure to the patient.	To obtain the patients's consent and co-operation.
2 Perform the procedure using an aseptic technique.	To prevent infection. (For further information on asepsis, see the procedure on aseptic technique, pp. 5–8.)
3 Clean the surrounding skin with an appropriate sterile solution, such as normal saline.	To prevent infection.
4 Cut a hole slightly larger than the site in a stomahesive wafer and apply the wafer to the skin surrounding the drain.	To protect the skin from the drainage which may cause excoriation. The wafer should fit as close to the drain as possible without interrupting the flow of effluent.
5 Leave the stomahesive wafer in position until the drain is removed.	To continue to protect vulnerable skin.
6 Cover the drain site and the stomahesive wafer with a keyhole dressing and sterile dressing pad. Tape securely.	To prevent spillage of drainage. To prevent infection.
7 Change the dressing whenever it becomes soiled.	To prevent infection.
8 Describe the wound and type of drainage in appropriate documents and amend the care plan accordingly.	For accurate evaluation of progress of drainage.

COPIOUS DRAINAGE

Action	**Rationale**
1 Follow steps 1–5 above, i.e. to the stage where the stomahesive wafer has been applied.	
2 Cover the drain with a drainage stoma bag.	To allow effluent to drain into the bag.
3 Ensure that the drain is enclosed by the aperture of the bag.	To prevent excoriation of surrounding skin. To contain any odour.
4 Secure the bag with suitable tape if necessary.	To prevent the bag from becoming detached from the skin.
5 Empty the contents of the bag regularly and record the amount in appropriate documents.	To prevent accumulated fluid from detaching the bag from the skin due to its weight. To maintain an accurate record of drainage.

GUIDELINES: SHORTENING OF DRAIN (PENROSE, ETC. DRAINAGE SYSTEMS)

Equipment
1   As for aseptic technique (see p. 7)
2   Sterile scissors or suture cutter
3   Sterile safety pin
4   Drainage stoma bag.

Procedure

Action	Rationale
1 Check the patient's operation notes.	To establish the length of drain to be shortened.
2 Explain the procedure to the patient.	To obtain the patient's consent and co-operation.
3 Remove the dressing or stoma bag and measure the contents.	To record accurately the amount of drainage.
4 Perform dressing using an aseptic technique.	To prevent infection. (For further information on asepsis, see the procedure on aseptic technique, pp. 5–8.)
5 Only clean the wound if necessary, using an appropriate sterile solution, such as normal saline.	To prevent micro-organisms invading the wound.
6 Hold the knot of the suture with forceps and gently lift upwards.	To allow space for the scissors or suture cutter to be placed underneath.
7 Cut the shortest end of the suture as close to the skin as possible.	To allow the suture to be liberated from the drain without any part of the exposed suture travelling through subcutaneous tissue.
8 Using forceps, gently ease the drain out of the wound to the length requested by the surgeon (usually 3–5 cm).	
9 Place a sterile safety pin through the drain as close to the skin as possible.	To prevent retraction into the wound.
10 Cut 3–5 cm from the distal end of the drain.	To ensure that there is not an unnecessary amount of drain in the drainage bag. To ensure patient comfort.
11 Place a clean, suitably sized drainage bag over the drain site.	To allow effluent to drain into the bag. To prevent excoriation of the surrounding skin. To contain any odour.
12 Secure the bag with a suitable tape if necessary.	To prevent the bag from becoming detached from the skin.

GUIDELINES: REMOVAL OF DRAIN (PENROSE, ETC. DRAINAGE DRESSING)

Equipment

1   As for aseptic technique (see p. 7)
2   Sterile scissors or suture cutter.

Procedure

Action	Rationale
1 Explain the procedure to the patient.	To obtain the patient's consent and co-operation.
2 Check the patient's operation notes.	To establish the number and site(s) of sutures.
3 Perform the procedure using an aseptic technique.	To prevent infection. (For further information on asepsis, see the procedure on aseptic technique, pp. 5–8.)
4 Only clean the wound if necessary using an appropriate sterile solution, such as normal saline.	To prevent micro-organisms invading the suture pathway at removal.
5 Hold the knot of the suture close to the skin as possible.	To allow space for the scissors or suture cutter to be placed underneath.
6 Cut the shortest end of the suture as close to the skin as possible.	To allow the suture to be liberated from the drain without any part of the exposed suture travelling through subcutaneous tissue.
7 Using sterile forceps, gently remove the drain.	
8 Cover the drain site with a sterile dressing and secure.	To prevent infection entering the drain site.
9 Record removal of the drain in the appropriate documents and alter the nursing care plan.	To maintain an accurate record.

INDEX